SPRINGER SERIES IN NEUROPSYCHOLOGY

Harry A. Whitaker, Series Editor

Springer Series in Neuropsychology

Harry A. Whitaker, Series Editor

Phonological Processes and Brain Mechanisms
H.A. Whitaker (Ed.)

Contemporary Reviews in Neuropsychology
H.A. Whitaker (Ed.)

Neuropsychological Studies of Nonfocal Brain Damage: Dementia and Trauma
H.A. Whitaker (Ed.)

Linguistic Analyses of Aphasic Language
W.U. Dressler and J.A. Stark (Eds.)

W.U. Dressler J.A. Stark
Editors

Linguistic Analyses of Aphasic Language

With 20 Figures

Springer-Verlag
New York Berlin Heidelberg
London Paris Tokyo

Wolfgang U. Dressler
Department of Linguistics
University of Vienna
1090 Vienna, Austria

Jacqueline A. Stark
Workshop on Neuropsychology
and Neurolinguistics
Brain Research Institute
Austrian Academy of Sciences
1010 Vienna, Austria

Library of Congress Cataloging-in-Publication Data
Linguistic analyses of aphasic language.
(Springer series in neuropsychology)
Bibliography: p.
Includes index.
1. Aphasia. 2. Linguistic analysis (Linguistics)
I. Dressler, Wolfgang U., 1939- . II. Stark,
Jacqueline A. III. Series. [DNLM: 1. Aphasia—
psychology. 2. Linguistics. 3. Phonetics.
WL 340.5 L755]
RC425.L56 1988 616.85'52 87-36946

Typeset by Ampersand Publisher Services, Rutland, Vermont
Printed and bound by Halliday Lithograph, West Hanover, Massachusetts
Printed in the United States of America.

9 8 7 6 5 4 3 2 1

ISBN 0-387-96692-7 Springer-Verlag New York Berlin Heidelberg
ISBN 3-540-96692-7 Springer-Verlag Berlin Heidelberg New York

Preface

The idea for this volume originated during the summer Linguistic Institute of the Linguistic Society of America, held at the University of Maryland, College Park in July of 1982. The Institute was dedicated to linguistics, psycholinguistics, and neurolinguistics. Both of us attended. From discussions with Harry A. Whitaker, the organizer of this summer course, emerged the concept of summarizing aphasia research from Vienna in one volume. We express our thanks to Professor Whitaker as the stimulus for publication of this book.

The research and editorial work of J. Stark was supported totally by the Austrian Academy of Sciences, Vienna. Much of the data discussed in this volume stems from an ongoing aphasia project financed by the Austrian Research Foundation (Fonds zur Förderung der wissenschaftlichen Forschung, Project No. 3632). We are deeply indebted to both of these scientific organizations.

The results summarized here have been obtained by testing aphasics. We are grateful to the clinic chiefs for permission to test their patients and for provision of the neurological examination reports (e.g., computed tomography scans). In particular, we would like to thank Dr. J. Bruck, Professor G. Schnaberth, Professor E. Sluga, Dr. J. Donis, Dozent H. Budka, and Professor C. Spunda. We also thank the aphasic patients for their willingness to undergo testing. We learned a great deal from them, and we hope that we were able to improve their situation a little.

In addition we wish to thank all contributing authors for their support, and Ruth Kramer Ostrin and Heinz Karl Stark for their help and very constructive criticism. Further thanks go to Otto Schlögl, Adrienne Günther, Gloria Carlson, Alberta Aug, Hannelore Kranner, and Eva Horvath for their editorial assistance, as well as to the staff at Springer-Verlag. We of course take full responsibility for any errors and shortcomings that remain.

We would like to dedicate this book to the memory of our colleague and teacher, the late Professor Karl Gloning (1924–1979), who introduced us to the study of aphasia.

October 1987

WOLFGANG U. DRESSLER
JACQUELINE A. STARK

Contents

Contributors

GIANFRANCO DENES Neurological Clinic, University of Padua, 35100 Padua, Italy

WERNER DEUTSCH Department of Sound Research, Austrian Academy of Sciences, 1010 Vienna, Austria

WOLFGANG U. DRESSLER Department of Linguistics, University of Vienna, 1090 Vienna, Austria

SYLVIA MOOSMÜLLER Department of Linguistics, University of Vienna, 1090 Vienna, Austria

CSABA PLÉH Department of Psychology, University of Budapest, 1064 Budapest, Hungary

HEINZ K. STARK Ludwig Boltzmann Society, Institute for Cerebral Blood Flow Research, 1130 Vienna, Austria

JACQUELINE A. STARK Working Group on Neuropsychology and Neurolinguistics, Brain Research Institute, Austrian Academy of Sciences, 1030 Vienna, Austria

RUDOLF WYTEK Computer Center, University of Vienna, 1010 Vienna, Austria

Introduction

WOLFGANG U. DRESSLER and JACQUELINE A. STARK

Linguistic research on aphasia may follow different paradigms. This volume presents examples of two approaches. In one approach, concepts of linguistic theory are the starting point and are then related to aphasic language. Language data from aphasics thus provide one type of substantial data for linguistic theory.

In the second approach, the emphasis is on the aphasic's language-processing abilities. Within this framework of research, linguistics is viewed as a necessary tool for describing the aphasic's intact processing abilities and processing deficits.

In both approaches, linguistic concepts are integrated with (neuro)-psychological ones, either for designing language tests or for interpreting the aphasic's spontaneous speech. The results from both approaches should ultimately contribute to the development of more adequate, linguistically founded diagnostic tests and therapeutic procedures.

When integrating linguistic analyses within an interdisciplinary framework of neuropsycholinguistics, linguists should not throw away time-honored methodological standards. The linguist's role in such an interdisciplinary area of research is to provide the specific linguistic expertise that the other specialized professions lack. In this context, when the linguist is confronted with the task of analyzing aphasic data, the first issue is identification of the aphasic's errors in terms of linguistic levels and categories. This is not possible without a reconstruction of the linguistic "target" the patient was attempting to produce and the "path" leading from the target to the actually produced form or utterance.

Depending on the complexity of the task (e.g., object naming versus discourse production) and the type of language impairment (e.g., agrammatic versus jargon), the reconstructing step may be more or less problematic. In case of conceivable alternative reconstructions, the linguist should be able to substantiate his or her choice on the basis of overall linguistic context. Thus, the linguist's task is to provide a qualitative, in-depth account of the aphasic's language performance. This is the indispensable prerequisite for any sound quantitative analysis of aphasic language performance. The ultimate goal of both aforementioned approaches is to arrive at a comprehensive understanding of the aphasic's abilities on all linguistic levels. Since no model of language processing currently exists that encompasses all linguistic levels, the treatment of linguistic levels as separate entities—as is the case in this volume—seems justified. By the time the interaction between/among the various linguistic levels is well understood, these separate analyses will have been refined and will be available for integration in a model of language processing.

Although the contributions in this volume necessarily reflect the authors' main areas of research, the chapters encompass almost all linguistic levels: phonetics and phonology, morphophonemics, word formation as part of morphology, syntax and semantics, and discourse. Furthermore, language data from German-, Italian-, and Breton-speaking aphasics are interpreted.

Chapter 1 presents a cumulative survey of previous work done on phonological paraphasias. The paraphasias are analyzed within the framework of the theory of natural phonology the author has been developing over the years. In Chapter 2, improvement in coarticulation is phonologically and phonetically described in a single case study of Broca's aphasia. The aim of this chapter is to define objective means of analysis for determining the process of recovery in coarticulation. The third chapter, on sociophonology, demonstrates the first systematic application of sociolinguistics to aphasia. The differential use of standard language and dialect in the same communicative situation by different types of aphasics was investigated.

Morphophonemics, the area relating morphology to phonology, is the subject of the fourth chapter. In this chapter the theories of natural phonology and natural morphology interact. This is the first and possibly last study of aphasia in a Breton-speaking population, because this Celtic language is rapidly being replaced by French. The level of morphology is represented in Chapter 5 by a study of Italian word formation (derivational morphology and compounding studied in terms of the framework of natural morphology). Agent noun and instrument noun formation are investigated in particular.

In Chapter 6 the role of semantic and syntactic factors in auditory sentence comprehension is interpreted with respect to the possible processing deficits demonstrated by the various aphasia types. Chapter 7 deals with grammatical and pragmatic phenomena of the discourse level in an attempt to differentiate primary from secondary impairment of the discourse level. This allows new insight into the nature of agrammatism and into the differentiation of grammar and pragmatics.

The final chapter deals with more basic issues of linguistic processing, which pertain to all linguistic levels—namely, the distinction between automatic and controlled processing, monitoring, and metalinguistic phenomena as they can be applied to aphasic data.

Throughout this book the subjects are described as demonstrating

Broca's, Wernicke's, anomic, or global aphasia. The classification of subjects was based on the "classical" descriptions of these aphasia types delineated in Goodglass and Kaplan (1972, 1983), Benson (1979), and Albert, Goodglass, Helm, Rubens, and Alexander (1981). In many cases the Aachen Aphasia Test was administered. The aphasics discussed in the various chapters fulfilled the following criteria: They had left hemisphere lesions that were predominantly of vascular etiology, they were right-handed, their vision was corrected for, and they were all in a stable condition at the time of testing. Other patient variables are discussed in the respective chapters.

Many of the analyses presented in the various chapters are tentative and at times speculative. The aim of the discussions can thus be viewed as departure points for further research—to arouse interest in the particular areas of research and in linguistic analyses of aphasic language in general.

1
A Linguistic Classification of Phonological Paraphasias

WOLFGANG ULRICH DRESSLER

Introduction

Any classification must have a purpose and must be based on an underlying theory. The classification presented here has a threefold purpose:

1. To differentiate and compare normal speech errors (lapses, slips of the tongue) and aphasic (= pathological) phonological disturbances.
2. To differentiate phonological paraphasias produced by Broca's, Wernicke's and anomic aphasics (in the hope that phenomenological description can serve diagnostic and, albeit indirectly, therapeutic purposes; cf. Dressler, 1980b; Kotten, 1984).
3. To show how a phonological approach may contribute to a better understanding of aphasic disturbances of sound structure, that is, to convince the reader that there is much more to phonology than is often thought. Phonology seems to be gravely underrated not only by neurologists, neuropsychologists, and speech therapists, but also by neurolinguists. Phonological concepts or criteria currently used are few and rather superficial; otherwise phonology is reduced to, and replaced by, phonetics (cf. Dressler, 1984a,b). The (interdependent!) relationship between phonetics and phonology will be discussed in the section on competence and in the conclusions; however, one example of this reductionism begins the section on the history of research.

Before proceeding further, the term *phonological paraphasia* must be defined. The term encompasses the following conditions:

1. There is an aphasic disturbance of the phonemic setup of a (morphologically simple or complex) word.
2. The target word or morpheme is identifiable.
3. The produced erroneous sequence can be derived from the target sequence via one or more phonemic replacements (including sequential replacements [movements] and replacement with zero or of zero [omissions and additions, respectively]).
4. The describer can classify and justify the assumed error path from target to produced sequence.

The second and third conditions are descriptive criteria which effect a phenomenological differentiation from morphological and verbal paraphasias (where morphemes or words replace each other).[1] On the underlying explanatory level, the critique of the segmental and phoneme-count view of phonological deviations (Niemi, 1983, p. 529) is rejected. The fourth condition demands classificatory consistency (differentiation of paraphasias from neologisms) and, if possible, a psycholinguistic account. The first condition presupposes the distinction between phonemic[2] and allophonic and/or phonetic replacements.[3]

A Brief History of Research

Starting Point

Although the great forefather of phonology, Baudouin de Courtenay (1886,1972) was the first linguist to publish on phonological paraphasias, his contributions were entirely forgotten in later decades. Therefore, 1939 may be a good starting point for this brief sketch. This year saw the publication of the first neurolinguistic (i.e., interdisciplinary) monograph: *Le syndrome de la désintégration phonétique dans l'aphasie* (Alajouanine, Ombredane, & Durand, 1939). This work is often also cited in the history of phonological research on aphasia. Its title, however, refers to phonetic disintegration, and its linguistic coauthor (Marguerite Durand) was a phonetician, not a phonologist. Therefore, it is relevant for our purposes only insofar as (a) phonetic research is basic for phonology and (b) many areas—including phonological paraphasias—are of common interest to both phonetics and phonology.

Jakobson

In the same year (1939), Jakobson, one of the protagonists of structural phonematics, prepared his first talk in which he compared phonological acquisition and disturbances (Jakobson, 1939). This was followed by his pioneering book (Jakobson, 1941; English translation 1968) and more sophisticated later studies (Jakobson, 1971). In 1941 Jakobson emphasized the disturbance of phonemic systems (inventories) as a main feature of aphasia. This is quite incorrect, as shown by Lebrun (1970; Lebrun, Lenaerts, Goiris, & Demol, 1969; cf. also Kotten, 1984, p. 86), for only in the limited recordings of severe aphasics may phonemes be entirely missing, for example, the rather rare affricate /pf/ in German. (Of course, in total aphasia only one or a few syllables may be uttered, such as the "tan" of Broca's famous patient.) Also, the production of phonemes that do not exist in the patient's language is rare.

Jakobson (1971) proposed the dichotomy between paradigmatic similarity/selection disorders (i.e., those in which substitution of phonemes in the same position occurs, e.g., *day–tay*) and syntagmatic contiguity combination disorders (e.g., perseverations such as *dog–dod,* or phonotactic disorders). This distinction was highly valued in Luria's neuropsychological/linguistic model (e.g., Luria, 1973, 1976); elsewhere it has been used as one phenomenological criterion for classification of paraphasias and for statistical analysis. (For a similar approach see Guyard, Sabouraud, & Gagnepain, 1981).

Jakobson (1971) also introduced distinctive phonological features and the notion of markedness, that is, that marked feature values (e.g., voiced consonants) tend to be replaced with unmarked feature values (e.g., unvoiced consonants).

The later development of aphasiological studies in terms of structural phonematics may be characterized by the systematic account of phonological substitutions in terms of phonematic oppositions (with or without the use of distinctive features) and markedness theory (cf., e.g., Blumstein, 1973, 1981; Lecours & Lhermitte, 1969; Mierzejewska, 1977; Nuyts, 1982, p. 47; Pilch & Hemmer, 1970). All of these investigators found that the more similar phonemes are (especially those that are distinguished by a single distinctive feature, e.g., (± voiced) *p* vs. *b, s* vs. *z* etc), the more likely they are to be substituted by one another. Lecours and Lhermitte (e.g., 1969) measured (and treated statistically) the distance between substituted and substituting phonemes, so that the distance between /t/ and /p/ or /d/ were 1, the distance between /t/ and /b/ were 2 [as if the distance between /p/ and /b/ were identical to the distance between /p/ and /t/, and so on.] The reason was that these distances could then be added together. Their measurement of the sequential distance between phonemes in sequence (combination or contiguity) disorders presupposes the irrelevance of syllable structures and prosodic feet. For example, if the sequential distance between /p/ and /n/ in *paints* and *Pinocchio* is considered to be identical (i.e., the distance of 2), then the difference of syllabic distribution (onset and coda of the same syllable vs. onsets of two subsequent syllables) is disconsidered. (Cf. also Nuyts, 1982, pp. 66ff, and more critical discussion in Dressler, Tonelli, & Caldognetto, 1987)

As far as distinctive phonological features are concerned, Blumstein (1973) concluded that aphasic substitutions point to the necessity for changes in the specification and hierarchy of Jakobsonian features. However, except for aphasiology, phonologists and phoneticians have proposed quite different changes in the distinctive feature model. Thus, an undifferentiated use of distinctive feature theory, or of markedness theory, is not warranted.

The only rather undisputed heritage of structural phonematics in current neurolinguistic work is the notion of phoneme and the segmentation of sound sequences into phonemes, but even this has been criticized by Lebrun et al. (1969) and relativized by phonetic work on transitions such as voice onset time (VOT) (Blumstein, Cooper, Goodglass, Statlender, & Gottlieb, 1980).

Generative Phonology

The only major published attempt to explain aphasic phonology in terms of generative phonology (Schnitzer, 1972) fails on several accounts. Schnitzer investigated only reading errors of a single patient, and these errors were of a lexical and morphological nature. He claimed, for example, that the mispronunciation of *compulsory* as [kəm'pʌlsōriy] resulted from a disturbance of the "trisyllabic laxing rule" (which shortens long-vowel phonemes in the second-to-last syllable of Latinate English words), so that the putative underlying /ō/ could surface. However, surprisingly few errors in the application of generative phonological rules can be found in this or any other patient from whom data are available. Nearly all phonological "errors" would have to be described as resulting from the application of optional pathological rules. It is therefore not surprising that Schnitzer later gave up applying the model of generative phonology.

Natural Phonology

The unsatisfactory account of phonological paraphasias in terms of both generative and structural phonology has prompted me to apply natural phonology (cf. Donegan & Stampe, 1979; Dressler, 1984b, 1985; Dressler & Tonelli, 1985; Stampe, 1969) to the study of paraphasia, first in the 1970s (Dressler, 1974, 1978); larger studies have been published by Wurzel and Boettcher (1979) and particularly by Kilani-Schoch (1982). For a combination of generative and natural phonology see Dogil (1985) and Stark (1974).

First, there cannot be any unitary explanations for phonological paraphasias because aphasia is neither a disturbance of performance alone nor of language-specific competence combined with performance. Instead it is necessary to operate with E. Coseriu's quintuple: *faculté de langage* (language faculty and language universals), language *type, langue* (language-specific competence), *norme* (sociolinguistic norms of realization) and *parole* (actual performance).

Universal human language faculty may be said to be disturbed in cases of total aphasia when patients seem to be unable to respond to language therapy but are able to learn a simple artificial symbol system (Glass, Gazzaniga, & Premack, 1973). Such patients' capacity for communicative learning thus seems more comparable to that of chimpanzees than of normal human beings.

Disturbances of language type can be asserted only when current cross-linguistic aphasia studies have given more results.

Competence and Performance

In tackling the vexing questions whether and to what extent performance only or competence as well can be disturbed,[4] we must first refer to Whitaker's (1971a, p. 16; 1971b, p. 143) often-cited witty rebuff of equation of all aphasic disturbances with performance disturbances (even in the case of hemispherectomy). We must also exclude from consideration Saussure's social concept of *la langue* and Chomsky's comparable but excessively abstract notion of competence, because both notions cannot be operationalized in a real-time model of language. Dubious interpretations of competence are, in my opinion, its equation with:

1. "Inner speech" (*innere Sprache* in the German aphasiological tradition, cf. Leischner, 1979), because patients' ability or inability to correctly evaluate utterances of their mother tongue is just another type of performance—evaluation performance (cf. Ringen, 1975).
2. "Ideal performance" (Keller, 1981), since this is again performance.
3. Patients' variable, day-to-day availability of linguistic information (Keller, 1981), because this typically depends on performance factors (such as level of attention, of activation, etc.).

However, all of these interpretations go in the right direction insofar as they refer to "higher," that is, more central, levels of performance. (Cf. the notion of "intermediate competences" such as competences for oral speaking vs. auditory comprehension, etc., Lesser, 1978, pp. 50ff.)

More promising interpretations of competence are the following:

1. Competence represents the types, performance represents the respective tokens (Herdan, 1966). Thus, if the tokens of a given type, for example, realization of a given phoneme, are never produced, one might assume that the type itself is unavailable. But this is rarely the case, at least for the structuralist concepts of phonemes and phonemic representations, and lack of production does not imply lack of comprehension (cf. Kohn, Schoenle, & Hawkins, 1984), for example, distinguishing and/or identifying a given phoneme.
2. Thus, across-the-board disturbances of all types of performance (modalities of speaking, writing, comprehending, evaluating) can be taken as disturbances of competence, if competence is understood as the central capacity that underlies all types of performance (Peuser, 1978a, pp. 114, 144, 176, 275ff).
3. Since linguistic competence must be defined as language specific (as opposed to universal language faculty), differential language disturbance of bilinguals, at least of coordinate bilinguals whose competences are supposed to be stored separately, is relevant (Paradis, 1983, especially pp. 803, 808ff). That is, if language L1 is rather well preserved and language L2 is severely disturbed in all types of performance, one

is led to believe that competence of L2 is disturbed. However, Peuser (1978, pp. 322ff) objected that if therapy leads to improvements in one language, there is a transfer to improvements in the other language (cf. Voinescu, Vish, Sirian, & Maretsis, 1977; Watamori & Sasanuma, 1976). This leads to the next point.

4. Spontaneous recovery points to improved performance or intact competence. The same holds for successful deblocking techniques, which presuppose differential disturbances of different performances (modalities). However, if therapy consists of new learning (or relearning), then competence is improved. And since improvement of competence in one foreign language may transfer to another foreign language in normal learning, the objections in point 3 are refutable.
5. All of these points suggest the possibility of identifying both loss of language knowledge competence and processing deficits (of performance) in phonological disturbances.

Methodological Prerequisites

Before I try to show what my approach may contribute to the differentiation of disturbed competence vs. norm vs. performance, certain types of errors must be excluded to ensure that only phonological disturbances are being investigated (cf. Dressler, 1974, 1978; Kotten, 1984):

1. Data from patients with dysarthria (cf. Dogil, 1985; Lehiste, 1965) must be excluded, because dysarthria is due to a disturbance of the peripheral control of articulatory organs outside the "language center" in the brain.
2. The same holds for data from patients with apraxia, as distinguished from those with Broca's aphasia (cf. Blumstein, 1981, p. 134; Buckingham, 1983; Lebrun, 1983, pp. 244ff).
3. If we want to focus on phonological paraphasia, we must, at least initially, exclude data in cases where morphological and lexical errors may be involved; for example, the misreading of *abandon* as *abandomen* by Schnitzer's (1972, p. 95) patient probably contains a lexical contamination with *abdomen.* Thus also simultaneous phonological and semantic confusions (cf. Burns & Canter, 1977; Lecours & Caplan, 1975) must be excluded to guarantee a minimum homogeneity of the data basis.
4. Data from writing and reading errors must be excluded because visual apractic disorders may be involved and because dyslexias often represent syndromes of their own.
5. Phonological errors must be differentiated from morphonological and morphological ones (cf. Dressler, 1985, and chapters 4 and 5 of this volume).

Paraphasias Versus Slips of the Tongue

Since normal slips of the tongue are universally held to be errors of performance, all paraphasias that resemble normal slips can best be classified as disturbances of performance. However, there are significant quantitative differences,[5] often of a polar nature, and also qualitative differences, some of which also involve language-specific competence constraints on phonological productions possible in other languages (and thus belonging to the realm of phonological universals). The normal speech-error data cited here come from Meringer (1908) and Meringer and Mayer (1895) for German, from Fromkin (1973) and Garnham, Shillock, Brown, Mill and Cutler (1982) for English, and from Dressler, Magno Caldognetto, and Tonelli (1986) for Italian.

Main Types of Slips

Normal speech errors (slips of the tongue) consist mainly of anticipations, perseverations, and metatheses. The first two are either replacements (movement errors), copying replacements, or copying errors (without replacement).

An example of metathesis is *Piprikaschnatzel* for German *Paprikaschnitzel,* with a violation of the crossover constraint (Dressler, 1979a). English examples for the other types are (a) anticipatory replacement: [insen] for *intense,* with anticipation of /s/ replacing /t/ (classified by Garnham et al., 1982, p. 809, as substitution); (b) perseveratory movement: *lumber sparty* for *slumber party* (Fromkin, 1973, p. 249 no. 20); (c) anticipatory copying replacement: [r∧n] corrected to *one rouble,* with replacement of [w] by [r] (classified by Garnham et al., 1982, p. 810, as substitution)—it could also be a blend (contamination) of [r∧n] and *rouble;* (d) perseveratory copying replacement: *the one that* [r∧n] for *rung,* with perseveration of /n/ (classified by Garnham et al., 1982, p. #809, as substitution); (e) anticipatory copying (without replacement): *to* [brai] *the Irish press* for *buy* (classified by Garnham et al., 1982, p. 810, as addition).[6]

Such errors in aphasia (of all types)[7] are simply more frequent than errors in normal speech—a quantitatively significant but not important difference.

Syllable Position

As many authors[8] have emphasized, normal slips of the tongue nearly always respect position in the syllable and in the foot. For example, metathesis occurs only between elements in the same syllable position and between two stressed (or, more rarely, two unstressed) elements, as in *Piprikaschnitzel* (see above).

This holds to a far lesser degree in all types of aphasia, for example,

German *Korporal* → [lɔkɔ'ra:l] (anticipatory replacive copying of /l/ from word/syllable-final to word/syllable-initial position), *Soldat* → [lɔl'da:t], *Text* [tɛkst] → [kɛst], and so on, where syllable position is not respected. This is an important quantitative difference. In the Italian material of Dressler et al. (1986), 6% of the paraphasias but only 1% of the slips do not respect syllable position identity. Of 19 German metatheses, 6 do not respect syllable position identity, for example, *Pfeifer* → *Feipfer*.

Phonological Blends

Phonological blends (contaminations; cf. Stemberger, 1984, pp. 301ff.) occur frequently in normal speech errors, for example, [glez] from *girl* + *lesbian*, immediately corrected to *lesbian* (Garnham et al., 1982, p. 813).

Phonological (though not morphological) blends are extremely rare in aphasia other than very mild ones—in fact, I have been unable to detect any in severe aphasias. Many instances reported by Buckingham (1980, p. 203) should rather be classified in other terms: his example *key, button, spoon, fork* → *key, cutty, skoon, sfork,* should be classified as perseverations of /k/ and /s/.

This is a very important quantitative difference, which goes with morphological editing.[9]

Morphological Editing

Morphological editing (rescue) often occurs in normal speech errors, that is, a control mechanism replaces phonologically wrong sequences (due to slips) with a morpheme of the language. This happens rarely in aphasia. An example is German *Kapellmeister* ([musical] conductor) [ka'pɛlmaestəʳ] replaced by [ka'me:lmæstɐ]. This paraphasia is due to replacive copying anticipation of /m/. But is there, in addition, a paraphasic lengthening and tensing of stressed [ɛ] to [e:]? Since *Kamel* [ka'me:l] (camel) (but not [ka'mɛl]) and *Meister* (master) are existing German words, *Kamelmeister* (camel master) is a possible word in German, although so far a nonexistent (morphological!) neologism (or nonce form). Therefore this particular paraphasia may have involved morphological editing.

This is another very important quantitative difference, which seems to show that morphology, on the whole, is unable to interfere in the production of phonological paraphasias (cf. Kilani-Schoch, 1982, pp. 461).

Repair

Successive approximations are often unsuccessful in all types of aphasia.[10] However, when a healthy person notices production of a slip he or she corrects it immediately (often during production.). This correction is rarely wrong—and is then followed by a second correction which is usually successful (always successful in German and Italian slips in the work of Dressler et al., 1986). In Levelt's (1983b) Dutch material the attempts at repair are more staggering, because he includes syntactic and semantic inappropriateness of corrections, but he did not report a single case of unsuccessful phonological correction of a target word, if the target word was retrieved at all.

Thus, with normal speech errors, failure to produce the target word correctly (in one or more attempts to correct the error) is extremely rare; there is no example in Meringer (1908) and Meringer and Mayer (1895); none in Garnham, Shillock, Brown, Mill, and Cutler (1982); and only two instances in Fromkin (1973, p. 247, F 19, G 15).

This is again a very important quantitative difference (if not a qualitative one, because only two counterexamples in normal speech errors may be due to causes like despair,[11] other than lack of competence), and it sheds light on the distinction between competence and performance (cf. Keller, 1981): Successful correction of slips by healthy persons points to intact competence, whereas lack of success by aphasics points to disturbed competence.

Multiple Interdependent Substitutions

If we exclude morphological editing, then the way from the target word to the phonological speech error can nearly always be bridged by a single step or by simultaneous steps, that is, the "error path" (Dressler, 1984a) between target phoneme (or phoneme sequence) and actually produced phoneme (or phoneme sequence) involves a single substitution (or independent simultaneous substitutions in the case of phoneme sequences). No counterexamples are to be found in Meringer's corpora or in Garnham et al. (1982), and only between four and six in Fromkin (1973), for example, *hypothesis* replaced by [pə̯ɪ̆θə̯s] where the final *-esis* can only be deleted after /s/ has been anticipated into the position after the second vowel. And if we do not allow a simultaneous replacive anticipation of the 3 consonants /p, θ, s/ to the position before the vowels preceding them, multiple successive (or interdependent) steps are needed to produce the parpahasia.

This is yet again a very important quantitative difference (already noted in Dressler, 1973). In the Italian material of Dressler et al. (1986) there are, within the slips, 16 cases of multiple simultaneous (independent) substitutions, but 2 cases of multiple successive (interdependent) substitutions. However, Wernicke's patients produced 83 cases of simultaneous (independent) and 41 cases of successive (interdependent) multiple substitutions.

Other Substitutions

Substitutions that cannot be classified as anticipations, perseverations, metatheses, or blends are rare in normal speech errors (cf. note 5) but are frequent in all types of aphasia except anomic aphasia.

This is an important quantitative, if not a qualitative, difference, because speech error collections usually do not present enough context to allow exclusion of anticipatory or perseveratory impacts. For example, Fromkins's (1973) appendix contains only seven such errors (e.g., *capacity → camacity*), but the reader cannot judge whether a preceding or subsequent nasal (preferably in the onset of a stressed syllable) may have been anticipated or perseverated.

The same methodological critique can be leveled against corpora such as Blumstein's (1973; cf. Lecours & Caplan, 1975), which is based on single-word file cards.

Meringer's (1908) and Meringer and Mayer's (1895) classification of phonological speech errors consists only of metatheses, anticipations, perseverations, blends, and omissions. Also Kaczmarek's (1984a, p. 38) statistics underdifferentiate errors, but show an essential difference between "normal" errors such as perseveration and "normal" errors such as phoneme "substitutions":

	Percent of "error"				
Type of "error"	Wernicke's	Anomic	Semantic	Broca's	Normal controls
Perseverations	6.9	3.6	12.2	15.9	1.6
Substitutions	3.0	0.8	2.9	6.0	0.6

Results of persons with anomic aphasia are closest to those of normal controls.

Quantitative Versus Qualitative Differences

Future research involving large-scale statistics will show whether these very important quantitative differences are in fact only highly significant quantitative differences between normal speech errors and phonological paraphasias or whether they represent qualitative differences, inasmuch as only a few counterexamples are left that can be explained in a different way.

Qualitative Differences

Qualitative differences between normal slips of the tongue and aphasiological errors falsify the view (held since Sigmund Freud) that all (phonological) paraphasias are generated by the same mechanisms as normal (phonological) speech errors and that the only difference is in the quantity of the errors. In very severe aphasia, rarely, phonemes may be missing (cf. the above section on Jakobson).

Neologisms

Phonological neologisms, that is, phonological words that do not contain morphemes of the language in question, are typical of jargon aphasia (Buckingham & Kertesz, 1974), but also occur in other types of aphasia.

This is never the case in normal speech errors: They can always be derived from target forms by means of anticipations, perseverations, metatheses, blends, or less frequently, other substitutions.

Monophonemic Affricates

Monophonemic affricates can be dissociated (very rarely) in severe aphasia. This is never the case in normal speech errors. German *Peferts* for *Pferd* (horse) illustrates the dissociation of monophonemic /pf/ into two segments /p/ and /f/, with an insertion between them. In ['ɔfb̥ɔ] for German *Apfel* (apple), /pf/ is dissociated and then metathesized to /fp/ in its dialectal variant [fb̥]. Similarly, the monophonemic affricate /ts/ is dissociated and methathesized in German *Besatzung* (occupation force), as substituted by [bɪ'z̥axstʊx] (Mössner & Pilch, 1971, p. 400; cf. Sadowska, 1976).

Phonotactic Constraints

Another quantitative difference is the fact that phonotactic constraints on possible phoneme sequences seem to be nearly always respected in normal speech errors but not in aphasia. I have found only four clear counterexamples:

1. Meringer's German *stnudiert nicht* for *studiert nicht,* with copying anticipation of /n/:[ʃtn] is a prohibited sequence in German.
2. Fromkin's (1973) [æskəbæθkənz] for *Athabascans,* with the un-English sequence [θk].
3. [sli:pʃ] for *sleeps* in Garnham et al. (1982, p. 809), with the un-English sequence [pʃ].
4. Italian *eredistasrietà* for *ereditarietà* (hereditarity) with the un-Italian sequence [sr] (Dressler et al., 1986).

However, Stemberger (1983, pp. 31ff) found many counterexamples (e.g., *dlorm, bworn, sthough, rpin, atk*), but did not give the relative frequency within his corpus. Berg (1985, pp. 270ff) agreed with Stemberger, but also gave no information about either absolute or relative frequency.

In aphasia, such violations of phonotactic constraints are much more frequent: Blumstein (1973, pp. 71ff) claimed that 2.3% and 4.3% of all errors in Broca's and Wernicke's aphasics, respectively, are of this kind. The percentages in Lindner's (1985) German study are 9.2% and 5%, respectively. (Cf. Schnitzer & Martin, 1974, and Blumstein, 1978, p. 195, for

English; Mihailescu, Fradis, & Voinescu, 1968, p. 104, for Rumanian; Mierzejewska & Grotecki, 1982 for Polish; and Dressler et al., 1986, for German and Italian.)

These data refute the claim (e.g., Buckingham, 1980) that phonotactic constraints are always respected in aphasia, a claim contradicted by Buckingham and Kertesz' (1974, pp. 44,48) examples [fhæf] for *half* and the neologism [tʃpíktərz] with the incorrect word initial clusters *fh-, chp-*.

Markedness

Unmarked Syllables

The above-mentioned violations of phonotactic constraints consist of complications of syllable structures insofar as new unpermitted consonant clusters are formed (more in the syllable onset than in the coda; cf. Blumstein, 1978, p. 196). On the other hand, Blumstein (1973, 1978, p. 195) did notice the antagonistic trend toward simple, particularly open syllables (the ideal open syllable being consonant-vowel [CV]). Only monosyllabic words (or logatoms) of a CV structure are often produced as CVC, that is, with word-final consonant-addition which produces a syllable coda (cf. Lindner, 1985, Martin, Wasserman, Gilden, Gerstman, & West, 1975, p. 43). The trend toward consonant cluster simplifications is discussed in Trost and Canter (1974) and in Wurzel and Boettcher (1979).

The relative naturalness (unmarkedness) of syllables can be judged according to several parameters. The most conspicuous one (and the one most often referred to) is the parameter of syllable openness. (The possible preference for CV over V or for CV over CVC and thus also for CVC over VC is derived from two other parameters.)

We may think of a very simplified scale of degrees of difficulty in phonotactic combinations, where a CV syllable would be the easiest syllable form, V the next easiest, CVC and CCV the next easiest, and so on:

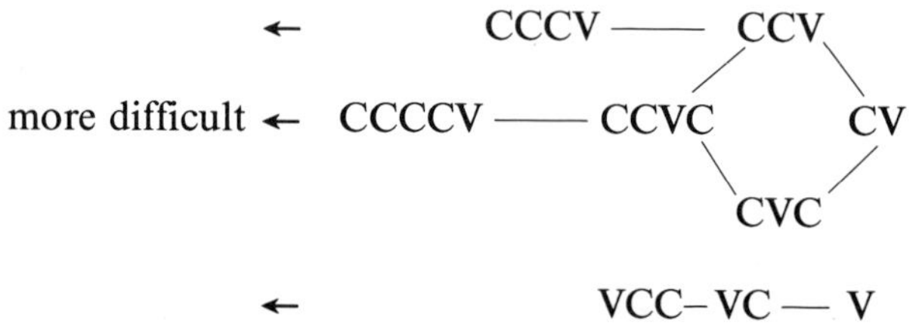

On this scale, languages such as Maori and Samoan would be placed to the right, because these languages have only CV and V syllables. Italian would have a larger range to the left, because it allows up to VC and

CCCVC syllables. German would have a still larger range to the left. However, in both Italian and German there are more easier syllables than difficult ones, for example, there are more CV syllables than any other syllable types, and this is truc of both type and token frequency.

Aphasic Deviations

Aphasia, I claim, causes two deviations from such language-specific distributions, both of them in the form of relaxations of language-specific regulations of universal phonology:

1. Easier/less marked/more natural phonotactic combinations are preferred; that is, aphasic production displays a higher token frequency of CV syllables (the most natural syllable type) than does normal speech or slips of the tongue (cf. Dressler et al., 1987).
2. Constraints on the most difficult combinations/syllables allowed in the respective language are relaxed. Aphasics sometimes produce phonotactic sequences that are allowed in languages farther to the left on the (simplified) scale of phonotactic difficulty. This relaxation of constraints on syllable types does not, however, challenge the preference for simple syllable tokens (first deviation).

German Examples

Lindner in her MA thesis (1985) tested these and other related hypotheses. Her findings support my first claim insofar as the ratio of consonant deletions/additions is higher in codas than in onsets:

Type of error	Broca's (n = 5)	Wernicke's (n = 6)	Total
Onset			
Additions	112	32	145
Deletions	77	45	122
Coda			
Additions	44	59	103
Deletions	49	74	123

This means a trend towards CV syllables rather than towards VC syllables. My second claim is also supported by the incorrect clusters (due to consonant additions): syllable-initial *bm-;* word-initial *bʃ-*, *ʃfl-*, *ʃfr-*, *ʃtl/ʃdl-*, *ʃtpr-*, *ʃtʃ/ ʃdʃ-*, *dʃn-*, *dʃr-*, *dʃd-*, *dspr-* (where *dʃ-*, *tʃ-*, *ds-* denote affricates); syllable- and word-final: *-çʃ*, *-xft.* (The question remains, why consonant additions are more frequent in the onset by Broca's and in the coda by Wernicke's patients.)

The qualitative similarity of errors in Broca's and Wernicke's patients refutes the hypothesis (cf. Alajouanine et al., 1939) that they may be due to disturbed neuromuscular planning in Broca's aphasics.

Summing up, we may say that aphasics violate language-specific syntagmatic (i.e., chaining) constraints on phonemes but prefer (syntagmatically) less marked sequences of phonemes.

Unmarked Segments

The same may be said about the paradigmatic axis of phonology, that is, about the selection of phonemes at the same position of the phonological chain, and thus about disturbances of the phonemic inventory. As far as the token frequency of existing language-specific phonemes is concerned, aphasics, more often than normals, produce relatively "unmarked" phonemes of their languages (Blumstein, 1973). (Cf. Lecours & Lhermitte, 1969; Nespoulous, Lecours, & Joanette, 1983; Nespoulous, Joanette, Beland, Caplan, & Lecours, 1984; and Ulatowska & Baker, 1977, with regard to Broca's aphasics).

On the other hand, they extend (at least in the case of anterior aphasics) their sound repertory to more "marked" sounds than are allowed in the phonological system of their language. For example, in German aphasics the "un-German" sounds [d̥, ɸ, θ, w̃] have been noted, for example, [ɸraeç] for *Fleisch* (meat). That is, the language-specific constraints on the phonemic inventory have been relaxed. This never seems to occur in normal speech errors.

Disturbances of Sociophonological Norms

Normal speech is characterized by sociophonological variation between formal and casual speech, slow and fast speech, and dialectal and sociolectal variants.[12] Are these norms violated in normal speech errors at all? For example, the Garnham et al. (1982) corpus contains radical vowel reduction in [fən] for *fantastic* (p. 809) and [sʌre] for *surreptitiously* (p. 809), and presumably excessive reduction in [britʃ] for *British* (p. 809). We also observe malapropisms that consist of choice of the wrong phonological styles for a given speech situation.

Aphasics, however, do not shift appropriately according to speech situations in a general way, a fact that has been confirmed in a study on one formal and one informal speech situation (Dressler, Moosmüller, & Stark, 1985). Aphasics did not differentiate phonological styles, as did healthy controls: informal compressed speech in the informal situation, more formal speech in the formal situation, as judged by a German variation comparable to English formal *reckon* [ˈrɛkən] versus informal [ˈrɛkŋ̍] with weak vowel deletion.

It is necessary to differentiate[13] between (a) the relative frequency of normal sociophonological substitutions (including deletions and additions) by aphasics in contrast to normals (the subject of this section and of Chapter 3) and (b) the relative frequency of pathological substitutions by aphasics in comparison with normal slips of the tongue. These are errors, whereas the first group of substitutions are part of the normal sociophonological repertory of which prescriptive norms of school grammar describe only a small subpart.

Phonological Naturalness in Prosody

Dogil (1981, 1985) found a universal natural tendency toward trochaic rhythm in language typology and child language. This natural tendency is manifested in aphasic speech as well, for example (V́ = primary stress, V̀ = secondary stress):

Spitálschwèster (hospital nurse) → [ʃtíp‡ʃvɛstɐ], or V V́ V̀ V → V́ V V̀ V
Primárius (chief doctor) → [brìnımá:rĭʊs], or V V́ V → V̀ V V́ V
Zúendnàdel (ignition needle) → [tsyntná:dəl], or V́ V̀ V → V V́ V
Soldátentùm (soldierhood) → [sóltəntàntʊm], or V V́ V V̀ → V́ V V̀ V (the alternating iambic rhythm replaced with an alternating trochaic rhythm)

Thus we see that a universal natural process that is absent in the collections of normal speech errors can be manifested in German aphasics much more than in the language-specific prosodic system of German.

Phonological Naturalness in General

Similarly, I have claimed since 1974 (Dressler, 1974) that a great part of phonological substitutions in aphasia are instances of universal natural processes of segmental phonology.[14]

My modified version of natural phonology (cf. Dressler, 1978,1984b, 1985) provides a dichotomy of two main types of universal natural phonological processes—backgrounding and foregrounding.[15] These are at the disposition of the language-acquiring child, who must restrict, suppress, or preserve them according to the language being acquired. For example, the universal process of syllable-final obstruent devoicing must be suppressed by English children, must be restricted to word-final position by Russian and Polish children, but is preserved by German children.

Now I claim that the great majority of segmental paraphasic substitutions (which are neither anticipations, perseverations, metatheses, nor blends) represent such backgrounding or foregrounding processes that normally would be suppressed in language acquisition. Their occurrence in aphasic speech represents another instance of language-specific constraints being relaxed or uninhibited. For example, English-speaking aphasics have been observed to devoice word-final obstruents (Mössner & Pilch, 1971, p. 397). In a sense, such substitutions can be described as markedness substitutions, insofar as the voiced obstruents [b, d, g, z . . .] are marked in word-final position in comparison with their unvoiced partners [p, t, k, s . . .]. Therefore, devoicing (but also deletion or assimilation, etc.; see below) of word-final voiced obstruents can be considered as a change in the direction of less markedness. However, intervocalic voicing of unvoiced obstruents is also a universal process toward less markedness. Thus, it is impossible to study markedness effects in aphasia (cf. Nespoulous et al., 1984) with the help of statistics that lump together, for example, obstruents in all word/syllable positions. The aphasics' disinhibition of language-specific suppressions of universal backgrounding and foregrounding processes has been documented in Dressler (1978), Kilani-Schoch (1982), and (for consonant cluster simplification) Wurzel and Boettcher (1979). Illustrations of these substitutions from Austrian aphasics follow.

Backgrounding Processes

Backgrounding processes are most frequent in Broca's aphasics (especially in unstressed = weak syllables), less frequent in global aphasics, and still less frequent in Wernicke's aphasics. Anomic aphasics can be grouped with normals. We can distinguish the following types of backgrounding processes.

Shortening Processes

Vowel shortening processes are found in ['nɛbɫ̩] for [' ne:bəl] *Nebel* (fog, mist), ['ʃnɛbal] for ['ʃne:bal] *Schneeball* (snowball). There are no long consonants in German, but in Italian these are frequently shortened in Wernicke's aphasia, for example, in ['bani] for *panni* (cloths).

Deletion Processes

Deletion processes can be found in ['ʃtɪpɫ̩ʃvɛstɐ] for *Spitalschwester* (nurse) with loss of /a/ and in consonant cluster reduction (Wurzel & Boettcher, 1979), both demonstrated in *Oktober* (October) → ['to:βɐ]. In material from Padua, Italy, there are many more omissions with Wernicke's than with Broca's aphasics (cf. Fradis & Calavrezo, 1976; Mihailescu, Fradis, & Voinescu, 1968).

Weakening Processes

Examples of weakening processes are vowel centralization, as in *Universität* → ['ʊnəbɛʳɖə] (with trochaic rhythm), together with spirantization of stops, such as in *(der) Kinder* (children) → ['xɪndər]; *Prävision* (prevision) → [frɛv̥ɪ'sĭo:n]; *Ball* (ball) → [βal]; and affrication of stops, for example, *April* (April) [a'pri:l] → [a'bfrɪl] (for substitution of affricates with fricatives in Polish [which are much more frequent in Wernicke's than in Broca's aphasia] cf. Sadowska, 1976). Replacement of oral spirants with laryngeal [h] is most frequent in Broca's aphasia, for example, *Schlüssel* (key) ['ʃlys(ə)l] → ['hysʃ], *Mechaniker* (mechanic) [mɛ'çɑ:nɪkər] → [ˌme'hɑ:nə].

Assimilation Processes

Assimilation processes are relatively frequent in Wernicke's aphasia. For example, in German only the apical nasal can be assimilated to neighboring obstruents in place of articulation. Not so in the following production of Wernicke's aphasics: *faengt* [fɛŋt] = /fengt/ (catches) → [fɛnt]; *faengt Ball* (catches [the] ball) → [fɛmbə[(also with vowel centralization and consonant deletion); *nimmt* (takes) → [nɪnt]; *gemalt* (painted) = dialect [gmɒ:lt] → [gŋɒ:l] (with assimilation of the labial to a velar nasal and cluster simplification).

Fusion Processes

An extreme case of assimilation processes is fusion processes as in *nein* (no) [naen] → [næ̃]; *gern* (gladly) = dialect and colloquial [gɛɐn] → [gɛ̃ɐ̃]; *Spielzeug* (toy) ['ʃpi:ltsɔek] → ['fi:ltsɛt].

Foregrounding Processes

Foregrounding processes can be identified in Broca's and global aphasia, but rarely in Wernicke's aphasia and never with anomics (and in normal slips of the tongue). Examples of subtypes are the following.

Lengthening Processes

Lengthening processes (antagonistic to the above-mentioned shortening processes) occur in [ki:nt] or [kI:nt] for *Kind* (child) [kɪnt].[16] Aspiration of unaspirated (Austrian colloquial/dialectal) stops has been found by Dressler and Stark (1981) in 28 instances in Broca's aphasia but in only one instance of Wernicke's aphasia (in a study of four patients from each group).

Vowel Insertion

Vowel insertion (antagonistic to vowel deletion) occurs in ['tse:bɐra] ← ['tse:bra] *Zebra,* ['mɪləx] ← ['mɪlç] *Milch* "(milk)" and in the Dressler and Stark (1981) analysis it occurred in 22 cases of Broca's aphasia but in only 2 of Wernicke's aphasia.[17] (Cf. Mihailescu et al., 1968.) Kaczmarek (1984a, p. 38) found 0.3% epentheses in Wernicke's aphasia but 2.2% in Broca's aphasia (the highest percentage within the five aphasia types differentiated by him). Lindner (1985) found consonant insertions especially with Broca's aphasics and in syllable-initial (=strong) position.

Strengthening Processes

Strengthening processes (antagonistic to the above-mentioned weakening processes) can appear, for example, as substitution of fricatives with affricates, as in *Hosentraeger* (suspenders) → ['χo:ʦntrɛgə]; *Hauptmann* (captain) → ['kaɔptman], *Musik* (music) [mu'tsi:k] (82 Broca's, 2 Wernicke's in Dressler & Stark, 1981); or as substitution of fricatives with stops, as in *Schwester* (sister) ['ʃvɛstɐ] → [ʃə'bɛstɐ] (notice the inserted vowel) (44 Broca's, 10 Wernicke's in Dressler & Stark, 1981). The voicing contrast with stops is largely neutralized in Austrian dialects and is thus not a good criterion in aphasia, but this is not the case in Italian. In the Padua, Italy, material, unvoicing of syllable-initial voiced stops is much more frequent with Broca's than with Wernicke's aphasics.

Another strengthening process is substitution of less sonorous by more sonorous vowels (/a/ being the most sonorous one). Keller (1978, 1981, 1984) found this substitution type especially with Broca's aphasics.

Polarization Processes

Polarization processes (antagonistic to the above-mentioned fusion processes) can be exemplified by diphthongization, as in [groʊs] for [gro:s] *gross* (great), [b̥aɔb̥] for [bu:p] *Bub* (boy), [fil'kɑɔst] for [li:p'ko:st] *liebkost* (caresses). The dissociation of affricates is another subtype of polarization.

Frequency of Foregrounding Processes According to Aphasia Type

Why should foregrounding processes be more frequent in anterior aphasia than in Wernicke's aphasia? The sociopsycholinguistic model of phonological variation as developed in Dressler (1978, 1985) and in Dressler and Wodak (1982) predicts that

1. Foregrounding processes are maximized in slow speech and minimized in fast speech. Anterior and particularly Broca's aphasics speak slowly and haltingly; Wernicke's aphasics do not (fluent aphasia).
2. Foregrounding processes are, in general, produced with more articulatory effort than backgrounding processes. Broca's (and anterior) aphasics enunciate with excessive articulatory effort.
3. Foregrounding processes are maximized in speech situations where much attention is paid to speech (great monitoring, effort for clarity) and are maximized particularly in strong positions, that is, in stressed syllables and in word- or syllable-initial position. The reverse holds for backgrounding processes.

Broca's aphasics are fairly well aware of their speech; they are often very attentive. Fluent aphasics have less awareness of their speech (especially those with severe Wernicke' aphasia with anosognosia); they monitor their speech production little.

Thus, this theory provides three connected reasons for the asymmetry in the distribution of many substitution types in Broca's versus Wernicke's aphasia. Since there is interdependence between tempo and attention and between attention and effort, and since attention experiments such as those described in Dressler and Wodak (1982, pp. 352ff) can hardly be performed with aphasics, the relative importance of these factors is difficult to isolate.

Conclusion

Obviously this classification does not cover all cases of phonological paraphasias (cf. note 14). It does, however, represent a step forward toward a consistent theory of phonological paraphasia. Furthermore, the distinction between quantitative and qualitative (or very important quantitative) differences between pathological paraphasias and normal speech errors offers the speech therapist a practical tool for assessing progress in the therapy of phonological disturbances in aphasia and for determining when the errors of a patient have stopped being pathological. Assessment can be done without the necessity of gathering enormous samples of the patient's speech. (Speech sampling would be necessary only if the difference between normal speech errors and the pathological phonological paraphasia was of an exclusively quantitative nature) (cf. Dressler, 1980b; Kotten, 1984).

Phonology Versus Phonetics

Phonology must not be reduced to phonemic representations with the result that all phonological rules/processes have to be assigned to phonetics (as Kohn et al., 1984, seem to believe necessary). Evidently phonological paraphasias do not comprise phonetic disturbances such as of VOT (Blumstein et al., 1980) or of other fine articulatory detail (e.g., Blumstein & Shinn, 1984; Harmes et al., 1984).

Although most neurolinguistic authors explicitly distinguish phonetics and phonology,[18] there are authors who propose phonetic explications for these phonological substitutions that I have accounted for in terms of natural phonology (cf. Blumstein, 1981, p. 138) particularly for those of Broca's aphasics.[19] And whereas Blumstein et al. (1980) and Shinn and Blumstein (1983) meticulously distinguished phonemic and phonetic errors in their VOT studies, Gandour and Dardarananda (1984) tried to subsume them into phonetic etiology. This strategy threatens to reduce phonology completely to phonetics.

Natural Phonology

Keller (1984) objected that explanations of aphasics' errors with phonological markedness would shift the weight of the question from the nature of the pathology to the nature of markedness. But this is a legitimate step, if we do not pay only lip service to the concept of a phonological component, and if we believe in both a phonetic and a psychological basis for phonology (as natural phonology assumes). With regard to Keller's objection, the question would have to be answered as to what cognitive or motoric aspect of unmarked sounds causes these sounds to be easier to produce than marked sounds under conditions of speech pathology. My answer is twofold:

1. The substitution of marked with unmarked sounds can be attributed to universal, natural phonological processes. This accounts for the directionality of substitutions.
2. I have tried to explain why foregrounding processes inhibited by the system of a given language are disinhibited in aphasia (and differentially in Broca's and Wernicke's aphasia). The "optional" fluctuating character of unmarked substitutions for marked sounds follows from the very notion of disinhibition.

However, Keller (1984) had still another objection: How does one account for the minority of substitutions that go in the opposite direction? I propose that these be lumped together with nondirectional (statistically bidirectional) substitutions, those famous confusions or selection errors of phonemes X,Y (cf. Jakobson, 1971; Kohn et al., 1984; MacNeilage, 1982; and Stark, 1974).

Final Classification

Thus I propose the following basic classification of phonological paraphasias:

1. Errors in selecting the correct phonemes, that is, nondirectional ($x \leftrightarrow y$) confusions in lexical access.
2. Disinhibition of phonological processes, that is, directional substitutions (substitutions with a preferred direction of substitution $A \rightarrow B$) presumably at a very early stage of production programming (similar to directional substitutions by young children).
3. Performance errors in linearization similar to normal slips of the tongue with different or differently weighted restrictions on linearization errors.

Sociophonological errors, that is, sociopsychological malapropisms or "misjudgments" in disinhibiting the application of variable phonological processes appropriate for certain styles/registers only, do not result in phonological paraphasias, but in inappropriate sociophonological styles.

Notes

[1]In practice paraphasias may be ambiguous.

[2]Be it in terms of more abstract input phonemes of generative phonology or of (taxonomic) phonemes of structural phonology, sound intentions of natural phonology, archiphonemes/archisegments of structural phonemics, quasiphonemes of natural phonology (cf. Dressler, 1985), or distinctive features of phonemes.

[3]"Replacements" on the phenomenological level, "deviations" on the psycholinguistic level.

[4]The best discussions are in Keller (1981), Lesser (1978, pp. 45ff), Nuyts (1982, pp. 85ff), and Peuser (1978a, pp. 275ff).

[5]See Borrell and Nespoulous (1977), Buckingham (1980), Freud (1891), Söderpalm (1979), Söderpalm-Talo (1980), and Stemberger (1984). These authors assume only quantitative differences and assume normal and pathological errors to be basically of the same nature. In contrast, Dressler (1978, 1980b, 1982) Dressler, Magno Caldognetto and Tonelli (1986), Dressler, Tonelli, and Magno Caldognetto (1987), and Magno Caldognetto, Tonelli, and Luciani (1987) have pointed to polar quantitative and to qualitative differences (accepted by Kotten [1984]); cf. also Blumstein (1978, p. 190).

[6]Garnham et al. (1982) presented no example of addition that was not either anticipatory or perservatory in nature. So far all subclassifications to be found in the literature are not detailed enough. But see Berg's PhD thesis (1985) and a monograph on corrections of slips versus paraphasias prepared by Dressler & E. Magno Caldognetto & L. Tonelli.

[7]Many examples can be found in Blumstein (1973), Kaczmarek (1984a, pp. 33ff), Kilani-Schoch (1982), Lecours and Lhermitte (1969), and Pilch and Hemmer (1970).

[8]For example, Berg (1985, pp. 23ff, 37ff, 79ff, 88ff), Buckingham (1980, pp. 210ff); Ellis (1980, p. 633); Magno Caldognetto and Tonelli (1985, pp. 80ff); Meringer (1908, p. 24ff); Shattuck-Hufnagel (1979, p. 30).

[9]Kilani-Schoch (1982, pp. 461ff) listed a somewhat higher number of blends from her aphasic patient. However, some examples are of rather doubtful nature because the target words are more similar to each other than is the case in German and English blends of normals.

[10]See Joanette, Goulet, Ska, and Nespoulous (1986), Kohn (1984); Dressler et al. (1986) (the latter authors are planning a monograph on corrections of slips versus paraphasias): of the Viennese approximately one fourth of the Broca's, one third of the Wernicke's and one half of the global patients were unsuccessful, in contrast to one half of the Italian Broca's and nearly two thirds of the Italian Wernicke's patients.

[11]At least in one of Fromkin's two examples (1973, pp. 249G.15): for "stick around and try to see"—"sick around and tie to tree—I near—trick around and sigh to tea—oh you know what I mean."

[12]See Lesser (1978, pp. 49ff). On the model and methodologies of studying sociophonological variation as developed in Vienna since 1971, see Dressler and Wodak (1982), and chapter 3 of this volume.

[13]For example confusion is not differentiated in Fradis & Calavrezo (1976).

[14]This claim has been enlarged by Wurzel and Boettcher (1979) to the view that all segmental substitutions in aphasia represent universal natural processes in the sense of Stampe (1969). However, performance errors do not represent natural

phonological processes, nor do intrusions (such as *papra* for *papa*) or other fairly infrequent errors that seem to be genuine selection errors, such as paradigmatic changes of place of articulation (cf. MacNeilage, 1982).

[15]These correspond roughly to lenition and fortition processes in Stampe (1969) and in Donegan and Stampe (1979).

[16]Differentiation of phonetic lengthening and hesitation phenomena is difficult. Clearly the labored pronunciation of Broca's aphasia (cf. Williams & Seaver, 1986) is not meant here.

[17]Instances with anticipatory or perseveratory vowel copying (intrusion) are not included, since they are classified as pure performance errors.

[18]See, for example, Blumstein (1973, p. 98) and other Blumstein references listed, Borrell and Nespoulous (1977), Buckingham (1982), Harmes et al. (1984), Keller (1984), Kohn et al. (1984), Kotten (1984), Nespoulous and Borrell, (1979), and Nespoulous et al. (1983,1984).

[19]For example, Berndt and Caramazza (1980), Canter, Trost, and Burns (1985), Keller (1978,1984), Kohn et al. (1984), MacNeilage (1982), Nespoulous et al. (1983).

2
Improvement of Coarticulation in Broca's Aphasia

HEINZ K. STARK, WERNER DEUTSCH,
JACQUELINE A. STARK, and RUDOLF WYTEK

Introduction

In the clinical setting, it often is necessary for therapeutic reasons to objectivize a patient's recovery process in a specific domain over time. This applies particularly to the articulatory abilities of the Broca's aphasic. In such a patient one perceives quantititative and qualitative differences in performance. However, it is difficult to describe the changes in performance in an objective manner. The purpose of the study reported here is to show in a single case study of Broca's aphasia how reliable information about improvement in language functions can be obtained without administering special tests. In this study, we analyzed and measured changes in coarticulatory speech behavior by applying direct and indirect measures and parameters not often used or described in the literature. Validity of the hypotheses and results were tested by means of statistical computations.

The reason for choosing coarticulation as the topic of the study lies in the fact that although our patient, H.B.—who received intensive and structured speech therapy—improved from severe to mild impairment, he showed remarkably less improvement in the modality "repetition" compared with the other tested modalities (reading, writing, naming, token test, language comprehension, and spontaneous speech). Even in his spontaneous speech and naming, the difficulties he encountered producing long words (e.g., compound nouns) or utterances were due to articulatory problems in addition to agrammatic deficits. That is, the execution of sound chains that build up words of more than two syllables was most difficult for our patient. For this reason, the articulatory difficulties were considered to stem from a problem of coarticulation, both in planning and in execution. Which of the two predominated, that is, was more severely affected, we could not discern.

Coarticulation

A very broad definition of the concept of coarticulation provided by Daniloff and Hammarberg (1973) was used by Johnston, Goldberg, and Mathers (1984):

> Coarticulation . . . is the influence of one speech segment upon another; that is, the influence of a phonetic context upon a given segment. The greatest variation of phonetic context is given in connected speech especially in discourse or "conversational speech." (p. 33)

Speech is thus viewed as a dynamic constant flow of overlapping, articulatory movements in which there are no clear boundaries between segments (cf. Johnston et al., 1984, p. 32).

Another basic feature of coarticulation is its bidirectionality. That is, a segment can exert influence in both directions up to three segments from left to right (L→R) or from right to left (R→L). In other words, we can have perseveratory (L–R) and anticipatory (R–L) coarticulation (cf. Johnston et at., 1984, p. 33). Accomodation is a form of coarticulation that should smooth out the differences between adjacent sounds. In terms of phonology, it is the application of natural processes such as assimilation, when two adjacent sounds have the same or different articulators (cf. Johnston et al., 1984). To explain the phenomenon of coarticulation properly we need an adequate model of coarticulation in the narrow sense, or better, an adequate model of speech production in the broad sense. Such a model should explain how speech is produced, taking as input discrete entities such as phonemes, which are transformed into a complex, overlapping, and variable articulatory output of the system (cf. Johnston et al., 1984).

Kent and Minifie (1977) developed a hierarchical model of speech production considered to account for the organization of speech motor control. We think that this model should be integrated into a model of speech production that starts from the intentional level as the highest level initiating speech production. It then works down from the semantic, syntactic, morphosyntactic level, constructing a hierarchical morphosyntactic representation, to the phonological phonetic level. It uses prosodic means to build up a prosodic hierarchy for the phonological representation of a word or an utterance, which is considered to be independent from the morphosyntactic hierarchy (cf. Van der Hulst & Smith, 1985). Sets of phonetic features are translated into articulatory patterns and finally into sequences of neuromotor commands as ". . . neutral instructions to the muscles, derived from transition requirements" (Johnston et al., 1984, p. 35). Such an integrated hierarchical model uses feedback, forefeeding, and short-term memory as components, as is the case in Laver's model (cf. Edwards, 1984).

Coarticulation has also been viewed as a form of co-production or as the result of it. The functional unit is assumed to consist of "different, though possibly overlapping sets of muscles" (Kent, 1983, p. 64), for example, the articulatory adjustments that take place for the vowel in co-occurrence with the articulation of the preceding consonant in a consonant-vowel (CV) sequence (cf. Kent, 1983). With reference to a coproduction model, there are different grades of overlapping of movements of the articulators. We can assume (a) minimal overlapping of coproduction units in a sound combination such as /bs/ and /xt/ in /ha:bsuxt/ (greediness); or /xtb/ in /axtbar/ (respectable); and (b) great overlapping as would be the case of "articulatory adaptation or accomodation between units that are highly similar in motor performance" (Johnston et al, 1984; Kent, 1983, pp. 63–65), for example, a sound sequence like /ist/ in /frist/ (time limit).

In articulatory planning, a continuum of variation can be posited between succession and synchrony, and overlapping is probably the form between these two poles. As the more natural form, overlapping allows articulation in an economical and unstrenuous manner, resulting in a smooth speech flow. This provides optimal perception for the hearer (cf. Dressler, 1985; Lindblom, 1983). "Articulatory movements seem to be programmed as coordinated structures so that movements of the tongue, lips, velum and jaw often occur in highly synchronous patterns" (Kent, 1983, p. 68). Motor control in healthy adults is refined and does not operate according to the principle of everything moves at once. This principle would mean total synchronization and would in fact be a breakdown of coarticulation, resulting in a very distorted, noncomprehensible sound sequence or in a blockage of the articulators. In fluent speech, a "fluent motor execution might depend on an overlapping of movements rather than synchronization of movements" (Kent, 1983, p. 71).

On the basis of these comments, a relationship between predominant type of coarticulation and type of speech style can be suggested, for example, casual versus very formal; even more concretely, a relationship between predominant type of coarticulation and phonological processes, as described in natural phonology, can be suggested. We claim that foregrounding (formal styles), corresponds with succession and overlapping and that backgrounding (casual, fast speech) corresponds predominantly with overlapping and synchronization. These two basic types are expressed articulatorily in strengthening processes, for example, /b/ → /p/ or, to the contrary, in weakening processes, /b/ → /β/, /p/ → /pf/(cf. chapter 1 and Dressler, 1985; Lass, 1985). The notions of backgrounding and foregrounding implicitly express that a segment, or in more general terms a figure, becomes more salient or less salient in relation to its surrounding context. This in turn is important for perception and is a basic principle in human perception (cf. Hilgard, Atkinson, & Atkinson, 1971).

Apraxia of speech (verbal apraxia or verbal dyspraxia) is one of the most common articulatory disorders and it co-occurs very often with Broca's aphasia. It affects coarticulation and is considered to be an impairment of the capacity to program the positioning of speech musculature and the sequencing of muscle movements for the volitional production of phonemes. The speech musculature shows neither significant weakness, slowness, nor incoordination when used for reflex and automatic acts. Prosodic alterations may be associated with articulatory problems, perhaps in compensation for them (cf. Deal & Darley, 1972; Rosenbek et al., 1984). Altered stress patterns or rhythmic patterns disrupting the hierarchical structure of the prosodic representation of an utterance have not been investigated thoroughly.

Verbal apraxia shows great variability, similar to the variability in children's speech patterns. Children need to acquire a certain level of refinement in motor execution to be able to perform a certain articulatory or phonetic goal that causes variation. However, in Broca's aphasics an impairment in this refinement causes variation in control of the durations of sound sequences, syllables, and words (cf. Kent, 1983). For example, a significant variance in sound duration in polysyllabic words can be expected, especially if we consider the position of the segment within the syllable. Syllables in certain positions within a polysyllabic word, for example, strong syllables in a metric foot, are expected to vary greatly in duration. (We will discuss our related findings later.)

Among various characteristic features of verbal apraxia, Shewan (1980) mentioned variation of difficulty in the stimuli, the range being from consonant clusters as the most difficult to single consonants and vowels. Place of articulation is considered the factor that is most susceptible: The most errors are with regard to place of articulation. Phonemic substitutions are considered the predominant error type. Errors increase with increasing syllable length of stimuli (cf. Kent, 1983). We will discuss and add a further related source of error, namely, number of syllables in the stimuli. Our results indicate that the overlapping or nonoverlapping of the prosodic and morphosyntactic hierarchy of a word or utterance is a possible source of planning and execution problem in coarticulation, which causes segment errors, an increase in sound and syllable duration, and pauses between syllables (e.g., covert repairs at the end of a planning unit). The increase of duration in polysyllabic words was investigated by Williams and Seaver (1986). If we consider verbal apraxia not primarily as an isolated impairment on a certain lower processing level, but rather as a "decay of efficiency" (cf. Martin, Wasserman, Gilden, Gerstman, & West, 1975) also on higher levels, then components must be taken into account, such as short-term memory and the complexity of information, that stem at least from the phonological and morphosyntactic hierarchies or representations to be processed.

In our analysis of Broca's aphasia, apraxic difficulty in coarticulation is viewed as one of the issues. Preliminary acoustic analysis led Kent and Rosenbek (1982) to the assumption that "verbal apraxia involves a difficulty in transitionalizing as well as a difficulty in sequential ordering of the segments" (p. 78). Mistiming in phonation, and initiation difficulties expressed in false and labored starts, are further features of apraxic speech. The distortion of temporal organization of speech expressed in articulatory prolongation, syllable separation, lengthening of the transitional or steady-state phase in an otherwise unimpaired speech pattern, stair-step formant movements, and the tendency to equalize single-sound duration is for Kent and Rosenbek (1982) a result of segmental decomposition. These features result in an overall picture of lengthened and rather inflexible sound durations. Decomposition of syllables in apraxia of speech is indicated by a significant increase in syllable duration and marked interruptions between syllables. "These widely spaced syllables in apraxia of speech can be seen as an exceeding of considerable time in preparing or programming each syllable. Each syllable interval between successive items can be a measure of programming complexity" (MacKay, 1974). In contrast to MacKay, Kent (1983) interpreted the interval between repeated syllables as "read out time," that is, as the time required to read out a program already prepared, rather than as programming time per se.

Articulatory prolongation defined as "the lengthening of transitional or steady state components in an otherwise uninterrupted speech pattern can be measured in voice onset time VOT or in the trajectories" (Kent, 1983, p. 78). Syllable segregation is defined as temporal separation or isolation of the syllables in a syllable series (cf. Kent & Rosenbek, (1982). An apraxic speaker has a considerably longer duration of utterance and a remarkable lengthening of the transitional and steady-state segments. A speaker acquires generalized spatiotemporal schemata for speech articulation. Individual motor programs are specified from these internalized general schemata. The schemata can become deteriorated. A breakdown in the processes of using the space coordinate system for speech shows up in place errors (cf. Kent, 1983)

Aphasia Studies on Coarticulation

Voice onset time (VOT) has been intensively investigated as a parameter in the aphasia literature (cf. Blumstein, Cooper, Zurif, & Caramazza, 1977; Blumstein et al., 1980). VOT was used as an operational measure for the distinction between phonemic and phonetic disintegration in aphasia. Broca's aphasics demonstrate both types, and anterior aphasics have a deficit in the articulatory programming of speech sounds. They make phonetic errors in VOT but also mistarget particular speech sounds. As a consequence, they shift into another phonetic category. The phoneme selection is largely correct, but the subsequent speech programming is impaired. In contrast, posterior aphasics have an impairment of phoneme selection in the context of appropriate articulatory programming (cf. Blumstein et al., 1977,1980). Broca's aphasics, however, make phonetic as well as phonological errors. Although their deficit is primarily a phonetic one, it is "rather a speech deficit than a low level motor control problem" (Blumstein et al., 1980, p. 153).

Ziegler and Cramon (1986) studied speech timing in apraxia of speech. They showed how overlapping and synchronization of different articulators fail in their timing. Shinn and Blumstein (1983) investigated the effect of phonetic disintegration of speech on spectral characteristics of speech sounds. They found an impairment of the dynamic aspects of speech production insofar "as their productions reflected problems with the source characteristics of speech sounds and with the integration of articulatory movements in the vocal tract" (p. 90). In a study on anticipatory coarticulation, Ziegler and Cramon (1985) observed delayed onset of coarticulatory gestures such as lip rounding, in particular in patients with apraxia of speech.

The interaction of phonological and morphological levels in aphasic performance in a repetition task was demonstrated by Martin et al. (1975). They found that the number of cognitive units to be processed within one stimulus word plays a role in the number, type, and position of errors. Stimulus words consisting of only one syllable but of two morphemes, for example, show more errors than one-syllable words only, even with an identical segment chain. They considered the errors not as reflecting a loss of particular skills but rather as reflecting reduced efficiency within the entire system. For them, articulatory impairment in aphasia expresses possible difficulties on all levels of language processing. They concluded that the presence or activation of "other aspects of language could not help but influence performance on an articulatory level" (Martin et al., 1975, p. 435).

Treiman (1983) pointed out that errors of speech production are influenced by syllable structure. She viewed the errors as evidence for a hierarchical syllable structure. Syllable constituents (onset-rime) might also have an influence on retrieval and perception. For Williams and Seaver (1986) it was not obvious whether the durational characteristics of speech sound production—found at least in some Broca's aphasics—are a primary component of a motor speech programming disturbance or a secondary characteristic resulting from difficulty or uncertainty in programming the segmental aspects of speech. The Broca's aphasics they judged as demonstrating labored articulation displayed longer sound durations; further—what is important for our study—the increases in duration were particularly marked for vowels and consonants in polysyllabic words. Williams and Seaver took into account the explanation suggested by Kent and Rosenbek (1982), that slowness of speech movements and prolongation of articulatory postures "are due, in part, to an impairment in retrieval and evaluation of information regarding the target" (p. 181).

Garnsey and Dell (1984) suggested that prolongation of segment and syllable duration or syllable segregation should rather be investigated from the assumption of a pre-editing component in the speech production model than from the programming view.

Goals of the Present Study

The aforementioned studies, although discussed only briefly, show the range of aspects investigated in the aphasia literature. In the present study we applied (a) the theories of metrical phonology (cf. Hogg et al, 1987) and natural phonology in combination with (b) measures of acoustic analysis (word duration mean value [WD], standardized syllable duration time per item [STSD]), and with (c) linguistic-prosodic measures such as metrical grid, stress pattern, and natural phonological processes, for analyzing and interpreting coarticulatory phenomena we think correlate with WD and STSD. The hypotheses addressed in this study were the following:

1. If speech is organized in a hierarchical and rhythmic prosodic structure with duration of segments and syllables determined by degrees of salience to convey information, then changes in the mean duration of words (WD) and in the standardized syllable duration of words (STSD) must indicate changes in the rhythmic pattern in general and in the stress pattern of a polysyllabic word or an utterance in particular, and vice versa.
2. A significant change in the mean values of WD and STSD correlates with improvement or worsening of coarticulation.
3. Significant lower mean values of WD and STSD indicate improved coarticulation.
4. Significant higher mean values of WD and STSD indicate deteriorated coarticulation.
5. Significant lower values in standard deviation of WD and STSD indicate stabilization of word and syllable duration, which in turn accounts for improved coarticulation.
6. Significant higher values in standard deviation of WD and STSD indicate increased fluctuation of word and syllable duration, which in turn can be interpreted as a sign of impaired coarticulation.
7. Intact coarticulation is a prerequisite for rhythmic patterns and stress patterns in speech.
8. Succession, overlapping, and synchronization—which are main categories of coarticulation in varying combinations in connection with intensity and pitch—facilitate the use of different speech styles according to their socially conventionalized pragmatic functions.
9. Impairment in coarticulation restricts the language user's capability of variation in the prosodic functions to a small range of possibilities for expressing semantic and connotational information.

10. The same stress pattern or metrical grid produced by a healthy person and by a Broca's aphasic may not serve the same pragmatic function.

Subjects

Patient H.B.

Our patient, H.B., a right-handed man with 12 years of schooling, suffered a cerebral-vascular accident (CVA) at age 49. By profession he was first a master baker and later an ice-cream maker who ran his own business. Eight months after his stroke he was able to go back to work. His premorbid language competence was assumed to comprise a local dialect of a small town in Lower Austria within the Middle Bavarian dialect group, Austrian Standard High German as it is taught in school, and Viennese dialect as the last acquired variety of German. Only Standard High German was acquired as a written language. In his communicative settings, the subject interacted with people of quite different social strata (customers, clerks of city and federal offices, etc). Therefore, it was necessary for him to be very flexible—on a small scale at least—in his language behavior. Use of hypercorrect forms was probably common for him. H. B. was not a fast speaker premorbidly.

CT Scan

The computed tomography (CT) scan performed 3 weeks after onset of the CVA showed a contrast-medium-enhanced lesion of the left frontal operculum and the insula (Fig. 2.1). The CT scan made 3 months later showed a large cystic lesion of the frontal operculum and the insula.

Language Testing

H.B. was intensively tested six times within 31 months after the CVA. We administered our own test battery—developed for research purposes—for the testing at 4 and 6 weeks post onset, and then also the Aachen Aphasia Test (AAT, cf. Huber, Poeck, Weniger, & Willmes, 1983) for testing 4, 9, 23, and 31 months post onset. H. B. was classified as a severely impaired Broca's aphasic 4 weeks post onset. He received intensive linguistically structured language therapy, and by 9 months post onset he had recovered to a mildly impaired Broca's aphasia. The AAT test results are summarized in the test profiles in Figure 2.2.

Language comprehension was H.B.'s best-preserved language modality from the beginning. His performance in the other modalities showed significant improvement; however, the repetition capability did not recover the same quantitative/qualitative amount as writing and naming. In his spontaneous speech there was significant improvement in coherence,

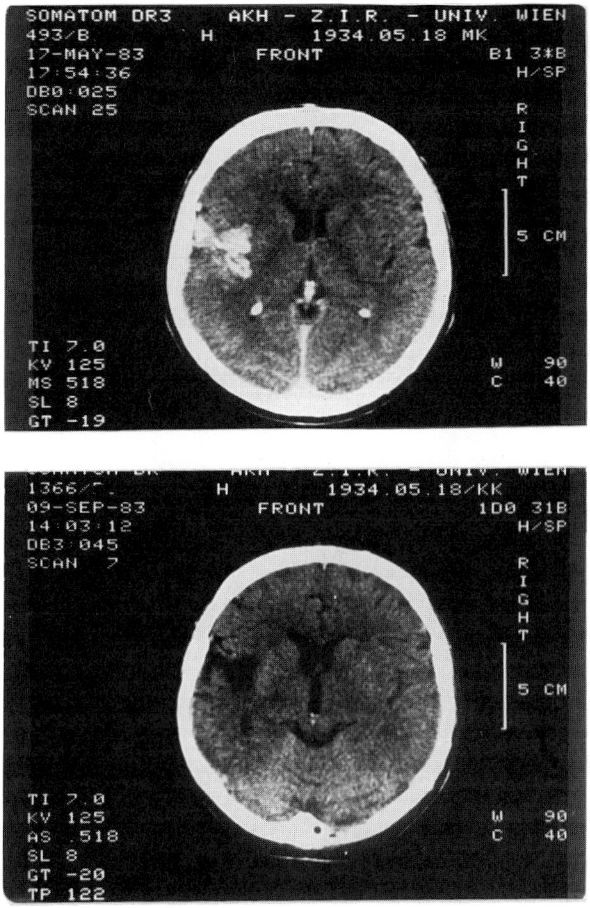

FIGURE 2.1 Representative CT Scan Sections of Patient H.B. (1) At three weeks post onset. (2) CT scan at 4 months post onset.

cohesion, informativity, and intertextuality (cf. Beaugrande & Dressler, 1981). Agrammatism, phonological impairments, and labored speech (e.g., coarticulatory difficulties, starts) were obvious on the sentence and text level and they seemed to interact with planning and reading out of plans. Language comprehension and naming were about normal at 23 months post onset (as determined by the AAT; however, H.B. displayed asyntactic comprehension. Cf. chapter 6).

Control Subject

The control subject was a 52-year-old, Viennese-born, male cartographer employed by the federal government. He acquired Viennese dialect orally

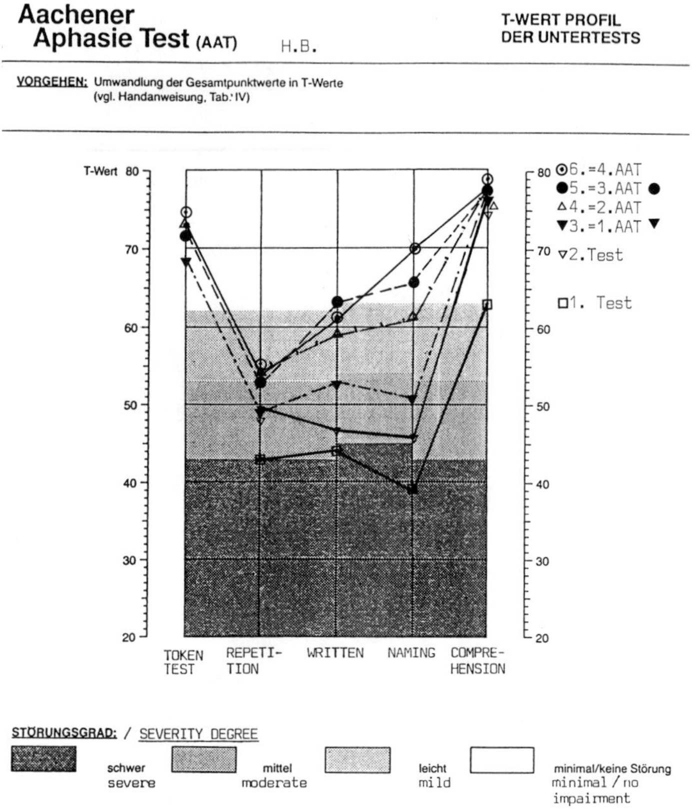

Figure 2.2 Aachen Aphasia Test Profiles of Patient H.B.

and Austrian Standard High German both orally and as a written language. His work required that he communicate with very different people (sociologically speaking) including superiors and clients. He also had to be relatively flexible in using different codes and in translating technical terms into everyday language. In his private life he preferred Viennese dialect or a mixture of dialect and Austrian Standard High German, typical of middle-class people with the same amount of schooling. He was a rather slow speaker.

Procedures

Recording Procedures

The two subjects and the tester were tape recorded on an Uher 4200 Report Monitor Stereo. The tape speed was 9.5 cm/s for the patient's tape recording and 19.0 cm/s for the control person's. (This difference was due to clinical conditions.)

Transcription

The tape recordings of the AAT were transcribed in a narrow phonetic transcription the international phonetic alphabet (1979 revised) using diacritics and marking of the stress pattern on each polysyllabic word. Narrow transcription was used mainly because we always try to extract linguistic-phonetic information from the tape recordings in as differentiated a way as possible. In the present study it was particularly important in order also to take into account apraxic speech patterns.

Acoustic-Phonetic Analysis

We produced two different types of spectrograms:

1. Wide-band spectrograms (300 Hz) made by a Digital Sonograph 7800 Kay. The dynamic range of this instrument is 8 kilohertz, the scale magnifier is 5 kilohertz, and the frequency marker is 500 kilohertz; it has 3D amplitude and a sonograph printer type 700.
2. Spectrograms based on (a) fast Fourier transform digitalized and (b) cepstrum analysis (according to Deutsch, 1985, pp. 98–102). Cepstrum analysis is used to extract fundamental frequency (f_0) from a speaker's sound signal. This analysis allows separation of the periodic parts of a speech signal, which is important for extracting fundamental frequency and the corresponding formants.

An example of a spectrogram made by cepstrum analysis is given in Figure 2.3. It consists of 384 spectras smoothed out by cepstrum analysis. The black dots within the dark printing of the speech signal correspond to the peaks of the single spectras; the dots compose traces that can be viewed as "candidates for formants" (cf. Deutsch, 1985).

The spectrogram basically contains information about (a) the time function (on the bottom), (b) the spectral analysis of the speech signal proper (formants, etc.), (c) the intensity of the speech item, (d) the fundamental frequency displaying the intonational pattern of the speech item, and (e) the values of the single formants printed out in numbers. (For further information about this method the reader is referred to Deutsch, 1985, pp. 95–103).

In our study, the spectrograms were used for duration time measurement and comparison of metrical grids with their acoustic correlates, intensity, and pitch (f_0). The stress pattern was one of our main measurements of change in coarticulation from the point of view of perception. Duration of sounds, syllables, and words was measured by using a scale corresponding to the spectrogram type, 1 millimeter equaling 10 milliseconds. For this reason we could measure only manually and in whole numbers.

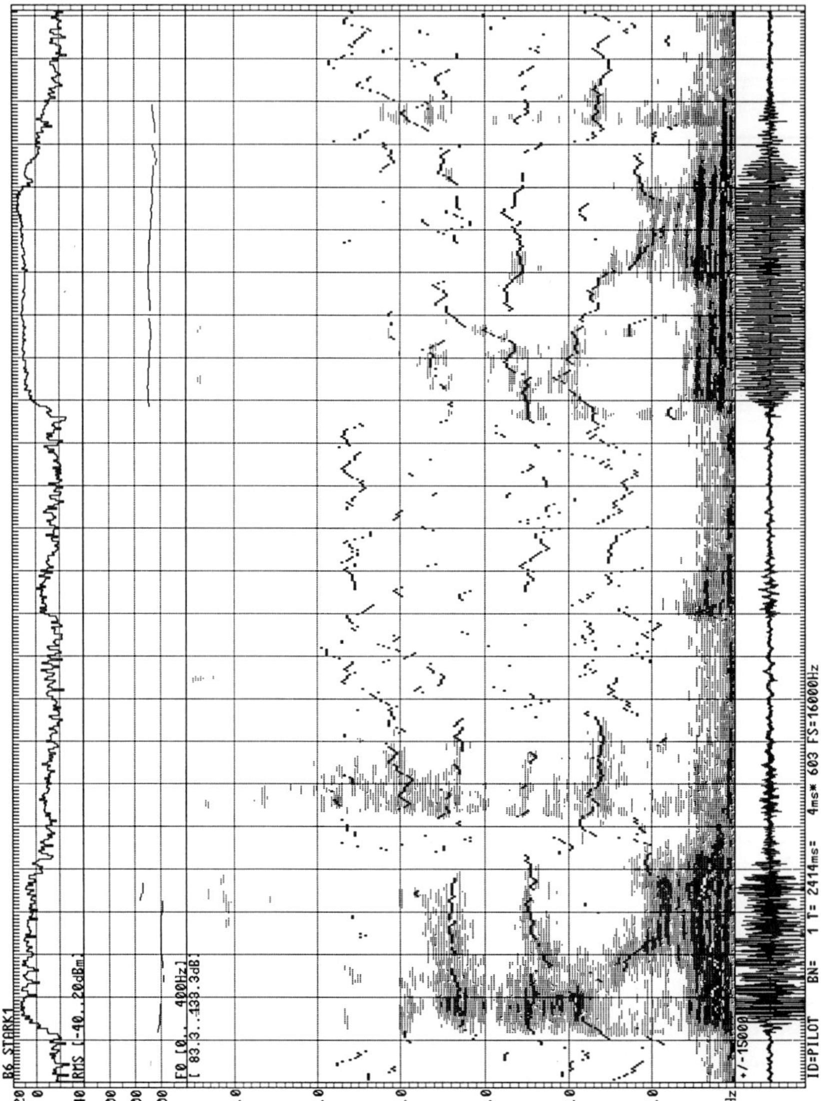

FIGURE 2.3 An Example of a Cepstrum Analysis Spectrogram

Variables Analyzed

For our analysis we chose the modalities of repetition and naming, but on the word level only. We used data from the repetition and naming subtests from the AAT given at 4 months and at 23 months post onset. Only those items H. B. produced in both tests without phonological mistakes (e.g., addition of segment) and without assumed covert repairs (marked by pauses between syllable or morpheme boundaries) were included in the analysis. The control person was tested in these two modalities only once. The tester's data from three tests were analyzed also. He had to pronounce each item once in each test session and the patient and control person repeated the particular word immediately after presentation. The tester spoke at a slower rate in the first test than in the second and third tests.

Repetition Task

For our analyses, the 23 (out of 30) correctly produced test items from the repetition subtest were divided into four groups according to the number of syllables: (1) one-syllable words (n = 11); (b) two-syllable words (n = 5); (c) three-syllable words (n = 4); and (d) four-syllable words (n = 3) (Table 2.1). German compound nouns and loan words were mixed together according to the number of syllables of each item.

Naming Task

This confrontation task required responses of one- to four-syllable words, like the repetition task. The tested items were grouped according to their number of syllables. The items in this subtest were different from those in the repetition subtest. Since the two subtests were administered within one testing session, a possible learning effect or generalization—which could have been induced by use of the same test items in the two subtests—was thus avoided. One shortcoming of the test design was that the groups did not contain the same number of items, for the reason that they were taken from a standardized test battery (i.e., screening test) and not from a specially designed, modality-oriented test (cf. Table 2.2, p. 41).

Statistical Analysis

We computed the following variables: word duration (WD), mean value and standard deviation; standardized duration of syllable per syllable group (STSD), mean value and standard deviation; and duration of each syllable in each syllable group, mean value and standard deviation. The statistical significance of the mean value and standard deviation of these variables was computed so that H. B.'s test 1 could be compared with his test 2. Further comparisons were (a) patient test 1 with test of control person, (b) patients test 2 with test of control person, and (c) test of control

TABLE 2.1 List of Test Items for the Repetition Task (n = 23)

One-syllable words (n = 11)	
Ast	(branch)
Floh	(flea)
Fürst	(prince)
Glas	(glass)
Knirps	(little boy)
Kur	(spa or cure)
Mund	(mouth)
Spruch	(spell or proverb)
Stern	(star)
Strumpf	(stocking)
Zwist	(quarrel)
Two-syllable words (n = 5)	
Haustür	(house door)
Kanu	(canoe)
Pilot	(pilot)
Püree	(mashed potatoes)
Verbot	(prohibition)
Three-syllable words (n = 4)	
Handschuhfach	(glove compartment)
Lotterie	(lottery)
Telefon	(telephone)
Umleitung	(detour)
Four-syllable words (n = 3)	
Hepatitis	(hepatitis)
Moderator	(talkmaster)
Schokolade	(chocolate)

person with tester's test. Tests 1, 2, and 3 of the tester were also compared and the mean of the three tests was compared with the mean of patient test 1 and test 2.

The purpose of this item-per-item comparison was to determine how H. B.'s performance changed from test 1 to test 2, in comparison with performance of the control subject. In other words, it was to determine whether the improvement due to therapy was significant. We applied the t-test for independent variables and the Mann-Whitney U test. We justified this because the patient improved to such an extent that we could, statistically speaking, analyze the data as if they stemmed from two different patients with the same aphasia syndrome but with a different degree of impairment (moderate versus mild).

Results

Repetition

Standardized Item Duration (STSD) or Standardized Mean Value of Syllable Duration

The STSD is the quotient of standardized item duration and number of syllables per item. Figure 2.4 gives the values for each item in milliseconds (vertical axis) and the number of the corresponding item (horizontal axis). Items of one-syllable words are the numbers 1 through 11; two-syllable words, 12 through 16; three-syllable words, 17 through 20; and four-syllable words, 21 through 23. The figure shows the patient's performance in the two tests. The difference of STSD between test 1 and test 2, that is, the amount of improvement, is displayed in the bottom line. There was a positive overall difference ranging from 250 milliseconds as the highest value to about 20 milliseconds as the lowest. The greatest differences or improvements in duration per item were in the one-syllable words. However, a decrease in improvement with increasing number of syllables per item is observed. The number of syllables and number of morphemes overlapping each other in the segment chain must be considered as sources for the higher values of duration in polysyllabic words. More processing time is needed to identify polysyllabic words that are compound

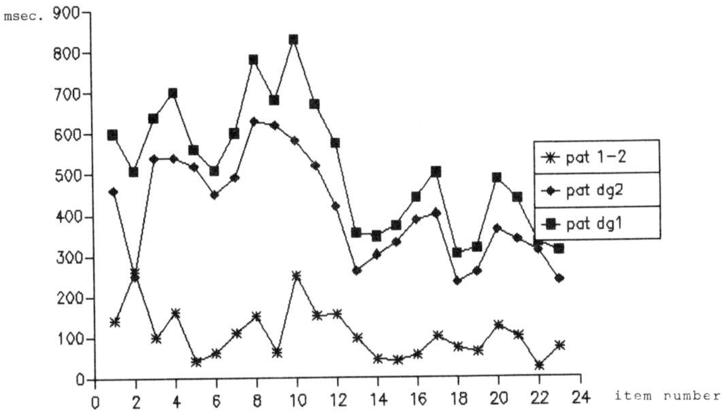

Legend:

pat 1-2 Difference between test 1 and test 2
pat dg2 Patient's test 2
pat dg1 Patient's test 1

FIGURE 2.4 Standardized Item Duration "STSD" or Standardized Mean Value of Syllable Duration

nouns in which the prosodic hierarchy and the morphosyntactic hierarchy are not in isochrony but overlap, that is, when syllable boundary does not equal morpheme boundary.

Comparison of STSD of Patient's Test 1 with Control Person's Test

The curve for the patient's first test clearly displays a longer duration for all items except one as compared with the control person's values (Fig. 2.5). However, in the second test the curves resemble each other. It is noteworthy that the patient spoke 7 out of 11 one-syllable words faster than the control person. The longer and the more complex the items were, the more the duration increased also within the patient's data. In nine items (39% in contrast to only 5% in the first test) the patient had better values than the control person. The better values were predominantly restricted to one-syllable words; only two polysyllabic words were repeated faster by H. B. than by the control person.

Comparison of Patient's Test 1 and Test 2 with Mean Values of Tester's Three Tests

There was a clear longer duration of items in the patient's first test (Fig. 2.6). Only three one-syllable words (13%) had a shorter duration. Comparison of the second test with the mean values of the tester's three tests shows a high resemblance of the curves. If we compare the values of the control person's test with the mean values of the tester's three tests (Fig. 2.7), they are about identical. The control person had better values (i.e., shorter duration) in 11 items, 8 of them one-syllable words. The control person's profile is very similar to the tester's, and the patient's profile resembles the control person's to a great extent.

Thus, the patient's improvement can be assumed to be due to therapy and not to conditioning by the tester during the second test: H.B. was able to produce the target item more often. One argument in favor of this conclusion is the fact that in the first test, although the tester spoke noticeably slower than in the second and third tests as one can see in the duration data, the patient articulated even slower. In summary, we can assume that therapy had a positive influence on the patient's skills to coarticulate words consisting of one to four syllables. H. B.'s performance declined greatly with items of more than six syllables, for example, the word ($ = syllable boundary) /ferantwor$tungs$lo:sigkait/, (irresponsibility), in which seven syllables overlap and the test item has a very complex morphemic structure /fer +ant + wort + ung + s + lo:s + ig + kait/, or another example /farb$fern$se:gerä:tever$kauf/ (sale of color TVs). It is noteworthy, however, that the patient had shorter durations in four-syllable loan words such as /hepati$tis/ (hepatitis) than in compound nouns or even three-syllable loan words like /lotteri:/ (lottery). These items are easier to pronounce than /hant$ʃu:$fach/ (glove compart-

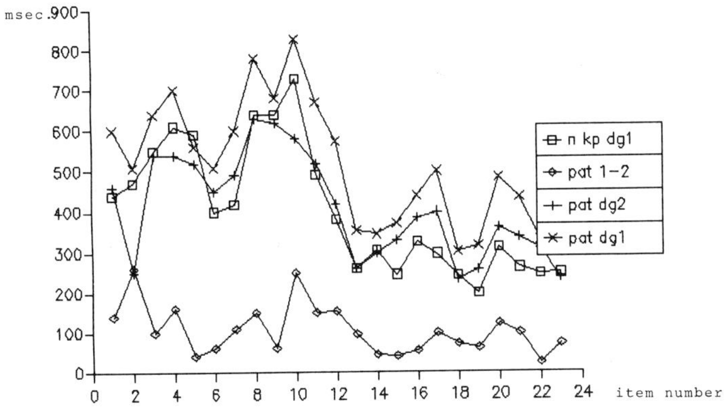

Legend:

kp Control Person
pat 1-2 Difference between test 1 and test 2
pat dg2 Patient's test 2
pat dg1 Patient's test 1

Duration (msec)

		pat dgl	pat dg2	pat 1-2	n kp dgl
Item Number	1.00	600.00	460.00	140.00	440.00
	2.00	510.00	250.00	260.00	470.00
	3.00	640.00	540.00	100.00	550.00
	4.00	700.00	540.00	160.00	610.00
	5.00	550.00	520.00	40.00	590.00
	6.00	510.00	450.00	60.00	400.00
	7.00	600.00	490.00	110.00	420.00
	8.00	780.00	630.00	150.00	640.00
	9.00	680.00	620.00	60.00	640.00
	10.00	830.00	580.00	250.00	730.00
	11.00	670.00	520.00	150.00	490.00
	12.00	575.00	420.00	155.00	380.00
	13.00	355.00	260.00	95.00	260.00
	14.00	345.00	300.00	45.00	305.00
	15.00	370.00	330.00	40.00	245.00
	16.00	440.00	385.00	55.00	325.00
	17.00	500.00	400.00	100.00	296.67
	18.00	303.33	233.33	70.00	243.33
	19.00	316.67	256.67	60.00	200.00
	20.00	483.33	360.00	123.33	313.33
	21.00	435.00	337.50	97.50	262.50
	22.00	330.00	307.50	22.50	247.50
	23.00	310.00	237.50	72.50	250.00

FIGURE 2.5 Comparison of STSD of the Patient's Test 1 and 2 with Control Person's Test on the Repetition Task

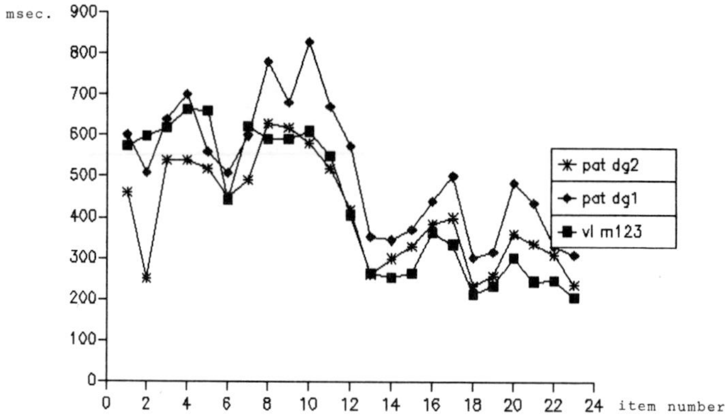

Legend:

pat dg2 Patient's test 2
pat dg1 Patient's test 1
vl m123 Tester's mean value for test 1,2,3

FIGURE 2.6 Comparison of Patient's Test 1 and 2 with the Mean Values of the Tester's Three Tests on the Repetition Task

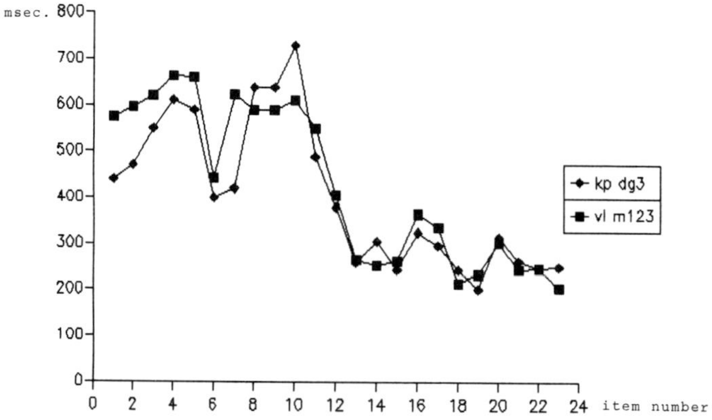

Legend:

kp dg3 Control Person
vl m123 Tester's mean value for test 1,2,3

FIGURE 2.7 Comparison of Control Person's Test 1 with the Mean Values of the Tester's Three Tests on the Repetition Task

TABLE 2.2 List of Test Items for the Naming Task ($n = 15$)

One-syllable words ($n = 2$)	
Buch	(book)
Tisch	(table)
Two-syllable words ($n = 8$)	
Besen	(broom)
Gürtel	(belt)
Kerze	(candle)
Koffer	(suitcase)
Kühlschrank	(refrigerator)
Nagel	(nail)
Rollschuh	(roller skate)
Waage	(scale)
Three-syllable words ($n = 3$)	
Eiskasten	(icebox)
Schuhlöffel	(shoe horn)
Staubsauger	(vacuum cleaner)
Four-syllable words ($n = 2$)	
Schraubenzieher	(screwdriver)
Taschenlampe	(flashlight)

ment), in which syllable boundaries and morpheme boundaries converge and consist of an identical number of segments. The word /umlaitung/ (detour) is another example of a German compound noun of three syllables that consists of three morphemes and overlaps in /laitung/. The syllable structure is /umlaitung/, whereas the morpheme structure is / um + lait + ung/.

Statistical Significances of the Repetition Task

H. B.'s results in test 1 and test 2 were highly significant ($p<.002$) in the difference between mean value of word duration (WD) and standardized syllable duration (STSD). Thus, the patient performed better in the second test. Standard deviation of the first syllable in two-syllable words was significantly lower in the second test ($p<.007$).

Comparison of Patient's Test 1 with Control Person's Test

The mean values of WD and STSD were significantly lower in the control person's results ($p < .032$). However, in two-syllable words there was nearly no significant difference in mean of STSD ($p < .049$) between H. B. and the control person. Only the mean duration of the first syllable was minimally significant ($p < .046$) in favor of the control person. The mean duration of the second syllable in two-syllable words was significantly longer ($p < .036$), nearly double that of the patient's items. Except for one item /haos$ty:r/ (housedoor), the first syllable was the strong syllable of the metric foot. The standard deviation of WD and STSD was significantly higher in the patient's items ($p < .028$). In four-syllable words the mean duration of the first and second syllable was much longer for the control person ($p < .016$) than in the patient's items.

Comparison of Patient's Test 2 with Control Person's Test

There was no significant difference in standard deviation and mean value for WD and STSD in one-syllable words. In two-syllable words there was a highly significant greater standard deviation ($p < .015$) for the second syllable in the patient's items. Three-syllable words showed no significant difference in all the tested parameters. However, there was a slightly significant higher standard deviation in WD and STSD ($p < .042$). However, mean value of WD and STSD and also mean duration of the single syllables in the four-syllable word group displayed no significant differences. On the whole, H. B.'s performance on the second test was statistically significantly better than on the first test and resembled the control person's values.

Naming

The patient improved on all items in the second test, the range being from 220 to about 15 milliseconds (Fig. 2.8). Compared with the control person, the patient had better values on six of the one-syllable words in his second test but on none of them in the first test. The tendency was—as pointed out for the repetition task—for performance to worsen proportionately to the increase in number of syllables and structural complexity of the items, for example, /rol$ʃu:/ (roller skates) or /ʃraobentsi:$er/ (screwdriver).

The greatest difference was observed for the word /ʃraobentsi:er/ (screwdriver). In German, this word consists of four syllables, two metric feet in its prosodic hierarchy, and four morphemes in the morphosyntactic hierarchy (two stems: schraub- and zieh-; one inflectional ending, -en; and one word formative, -er). In addition, the morphemes and syllables overlap in their relations to the phonemes: /ʃ raob + en + tsi: + er/ versus /ʃraobentsi:$er/. Both naming and repetition subtests present very similar processing difficulties that overtax coarticulatory programming and reading out of the program, that is, making of words. There is a complex interaction of different language and neuronal levels, starting from the intentional level and ending in the verbal utterance. For our patient, the main possibility for making errors appeared to be between the intentional level and the articulatory programming level (cf. Edwards, 1984). These findings support our main hypothesis that apraxia connected with Broca's aphasia is more than an isolated speech disorder, but is rather a matter of "decay of efficiency" (cf. Martin et al., 1975).

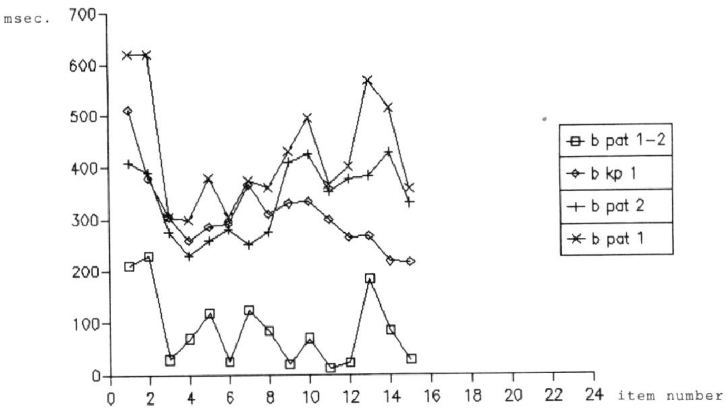

Legend:

pat 1-2 Difference between test 1 and test 2
kp Control Person
pat2 Patient's test 2
pat1 Patient's test 1

Duration (msec)

		b pat 1	b pat 2	b kp 1	b pat 1–2
Item Number	1.00	620.00	410.00	510.00	210.00
	2.00	620.00	390.00	380.00	230.00
	3.00	305.00	275.00	305.00	30.00
	4.00	300.00	230.00	260.00	70.00
	5.00	380.00	260.00	285.00	120.00
	6.00	305.00	280.00	290.00	25.00
	7.00	375.00	250.00	365.00	125.00
	8.00	360.00	275.00	310.00	85.00
	9.00	430.00	410.00	330.00	20.00
	10.00	495.00	425.00	335.00	70.00
	11.00	366.67	353.33	300.00	13.34
	12.00	400.00	376.67	263.33	23.33
	13.00	566.67	383.33	266.67	183.34
	14.00	512.50	427.50	217.50	85.00
	15.00	357.50	330.00	215.00	27.50
	16.00				
	17.00				
	18.00				
	19.00				
	20.00				
	21.00				
	22.00				
	23.00				

FIGURE 2.8 Comparison of Patient's Test 1 and Test 2 with the Control Person's Test on the Naming Task

Comparison of Patient's Test 1 with Control Person's Test

No significant differences could be expected in the one-syllable word group, since there were only two items.

Comparison of Patient's Test 2 with Control Person's Test

No significant differences existed in any parameter in one-syllable words. The same held for two-syllable words, except for a tendency in standard deviation of mean of WD and STSD ($p < .049$). In three-syllable words the patient's standard deviation of mean value in WD and STSD was significantly higher ($p < .003$). The greatest differences in mean of duration of syllables existed in the first and third syllables. Standard deviation of WD and STSD in four-syllable words was significantly higher ($p <$ .033) in the patient's results.

In summary, the naming results were similar to those of the repetition task, that is, no statistical difference with reference to one- and two-syllable words but a clear significant difference in three- and four-syllable items. The mean values and standard deviations of WD and STSD were not at all similar to the control person's. The difference displayed in Figure 2.8 was statistically significant, although the patient achieved better values in the second test on all items. The patient's coarticulation improved. However—as was true for the repetition task—if the patient had to produce a word (compound noun) that consisted of three or more syllables and had a fairly complex morphemic structure, coarticulatory processing slowed down. This was expressed by an increase in mean duration values of segments and syllables. It was also expressed by syllable segregation, which in turn was indicated by pauses between the syllables or at morpheme boundaries. Coarticulation was overtaxed and would break down to the extent that the patient even gave up repairing the target item he intended to produce. This can be taken as support for the hypothesis that coarticulation is brought about by a complex interaction of at least the phonological and morphosyntactic components as parts of the linguistic program, with the motor schema program, the neuromuscular program, and the articulatory program being supported by a feedback and forefeeding device and short-term memory (cf. Edwards, 1984; Laver, 1977).

Discussion

In our study we tried to show how parameters other than VOT, transjectories, steady-state duration, and so on can reliably be applied to evaluate changes in or improvement of coarticulation. It was our intention to determine whether data obtained under clinical conditions by administering a standardized aphasia test battery can provide objectively measurable information. Due to the difficulties involved in carrying out specific acoustic and linguistic experiments, we wanted to look for indirect parameters of coarticulation that we assumed would correlate highly with articulatory processes or speech production.

On the basis of empirically founded hypotheses, we selected mean word duration (WD) and standardized mean duration of syllables per item (STSD) as our two main acoustic parameters. Furthermore, the metrical grid pattern was viewed as a prosodic indirect measure for coarticulation, and natural phonological processes were viewed as a further indicator of variation in coarticulation. The statistical results of WD and STSD provide reliable support for our empirical impression that, on the whole, the patient's coarticulatory skills improved significantly in all of the tested items in both the repetition and naming tasks.

Improvement was indicated by an approximation toward the values of the control person and the tester. Although our patient improved, his performance was very dependent on

1. The number of syllables per item. An increase in the number of syllables resulted in poorer performance.
2. Increasing complexity of number and structure of syllables per word.
3. Increasing complexity of the morphosyntactic structure per word.
4. Increasing overlapping between the hierarchical prosodic structure and the hierarchical morphosyntactic structure of a word.

With respect to changes over time, the results show that improvement was much less in three- and four-syllable words in contrast to one- and two-syllable words, although the one-syllable words also had complex syllable structures such as CCVCC in /tsvist/ (quarrel) or CCCVCC in /ʃtrumpf/ (stocking). It must be stressed that these items have a one-to-one relation between syllable number and morpheme number. One syllable is at the same time one morpheme. For example, the item /ʃtrumpf/:

Prosodic hierarchy

Segment tier

Morphosyntactic hierarchy

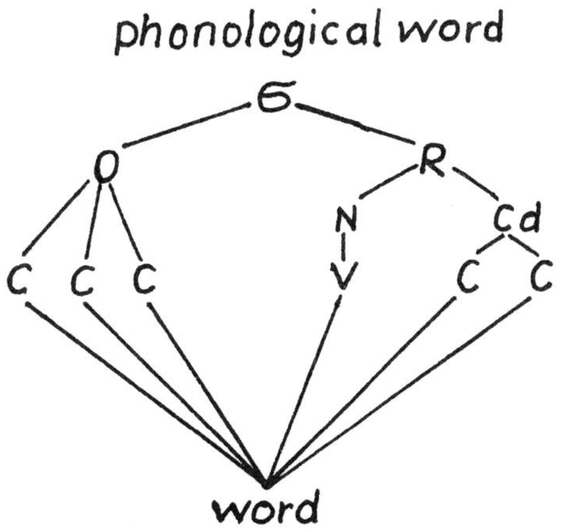

Comparison of the control person's rate of production with the rate of production on the second test revealed that the patient sometimes produced at a faster rate (e.g., for the word "glass" 540 msec, in contrast to 610 msec). On the patient's first test the rate of production was similar for the patient and the control person ("glass": 700 msec in contrast to 670 msec). The spectrogram shown in Figure 2.9 illustrates this similiarity in rate of production for a one-syllable word.

Another example of complex syllable and morpheme structure plus overlapping of both is the test item /umlaitung/ (detour):

Prosodic hierarchy

Segment tier

Morphosyntactic hierarchy

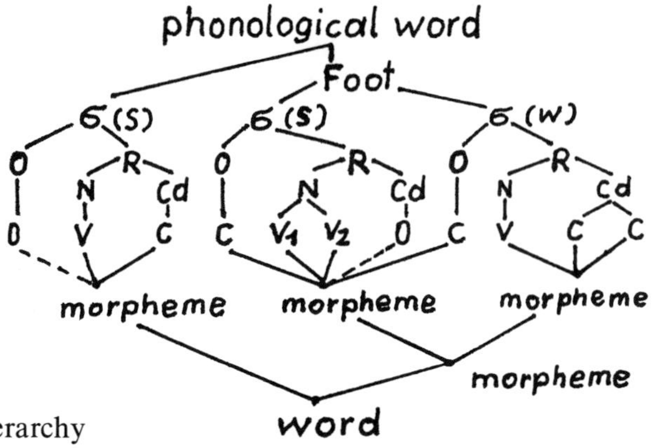

The complexity of these structures and their overlapping connections with the segmental tier has its correlate in the duration of strong and weak syllables. The complexity can be seen in the wide-band spectrogram for the word "Umleitung" (Fig. 2.10). Comparison of the patient's first and second test with the control person's test shows a great difference in the duration of the segments, the syllables, and the whole compound noun.

The spectrogram of the patient's first test displays an extraordinary lengthening of the phonemes /m,l,t/ and also of the three syllables, in comparison with the other spectrograms. It is important that the segment /m/ is the coda of the first syllable with the features /C, labial, nasal, continuant, voiced/. Segment /l/ is in the onset of the second syllable with the features /C, lateral, continuant, voiced/. Both segments are at syllable and morpheme boundaries. A further fact that complicates coarticulation at this point is the complex change from a bilabial sound to a lateral one. It is rather a succession of segments than an overlapping. A similar articulatory problem for the patient was found for the item /hu:bʃraober/ (helicopter) between the segments /b/ and /ʃ/. With reference to the word "detour," the next complex point is in /lai$tung/. It is not so much an articulatory problem in the transition from /ai/ to /t/, because overlapping and synchronization of the articulators is much easier than between /m/ and /l/. However, what is to be processed is the information about the

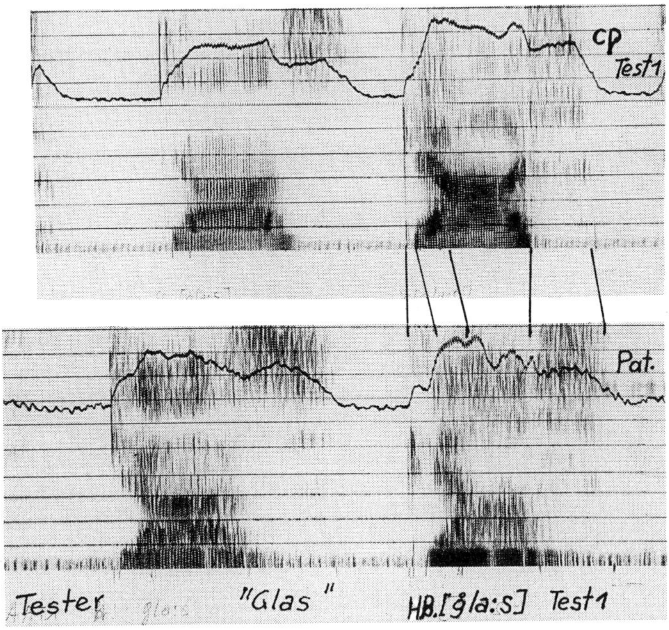

FIGURE 2.9 Spectrogram of Patient's Test 1 and Control Person's Test: Repetition of Word "Glass"

overlapping of the syllables /lai$tung/ with the morphemes /lait + ung/. This is further complicated by the fact that the syllable /lai/ is the strong one and /$tung$/ is the weak one. Thus, the information processing of the input, the planning, the reading out, and the execution of this word item are much more complex and a greater load for short-term memory than the item "Strumpf" (stocking).

If we consider all the above-mentioned facets involved in perception and production of polysyllabic words, then we cannot claim that the patient's problem is only one of motor programming. Rather, H. B.'s problem seems to be an insufficient operation of the components of the language system in connection with a decay of storage capacity of short-term memory and articulatory difficulties, which, however, are only slightly apraxic ones.

With respect to coarticulation and metrical grid, one of our basic assumptions and hypotheses in connection with coarticulation suggests that speech is organized in hierarchical rhythmic patterns. We decided to analyze and interpret our data by applying metrical phonology, because we were of the opinion that stress patterns must correlate with coarticulatory movements. We are aware, however, that the relation between stress patterns or rhythmic patterns and coarticulation is an indirect one,

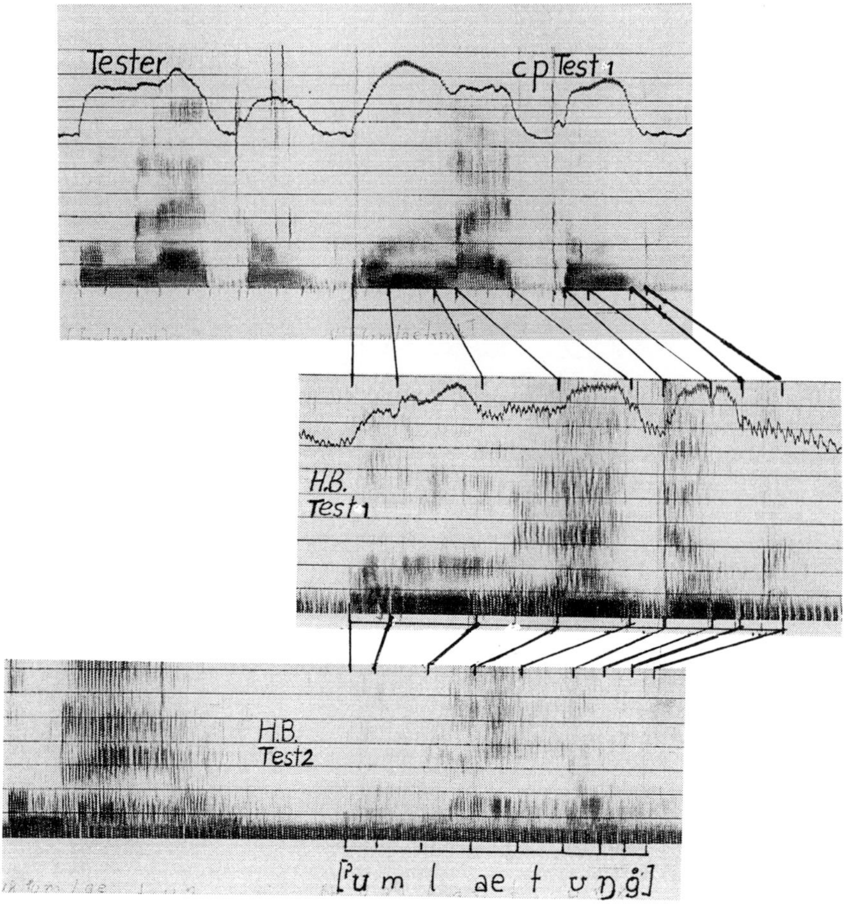

FIGURE 2.10 Spectrogram of Patient's Test 1 and Test 2 and Control Person's (cp) Test: Repetition of Word "Umleitung" (Detour)

because there are many possibilities of variation in intensity, pitch, and duration within one word item.

We applied a grid-cum-tree theory (cf. Hayes, 1984; Selkirk, 1984). The reasons were twofold: (a) A proper hierarchical phonological representation must consist of a binary tree structure, displaying the hierarchical relations between syllables, feet, and the phonological word, and (b) the stress pattern, as the other component, can be shown best in metrical grids, because stress relations between syllables within a word or utterance are n-nary in nature. Fine variation in the stress pattern or rhythmic pattern of an utterance can be captured by applying the TGA (text-to-grid-alignment) rules (cf. Hayes, 1984; Selkirk, 1984). This method is especially applicable to linguistic data of aphasic patients. In our analyses, changes in the rhythmic patterns were observed toward more rhythmicity, that is, shifts toward the control person's rhythmic patterns. Table 2.3 shows examples of changes in stress patterns in H. B.'s utterances.

Stress clashes as violations of the rhythmic alternation (RA) rule have to be interpreted with great caution (cf. Selkirk, 1984). If we take stress clash in the narrower sense—which Selkirk did not do—we will seldom find ideal rhythmic patterns. The comparison of metrical grids between our patient and the control person leads us to the conclusion that the n-nary nature of stress serves a communicative-pragmatic function. A healthy person has a wide range of varying stresses on syllables within a word or an utterance. Moreover, what is considered to be a stress clash might serve a certain communicative function. For example, if a person does not want to answer a question, he or she can show this reluctance by not using pitch accent and basic beat rules. At the other extreme, someone wanting to explain something clearly would use beat addition and pitch

TABLE 2.3 Examples of Metrical Grids from Patient H.B. and Control Person

	Patient H. B.	Control Person
Test 1	x x x x x x x [ˈˈhaɔsˈtyːʁ]	x x x x x x [ˈˈhaɔsˌty · ɐ]
Test 2	x x x x x x [ˈˈhaɔsˌty · ə]	
Test 1	x x x x x x x x x [ˈˈʔumˈlaeˌtʊŋk̥ʰ]	x x x x x x x x x [ˈˈʔumˈlaeˌtʊŋg̊]
Test 2	x x x x x x x [ˈˈʔumˌlaetʊŋg̊]	

accent rules, which would sound like spelling syllables. The Broca's aphasic has available only a limited range of purposeful variation in stress pattern.

Application of natural process rules as a function of foregrounding and backgrounding was also observed in H. B.'s repetition tasks. There was a remarkable tendency toward backgrounding in interaction with more rhythmic stress patterns in the second test. On some items the patient was even less formal than the control person, for example, on item /na:gel/ (nail):

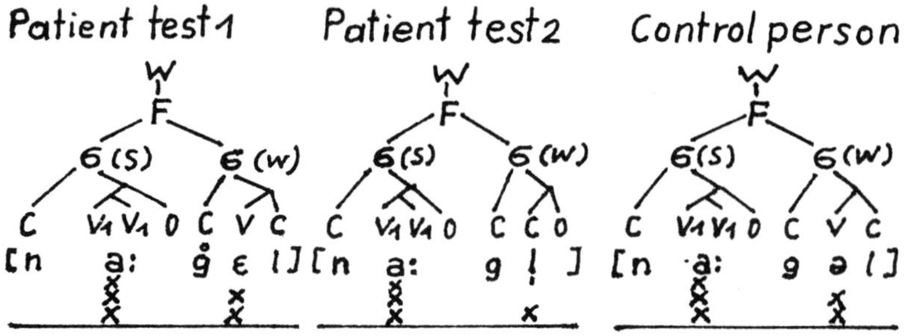

In test 1 the patient (a) devoiced intervocalic /g/ → [g̊] (onset); (b) did not apply vowel reduction in the unstressed syllable /e/ → [ə], and (c) did not apply Schwa deletion [ə] → ø. In test 2, intervocalic /g/ was not devoiced, but Schwa deletion and syllabification of /1/ (coda), which became the nucleus of the unstressed syllable, were applied. This test item also showed rhythmic alternation. In both tasks—repetition and naming—the application of backgrounding decreased within items of more than two syllables.

In summary, our results indicate that the chosen parameters, including WD, STSD, metrical grid, and natural processes, can be used in evaluating changes—in our case improvement—of coarticulation and in demonstrating the complexity of the processes involved in articulation of speech in various modalities in Broca's aphasia.

3
Sociophonology and Aphasia

HEINZ KARL STARK, WOLFGANG ULRICH DRESSLER,
and SYLVIA MOOSMÜLLER

Introduction

Sociophonological concepts or methods have not been applied to the study of aphasia in any systematic manner to date. We have combined two approaches—one developed in Vienna over the past 10 years and the other adapted to the study of aphasia—to enable such an application to language data collected on aphasic subjects in various test situations. These two approaches comprise the following:

1. The study of phonological disturbances in aphasia in terms of the framework of Natural Phonology (cf. Dressler, 1974, 1982, and chapter 1 of this volume).
2. The sociopsycholinguistic study of phonological variation as developed within the Department of Linguistics of the University of Vienna since 1972. In this approach, phonological processes and input switches, for example, are investigated in terms of social and psychological factors (cf. Dressler, 1975; Dressler & Wodak, 1982).

Crystal (1980) raised the question of style ranges in language pathology, but neither he nor any other researcher has approached this question seriously to date. Two of the reasons seem to be the following:

1. Sociolinguistics seems to be part of pragmatics, that is, of the relations among speaker, hearer, place, and time of the speech act; social and cognitive presuppositions of the interaction, and so on. Moreover, many aphasiologists have assumed that pragmatics is not impaired in aphasia (cf. Cohen, Kelter, & Woll, 1980; Reischies, 1984; cf. also a project announced in Bowerman & Eling, 1983).
2. Within aphasiology, the controversy has not been resolved whether aphasia affects competence or performance (cf. Keller, 1987; Weigl & Bierwisch, 1970; Whitaker, 1970; Zurif & Caramazza, 1976). However, L. Hjelmslev's and E. Coseriu's (1967) postulated intermediate level of (sociolinguistic) norms—which bridges the gap between the Saussurian levels of *langue* ("competence") and *parole* ("performance")—has

been overlooked (cf. Houston, 1969). That is, aphasia researchers have investigated structurally incorrect forms ("errors") but have not considered whether structurally correct forms are used in a sociolinguistically adequate way.

Dialect or Standard

In aphasia research, the use of dialect in the recovery process has been commented on mainly in studies on polyglot aphasics. The linguistic discussions are not extensive; they usually consist of brief descriptions of the aphasic's language skills in the various languages. In older literature this was often done in a phenomenological way.

Minkowski (1927), however, gave a comprehensive description—in particular of the recovery process—of two Broca's aphasics who premorbidly spoke Swiss German, and Standard High German. He discussed the possible reasons for the differential order of recovery of Swiss German versus Standard High German. In both cases the standard language, which was learned and used orally and in reading and writing, showed much faster and better recovery than dialect, which was acquired only orally. It must be noted that in the language therapy sessions the standard language form was used (Standard German in one case and Standard French in the other). Reading and writing exercises made up a substantial part of the patients' language therapy sessions. Minkowski stressed the significance of stored visual images of letters and words ("visuelles Bild der Druckschrift," p. 59) as a determining factor for the recovery of the standard language.[1] Dialect recovered in only one of the two Broca's aphasics. This was attributed to the patient's having learned how to read and write his Swiss dialect.

Weniger and Beck (1985) raised the question of the aphasic's differential susceptibility of symptoms in colloquial speech and standard language in a study of an aphasic's production of Swiss Standard German in comparison with colloquial Swiss German. They showed that a Wernicke's aphasic (moderately or mildly impaired) used different planning and description strategies in Standard German and Swiss German when producing picture stories. Descriptions were produced in both varieties of German (Standard German and Swiss dialect). Word-finding difficulties, which were more pronounced in the Standard German, were more easily compensated for in Swiss German. In Standard German descriptions there was a tendency to produce more precise and adequate descriptions of each picture, which resulted in greater word-finding difficulties. In dialect descriptions the patient tended to produce a coherent story based on the pictures.

Minkowski (1927) and Weniger and Beck (1985) both drew attention to important issues concerning the use of dialect versus standard language by aphasics. However, they did not explicitly deal with linguistic, especially phonological, rules and processes on a theoretical basis and did not discuss phonological phenomena.

Although the problem of whether to use dialect or standard language in therapy is well known to many therapists, it has been investigated only recently. Rekart and Buckingham (1979) reported on the use of Cuban versus Castilian Spanish.

In a discussion of the nature of the therapist's input language, Crystal (1984) emphasized the interactive or even constitutive role the therapist's language plays in defining the patient's symptoms. In this context, he considered an anlaysis of the linguistic level of the therapist's language in relation to the level at which the patient is functioning to be a central issue. In long-term studies pertaining to formal testing of conversational skills and the analysis of language samples collected over time, specific changes must be taken into account, in particular that the conversation will become more informal. This and other factors will determine the therapist's "choice of sounds, grammar, and vocabulary" (p. 148). Crystal discussed a detailed set of variety variables. (A summary of these variables and examples of the difficulties that could be encountered in therapy sessions is given in Crystal, 1984, pp. 152–153.)

The adequate use of dialect is just one case of style/register choice, and it depends on sociolinguistic norms of social class/stratum, social role, topic of interactive communication, social identification of the speech situation, and so on. Every speaker varies in speech production, and phonological variation has been successfully correlated with sociopsychological factors (e.g., in the above-cited studies on Viennese).

One important factor is the degree of formality of a speech situation, that is, whether the speaker interprets or defines the speech situation in which he or she is involved as (very) formal or (very) informal. According to this definition the speaker chooses more or less formal speech styles/registers.

With respect to aphasics, we have observed the following:

1. They use more formal styles/registers in therapy sessions than do patients whose speech is not impaired.
2. Whereas nonaphasics modify their styles/registers in the course of therapy, because of habituation to therapist and speech situation, aphasics remain formal.
3. Even in the framework of our ongoing aphasia project, aphasics remained formal when the same person (e.g., H. K. Stark) tested them with comprehensive language tests in four approximately 1-hour sessions, then administered ten 1-hour therapy sessions, and finally retested them again in four 1-hour sessions. The tester's and therapist's speech in terms of language style, that is, formality, consistency, and completeness of expression, is presently being analyzed.

Subjects

The 15 aphasic patients included in this investigation were evenly distributed among anomics, Broca's and Wernicke's; in each group of five, three were severely impaired and two were mildly impaired. These subdivisions into syndromes and degrees of severity were made according to the Boston Diagnostic Aphasia Examination (Goodglass & Kaplan, 1972, 1983) and/or the Aachen Aphasia Test (AAT) (Huber et al., 1983). All patients had left hemisphere lesions of vascular etiology. The average age of each aphasia group was, for anomics, 61.6 years, for Broca's, 57.4 years, and for Wernicke's, 57.8 years. A parallelization for sex was not possible; the male/female ratio was 1:4 (anomics, Wernicke's) and 3:2 (Broca's). Duration of school education ranged from 11 to 12 years for all. Social origin was either lower middle class or upper lower class. However, the professional position of the patients in their work life (tertiary socialization) was more important than their social origin (primary socialization), because all seemed to share social values and speech behavior typical of the lower middle class. Their premorbid jobs were all low white collar jobs. They all had school and job training in analytic and reflexive use of language (cf. Lempert, 1970).

The sociolinguistic properties of patients serving as controls were similar. Among the controls were three women with psychotic depression, two healthy women, and two healthy men. All subjects (aphasics and controls) were born and raised in Vienna and had lived there most of their lives.

Materials and Methods

The aphasics were tested twice. Between each testing they received a brief, intensive language therapy program consisting of ten daily 1-hour sessions. The tasks were developed/adapted on the basis of linguistic hypotheses for an aphasia project and included various types of naming, repetition, and comprehension tasks of words, sentences, and texts and the production/reproduction of various texts. All tests were tape recorded and transcribed using the narrow phonetic transcription system (international Phonetic Alphabet, IPA). The transcriptions served as the basis for various analyses of linguistic deficits.

The main purpose of the intensive testing was to arrive at a very comprehensive description of the aphasics' language symptoms on the basis of the results on the selected tests. Thus, the project was not directed at eliciting dialectal or standard speech. The testing can therefore be considered neutral in this respect.

The speech situations included in this investigation were (a) formal interviews and (b) reproductions of brief stories (DONKEY and RAIL; see chapter 7 by Dressler & Pléh on text production for elaboration of stories). The relative degree of formality of phonological style was measured by determining the use/nonuse of phonological casual speech processes. These are—according to the theory of natural phonology—backgrounding processes that serve for ease of articulation (cf. Dressler's chapter 1 on phonology). The various factors/processes discussed in this study are exemplified in the following sections.

Backgrounding

In speech situations that the speaker defines as formal, backgrounding processes are painstakingly inhibited, whereas in informal ones are rather disinhibited. For example, the two backgrounding processes of deletion and nasal assimilation:

1

$$\text{ə} \rightarrow 0/C\_\_ \begin{Bmatrix} n \\ l \end{Bmatrix}$$

2

$$n \rightarrow [\alpha \text{ place of articulation}] \ /C\_\_\_\_\_\_\_\_ \#[\alpha \text{ place of articulation}]$$

change the formal infinitives ['re:dən] *red* + *en* (to talk), ['le:bən] *leb* + *en* (to live), ['le:gən] *leg* + *en* (to put, to lay down) into the less formal outputs ['re:dn̩, 'le:bm̩, 'le:gŋ̍]. A third backgrounding process, lenis stop deletion before homorganic consonant:

3 = solid line: V____C

$$\begin{bmatrix} C \\ -\text{ continuant} \\ +\text{lenis} \end{bmatrix} \rightarrow 0/V\_\_\_\_\begin{matrix} C \\ [+\text{nasal}] \end{matrix}$$

derives the still more informal variants [re:n̩, le:m̩, le:ŋ̍]. We consider the lenis stop deletion to be a crucial process.

Dialect Use

Dialect use increases in Vienna with increasing informality of the speech situation, often in parallel with the aforementioned backgrounding processes. Dialect use was measured by means of the following two types of processes.

Input Switch Rules

Input switch rules between Viennese Standard German (st.) and Viennese dialect (dial.) input phonemes investigated in the present study consisted of the following:

4

/a/ ↔ /ɔ/

e.g., st.: /mat/ ↔ dial.: /mɔt/ *matt* (exhausted)

5

st. /ɪç/ ↔ dial. /ɪ:/

e.g., in st. [ɪç, mɪç, dɪç, sɪç] ↔ [ɪ:, mɪ:, dɪ:, sɪ:] *ich, mich, dich, sich* (I, me/myself, you/yourself, him/herself)

6

st. /nɪçt/ ↔ dial. /nɛt/, *nicht* (not)

Participle Prefix Reduction

Reduction of the unstressed past participle prefix is one of the dialect backgrounding processes that can appear in the midst of utterances derived from standard input phonemes. It can also co-occur with switches from standard to dialect inputs:

7

gə → g

as in *ge* +*leb* + *t* [g̊le:pt] (lived), *ge* + *nomm* + *en* ['gnɔmən] (taken)

Lateral Gliding/Vocalization

Other dialect processes consist of various processes of lateral gliding/vocalization such as

8

$$\mathrm{l} \rightarrow \breve{e} / \begin{matrix} \mathrm{V} \\ [-\text{ palatal}] \end{matrix} \; \_\_\_\_ \; (\mathrm{C})^{\$}$$

e.g., in *Holz* /hɔlts/ ↔ [hɔĕts] (wood), st. *als* /als/ = dial. [ɔĕs] (when, as)

9

$$\begin{matrix} \mathrm{V} \\ [+\text{ palatal}] \end{matrix} \rightarrow [+\text{ labial}] \, / \; \_\_\_\_ \; \mathrm{l}$$

e.g., in st. *will ich* = dial. [vy:lɪ] (. . . want I)

10

$$\mathrm{l} \rightarrow \breve{e} \rightarrow 0 \, / \begin{matrix} \mathrm{V} \\ \begin{bmatrix} +\text{ palatal} \\ +\text{ labial} \end{bmatrix} \end{matrix} \; \_\_\_\_ \; (\mathrm{C})^{\$}$$

e.g., *will* [vy:] (want), *selbst* [sœpst] (self)

Results

Lenis Stop Deletion

The application/nonapplication of the process of lenis stop deletion was analyzed. The results are given in Figure 3.1. The mean percentages for the five groups show that all patients (aphasic and psychotic) were more formal than the healthy controls, that is, they suppressed the casual speech process of lenis stop deletion more, which means that they identified the two speech situations as more formal than healthy controls did.

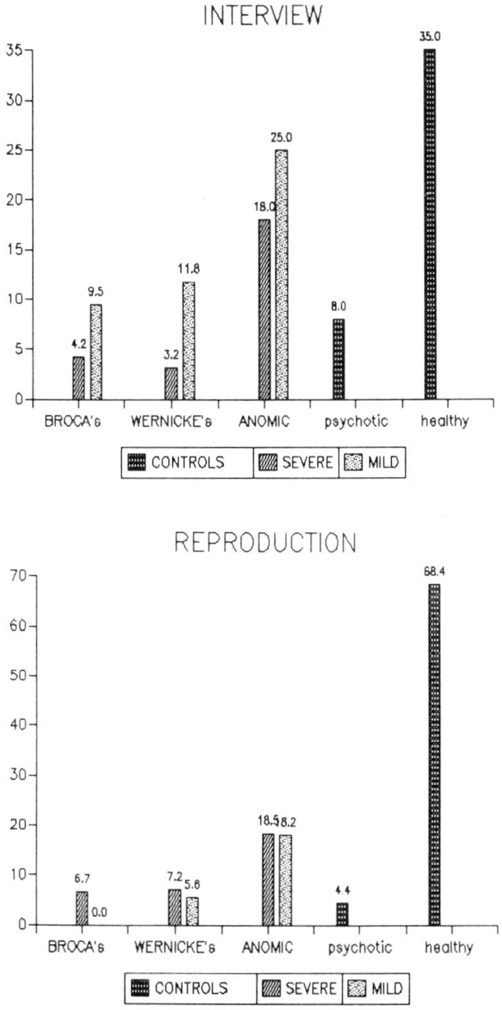

Figure 3.1 Lenis stop deletion in the interview and reproduction task.

Moreover, whereas healthy controls identified the task of reproducing stories as less formal than formal interviews, patients did the reverse. Apparently they identified reproductions as test situations, specifically as memory tests (this interpretation was confirmed by their remarks to the interviewer in cases of failure). In contrast to the situation with interviews, mildly impaired aphasics were at least as formal as severely impaired aphasics in reproductions.

The mean percentage of lenis stop deletion for interviews and reproductions together were, for Broca's, 15%; for Wernicke's, 14%; for anomic aphasics, 40%; and for healthy controls, 51.7%.

Input Switch Rules and (Loaned) Dialect Processes

It appears that the distribution of both input switch rules (4–6) and (loaned) dialect processes (7–10) co-vary. For this reason we considered the results in Figure 3.2 together. If we consider the severely impaired aphasics, we see that they clung to the standard, that is, they identified both interviews and reproductions as formal speech situations and avoided both casual speech processes and dialect. The mean percentages for the interviews were, for Broca's, 12%; for Wernicke's, 6%; and for anomics, 20% (almost as much as for healthy controls, 24.2%) (cf. Rekart & Buckingham, 1979). The mean percentages for reproductions are, for Broca's, 1.6%; for Wernicke's, 2.4%; for anomic aphasics, 19%; and for healthy controls, 24.5%. Thus, severely impaired aphasics seemed to avoid dialect even more in reproductions (identified as test situations). Healthy controls also identified interviews and especially reproductions as less appropriate for dialect use than for casual speech.

Discussion

When compared with casual speech, the dialect use of mildly impaired (MI) aphasics may come as a surprise. Whereas their speech behavior remains very formal in formal interviews and particularly so in reproductions, they use much more dialect in both of these speech situations than do severely impaired (SI) aphasics and even healthy controls (MI = 45.33%, SI = 10.74%, and healthy controls on the average = 29.35%). That is, in this study the mildly impaired aphasics appeared to consider the speech situations as formal but nevertheless appropriate for dialect use, although all of them had undergone language therapy (including structured conversational speech and reproduction) in which the therapists use formal Viennese Standard German rather consistently. Therefore, the much greater use of dialect by the mildly impaired aphasics cannot be an effect of therapy, but rather may be interpreted as a sociolinguistically in-

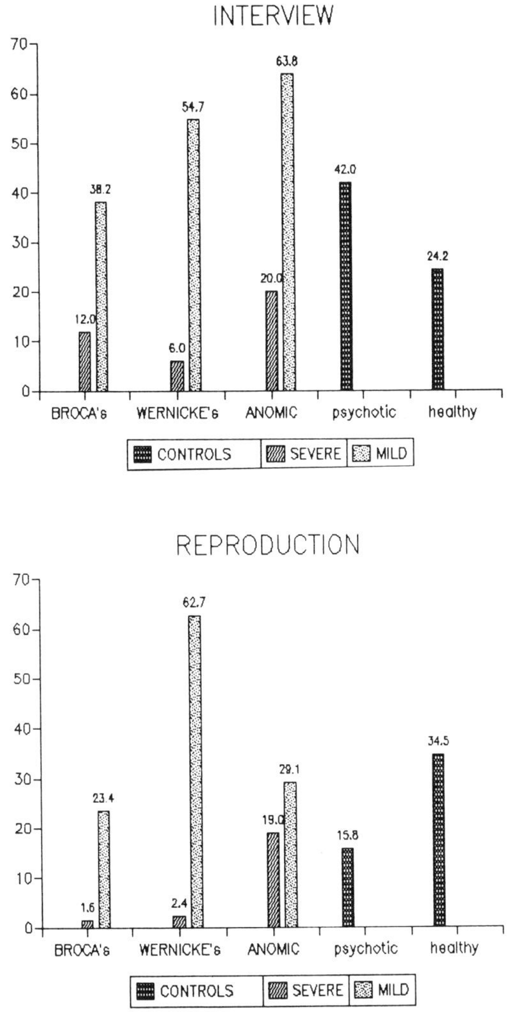

FIGURE 3.2 Use of dialect and input switches in the interview and reproduction task.

adequate interpretation of the speech situation with respect to established social norms (cf. Hartung, 1977).

Although definition of the situation as a more or less formal one is the decisive factor for the use of dialect versus standard language, the aphasia syndrome-specific symptoms must thus be taken into account when interpreting results.

The Broca's produced less dialect forms in both speech situations. The Broca's articulatory difficulties—present in both the severely and mildly impaired patients included in this study—must be considered as a main factor. Much attention is focused on the correct motor programming and production of sounds and words. For this very reason, code switching is made more difficult due to concentration on the correct production of linguistic targets.

Whereas Wernicke's aphasics use more dialect in reproductions, anomics produce more dialect in interviews. This may represent syndrome-specific effects: Wernicke's patients have less control over their speech production and can speak more spontaneously, that is, with less outside control, in reproductions than in interviews; therefore also their dialect use is less controlled. To a greater or lesser degree, anomics have word-finding problems, and this difficulty must show up more in spontaneous (re)production of texts than in interviews. In interviews anomics can direct the conversation, that is, they can turn the conversation on a subject/word they can momentarily produce. This is not the case in (re)-productions of specific texts; patients are more constrained. This may inhibit their dialect use in reproductions.

At the present time, conclusions must be drawn with some reserve because of the number of patients analyzed to date. We had only five patients in each aphasia group (two formal interviews and four text reproductions from each patient) and only four healthy controls. The three depressive psychotics were rather atypical patient controls; their speech behavior posed special problems (cf. Wodak, 1985, for a discussion of these problems). Furthermore, all of our subjects were classified as lower middle class, and the speech behavior of this class has been found to be more variable than that of other classes (cf. Leodolter, 1975).

Despite these reservations, the following conclusions can still be presented with some confidence:

1. As judged from their speech, all aphasic patients defined reproductions as test situations and as much more formal than did the healthy controls. Severely impaired aphasics even defined formal interviews as more formal than healthy controls. We cannot exclude the possibility that this reflects a general patient bias.
2. Dialect use—which can be better perceived and more consciously controlled than casual speech processes—is not evaluated in the same way by aphasics as by healthy controls. Whereas severely impaired aphasics underestimated the appropriateness of dialect use for both speech situations, mildly impaired aphasics overestimated it. In both instances the aphasics responded differently than the healthy controls. This behavior seems to reflect a sociolinguistic deficit of aphasics in identifying the sociolinguistic properties of speech situations.

This interpretation is corroborated by the evidence that the aphasics' dialect use cannot be an artifact of language therapy. (The lack of influence of therapy on dialect use is in striking contrast to therapeutic influence on tentative sex-specific textual strategies, which belong to pragmatic effects of socialization. Cf. chapter 7 on text production.)

The aphasics' control of structurally correct casual/formal speech and dialect/standard forms, as discovered in this study, cannot be derived from principles that govern the distribution of phonologically impaired (i.e. structurally incorrect) forms (phonological paraphasias), as discussed in chapter 1: Wernicke's patients produce only those phonological paraphasias that are to be classified as backgrounding substitutions, due to their deficit in speech monitoring and to their rapid speech. That is, they cannot inhibit backgrounding processes, which healthy adults have learned to inhibit consistently in their native language. However, Wernicke's patients can successfully inhibit stylistic backgrounding processes that are permitted in their native language but prohibited in formal speech.

In other words, the Wernicke's appear to have lost structural, but not stylistic, control over phonological processes. Their sociopsycholinguistic identification of speech situations, however, deviates from that of healthy controls. This becomes more evident in their use of dialect—and clearly production of dialect forms has nothing to do with production of pathological forms (phonological paraphasias).

Of course, our analysis must be extended to more aphasics and to more speech situations. With this study of the very neglected aspects of sociolinguistics in aphasia we have only touched on the subject. Future research will have to deal with interactions of various levels, such as the issue of rate of production, for example, in Broca's versus Wernicke's aphasia in connection with the production of formal/casual speech or dialect/standard forms. Not only the role of the therapist's or examiner's speech (or other input variables) must be considered, but much finer distinctions of the aphasic's language and speech production, to allow a more complete differentiation of the aspects (i.e. processing mechanisms) of speech production that merit consideration in terms of sociophonological concepts.

Note

[1]From a semiotic point of view one can say that with respect to the Broca's aphasic's semiotic competence (cf. Dressler, 1985; Scherer, 1984; H. Stark et al. in press) he had orally/aurally acquired the ability to recognize and use signs that made up his dialect (phonemes, morphemes, etc.). For Standard High German he had stored and enforced—by constant use—not only the phonemes but also the corresponding graphemes by learning to read and write. So these sign systems (phonemes and graphemes) were learned and also stored in a mainly associative manner, information for the motor programs for writing also being stored. In this context the strength of association seems to be an important factor (cf. Luria, 1982). The availability of such closely connected sign systems could facilitate the use of an impaired one (phonemes, words, etc.) or deblock it (cf. Weigl, 1979). In a case of global aphasia it could be demonstrated that the patient's articulatory gestures, coarticulation, and prosodic patterns improved after the patient read aloud single words and short sentences.

4
Phrasal Morphophonemics in Breton-Speaking Wernicke's Aphasics

WOLFGANG ULRICH DRESSLER

Introduction

Morphophonemics (or morpho[pho]nology) is an area that depends both on morphology (cf. chapter 4) and phonology (cf. chapters 1–3). For example, the phonemic alternations [ai] ~ [i] in *divine* ~ *divin-ity* or [k] ~ [s] in *electric* ~ *electric-ity* depend on morphological conditions such as the addition of a restricted set of suffixes (*-ity* in this case). These alternations seem to have some affinity to phonology as well, such as palatalization $k \rightarrow s$ before a palatal vowel in *electric-ity.* However, the delimitation and proper definition of morphophonemics is highly controversial (cf. Dressler, 1985). Some authors consider morphophonemics a proper component of grammar between morphology and phonology, whereas others assign it to either phonology or morphology. In my opinion (Dressler, 1985), morphophonemics (or at least the part of it defined as morphonology) is the area of interaction (or intersection and compromise) of morphology and phonology, and thus is not a component of grammar on an equal footing with morphology and phonology.

The first objective of this study is thus twofold:

1. To investigate whether aphasic disturbances shed some light on this basic question of the delimitation of morphophonemics.
2. To determine which competing linguistic framework(s) can best describe aphasic disturbances. (For this purpose the subpart "phrasal morphophonemics" is chosen.)

The second objective is to present aphasic data from a particular area of Celtic grammar, specifically Breton, which is still spoken in the westernmost part of France. Presumably this is the first and last linguistic study on aphasic disturbances of living mother-tongue Breton dialects. For only Bretons in the oldest generation learned their Celtic dialect before French and have used it throughout their life much more than French, and in fact even speak French with a marked Breton accent.

History of Research on Morphophonemics in Aphasia

Morphophonemic alternations within related words are of primary interest to generative phonology. Thus, the only generative monograph on aphasic disturbances of phonology (Schnitzer, 1972) concentrated on this topic in English (cf. chapter 1).

Disturbances of German umlaut, as in *Woche* (week), adjective *woch-ent-lich* (weekly) (lack of umlaut) instead of *wöch-ent-lich,* have been reported as a side issue in Kleist (1934, p. 892), Mugdan (1977, pp. 162ff., in tests of plural formation with nonsense words), and De Bleser and Bayer (1986, pp. 25, 27) but as a main topic in Dressler (1977b).

Results of a differential test of Polish palatalization rules of different types done by Mierzejewska and Grotecki are reported in Dressler (1985, p. 207). Both the Polish and the German data seemed to support my view of morphonology, depending on both morphology and phonology (see above).

Disturbances of morphophonemics in other languages have been mentioned in Traill (1970) on the Bantu language Ndebele, in Barkai (1980) on Hebrew spirantization, and in Peuser and Fittschen (1977) on Turkish, (cf. Nuyts, 1982, pp. 96ff).

So far I have mentioned only word morphophonemics, that is, morphophonemic alternations within related words. But we must also acknowledge morphophonemic alternations on the phrasal level, that is, alternations that are triggered by other elements within the phrase, as in "don't" as opposed to "do." The only publications on phrasal morphophonemics in aphasia are those by Kilani-Schoch (1982, 1983) on French liason and my prepublication on Breton (Dressler, 1977b), which is expanded in this chapter.

Breton Initial Mutations

As in other Celtic languages, in Breton initial consonants are shifted by preceding triggering elements of the same phrase. The structural description of each of the mutation rules (which follow) consists of a class of triggering elements (mostly function words) and a class of word-initial consonants that are shifted into other consonants (cf. Jackson, 1967).

Rule I. The most productive mutation rule (in terms of types and tokens) is lenition. It occurs after the possessive pronouns *da* (thy) and *e* (his), after certain verb phrase particles, after conjunctions, and after numbers, that is, its triggering elements are the most numerous of all mutations. It shifts the natural class of the voiceless stops *p, t, k* to the respective voiced stops *b, d, g,* as in *penn* (head), *da benn* (thy head); moreover, it triggers the following shifts: *b* → *v, m* → *v, d* → *z, g* → *h,* and *gw* → *w* (or to *v*, according to the dialect), for example, *mamm* (mother), *e vamm* (his mother). Feminine nouns and adjectives are lenited after the article and each other, for example, *mamm* (mother), *bihan* (small), *ar vamm vihan* (the small mother).

Rule II. Spirantization is triggered by the possessive pronouns *va* (or *ma* in other dialects) (my), *he* (her), and *o* (their), and by a few other function words. It shifts *p* to *f*, *t* to *z*, and *k* to *h*, for example, *va fenn* (my head), *tad* (father), *he zad* (her father), but *va mamm* (my mother), with *m* unchanged because it does not belong to the structural description of the rule.

Rule III. Fortition is triggered by the plural possessive pronoun *ho* (your) and by a few other function words, and shifts the natural class of voiced stops *b, d,* and *g* into the respective voiceless ones *p, t,* and *k,*[1] as in *dent* (teeth), *ho tent* (your teeth).

Rule IV. Finally, initial *k* is changed to [ç] after the possessive pronoun *hor* (our) and the definite article *ar* (the) (if the noun is masculine or is in the plural), for example, *kar* (car), *hor/ar* [ça:r] (our/the car).

Assumptions

If morphophonemics is the field of interaction between morphology and phonology (cf. Dressler [1985]) then the preservation of mutations in aphasia should be determined by morphological and phonological factors separately, that is, independently of each other.

If we look at the triggering elements, the only morphological principle that clearly divides them is existing versus nonexisting regularity: All possessive pronouns trigger mutations, whereas gender does only under certain circumstances; not all negations nor all verb phrase particles do, only a few numbers. Thus, if the initial phoneme of the following word is the right one (according to the structural description of the respective mutation rule), then all possessive pronouns regularly trigger mutations, whereas gender, negation, or other grammatical categories show much less regularity in triggering mutations (or in being signaled/symbolized by mutations).

Assuming that regular grammatical categories are better preserved in aphasia than are corresponding less regular ones, we may predict that mutations triggered by possessive pronouns should be better preserved than mutations triggered by other phrasal elements (prediction I).

As to the phonological aspect of mutations, we may assume (according to chapter 1) that mutations that better correspond to natural phonological processes should be preserved.

Hence one subtype of lenition (Ia: *p,t,k* → *b,d,g*) corresponds perfectly to a general lenition type that voices unvoiced stops in a regular way, that is, one natural class is shifted to another one by changing only one distinctive feature value in a uniform way. The same holds for the opposite mutation of fortition (Rule III: *b,d,g* → *p,t,k*).

All the other mutations either change more than one distinctive feature value in a nonuniform way, for example, in spirantization *p* → *f* (however, *t* → *z* instead of **s*) or in the other subpart of lenition (Rule Ib): *b, m* → *v* but *d* → *z, g* → (voiceless) *h, gw* → *w* (and not **hw*), or they do not apply to a whole natural class, such as Rule IV, where only *k* is affected after *hor* (our) in most dialects (but in some also *p* → *f*, and in a few even *t* → *z*). Accordingly, we should predict that fortition and lenition (subtype Ia) should be better preserved than the other mutations (prediction II).

Finally there is a general frequency effect: Lenition occurs after the greatest number of triggering elements and is applied to the greatest number of consonants. Thus it should be best preserved (prediction III).

Speech Samples

During my 1976 field research on a Breton dialect, I had the opportunity to study aphasics. It was, however, very hard to find patients who had learned a Breton dialect earlier, had always used it more than French, and were still in a Breton-speaking environment. I wanted to exclude other patients because I wanted to study the impact of aphasia on perfect competences of Breton but not on decaying Breton (cf. Dressler, 1972; Dressler & Hufgard, 1980).

Of the five aphasics whom I finally found,[2] two produced too little and one (with a mild Wernicke's aphasia) made hardly any errors with mutations. Thus, only two male Wernicke's aphasics were tested:

1. J.G., born 1915 in St. Thegonnec in Léon, the northwesternmost dialect area of Brittany; former mailman; 61 years old and living in Landivisiau in Léon at the time of my inquiry; 1 year post onset, then residual aphasia.
2. L.T., Born 1911 in Lothey near Briec in southeastern Cornouaille (Southern Brittany); former peasant; hospitalized old-age pensioner.

Bretons of the generation of these subjects would not know Standard Breton but only their local dialect, and would use the dialect (rather than French) only to speakers of the same regional dialect. Since I was fluent in only two dialects widely different from theirs, I had to use methods of inquiry that demanded little speaking. Therefore the speech samples consisted of serial speech (numbers, days of the week, months), reactions to a picture, and an object-naming test, plus intermediate spontaneous speech. These tests were administered twice to both patients.

Results

After possessive pronouns there were 24 correct cases without mutation because the following word-initial consonants did not fit the structural description of the respective rule, for example, *va mamm* (my mother), where spirantization triggered by *va* (my) must not apply to a consonant other than following *p, t, k* (see Rule II). There were 31 cases of correct mutation, and finally 8 excessive applications of mutations, that is, where the respective correct mutation would not be applicable to the initial consonant, for example, *va vamm* (my mother) with lenition instead of inapplicable spirantization, or *troad* (foot), *kutell* (knife) → [o 'drɔət, u 'gutl] (your foot, your knife) with lenition instead of fortition after *ho* (your), which is inapplicable to following word-initial voiceless stops. However, there never was lack of a mutation when it was applicable after the correct possessive pronouns to the following correct word-initial consonant. Thus, the morphologically regular class of possessive pronouns was generalized as a trigger for mutation rules.

However, mutations were generalized and degeneralized after other triggering function words or grammatical categories; for example, for gender signaling with mutations I counted three instances of wrong lenition, for example, ['labm 'viən] (small rabbit) (with lenition *b* → *v*) instead of *lapin bihan* (with no lenition because masculine singular), seven instances of wrong spirantization, and four instances of lack of lenition where it should have occurred.

Thus we can conclude that morphologically regular mutation after possessive pronouns is never suppressed, it is sometimes even overgeneralized; whereas morphologically irregular mutations can be even degeneralized. And this supports prediction I.

As to prediction III, I found 13 instances of lenitions instead of spirantizations, but only 3 instances of spirantization instead of lenition. This distribution can be explained by prediction III: The more productive mutation is better preserved and even may replace a less productive mutation, for example, in *va vamm* (cited above) or in *o benn* (their head) with lenition (of *penn*) instead of applicable spirantization (correct form: *o fenn*).

Regarding prediction II, instances of application or nonapplication of fortition were too few to allow a comparison. And as for lenition versus the other mutations, predictions II and III interact so that much more material would have been necessary to differentiate their hypothetical effects. But clear trends were visible with respect to the two types of lenition where prediction III is not applicable but where prediction II predicts better preservation of the phonologically more natural type Ia *(p,t,k → b,d,g,)*. In keeping with this prediction, in only one example was a voiceless stop not shifted to a voiced one: [mə 'fɔʊt 'kRap:] (my boy climbs) instead of *va/ma faotr (a) grapp* (with lenition *k* → *g* after the omissible verb particle *a*). In two instances an *m,* and twice a *b,* were not lenited to *v* (irregular phonologically subtype Ib).

Apart from highly irregular gender signalization, there were seven instances of morphologically unwarranted mutation, that is, of a phonological substitution of a word-initial consonant without a sufficient morphological reason, although all instances occurred in positions resembling those where a mutation might be called for. Interestingly enough, all seven cases of unwarranted mutations were cases of lenition sub-type (Ia), that is, of *p,t,k* → *b,d,g,* for example, ['noŋkə mem 'ga:d] (I am not even able) = (literally) *n'on ket mêmе* (French!) *kat.* Notice that not one of the aphasics otherwise produced word-initial voiced stops instead of voiceless ones, but only the reverse, for example, ##[pɛrn] instead of *bern* (heap) after a pause (without loss of any fortition-triggering function word), or similarly ##[kenvɛn] instead of *genver* (January) (with perseveration of *n*): There were phonological paraphasias the substitutions of which were identical with those affected by fortitions, but there were not any phonological paraphasias the substitutions of which were indentical with those affected by phonologically regular lenitions (subtype Ia). Hence, we may conclude that the above-mentioned seven instances of unwarranted lenitions should really be interpreted as excessive applications of the most productive mutation (prediction III). However, since all cases are instances of the phonologically regular subtype of lenition (Ia), this should be taken rather as support for prediction II.

Conclusion

A theory that considers morphophonemics as part of phonology (cf. introduction to this chapter) would predict that Breton mutations should be impaired in the same way as other phonological processes. However, other phonological processes of the language were rarely impaired. Instead, there were optional additional vowel processes (and, rarely, consonant processes, e.g., *e* → *i*) and generalized fast speech processes. A theory that considers morphophonemics as part of morphology does not account for plausible phonological substitutions being better preserved and even overgeneralized (and implausible phonological substitutions being degeneralized). The same observation holds for a theory that asserts that morphophonemic rules are dead, learned rules, that is, are rules that have no productivity (a claim that is wrong for independent reasons; cf. Dressler, 1985).

However, predictions derived from my basic hypothesis that morphological and phonological aspects of morphophonemics are relatively autonomous, that is, are mutually independent of each other, have stood the test. Furthermore, no results of this study are incompatible with the theory of morphonology developed by Dressler from 1977a to (1985).

Notes

[1]Some dialects have an extension of lenition and fortition called "new lenition" (*s* → *z*, *š* → *ž*, *f* → *v*) and "new fortition" (*z* → *s*, *ž* → *š*, *v* → *f*), but there were no examples in my patient sample.

[2]I would like to thank Dr. J. Gagnepain, Professor of Linguistics at the University of Rennes, for bringing me into contact with patient J. G., and Drs. Claquin and Conan for allowing me to investigate L. T. (and three other patients) at the Department Hospital at Quimper (South Finistere, western part of the dialect region Cornouaille).

5
Word Formation in Italian-Speaking Wernicke's and Broca's Aphasics

WOLFGANG U. DRESSLER and GIANFRANCO DENES

Introduction

GENERAL OUTLINE

The two main functions of word formation are:

1. Lexical enrichment via morphologically derived words, that is, the formation of new words from existing ones such as *dish-wash-er* from the bases *dish* and *to wash.*
2. Motivation of existing complex words, either compounds (e.g., *blackboard*) or derivatives (e.g., *to black-en, board-er*), by analyzing them into their bases[1] (e.g., *black, board*) and their affixes (e.g., *-en, -er*) with the help of word formation rules (WFRs). Within the framework of Natural Morphology (cf. Dressler, 1979b, 1985; Dressler, Mayerthaler, Panagl, & Wurzel, 1987; Schaner-Wolles & Dressler, 1985) we study how well these functions are served by specific WFRs according to universal parameters, two of which will be presented here (morphosemantic and morphotactic transparency).

For each parameter we establish relations of markedness (cf. Ulatowska & Baker, 1977; chapter 1) and predict that less marked forms or rules are better preserved in aphasia than more marked ones, and that more marked forms are more often substituted by less marked ones than vice versa.

MORPHOLOGICAL ANALYSIS

These general predictions presuppose that normal persons and/or aphasics are sensitive to morphologial complexity. First it must be ascertained that both groups analyze compounds or derivatives into their parts. According to psycholinguistic test results (e.g., Cutler, 1983; Freyd & Baron, 1982), morphological analysis is not necessary but is often done in learning, in the perception of or production of new or relatively new words.

Moreover, one type of speech error consists of anticipations, perseverations, or metatheses of affixes (cf. Fromkin, 1973; Garrett, 1982; Söderpalm, 1979). An Italian example of such a metathesis (from the Italian speech errors collected and studied by Magno-Caldognetto and Tonelli in Padua) is[2]:

(è un) gall-etto americ-ano → gall-ano americh-etto[3]
(it is an) Americ-an cock(-diminutive)

This metathesis presupposes relative autonomy of the bases (stems) of *gall-o* (cock) and *Americ-a* (America) within the derivatives *gall-etto* (diminutive), *Americ-ano* (adjective).

As far as aphasia morphology is concerned, Whitaker's (1972) patients replaced not only words with their derivations in repetition tests (e.g., *decide* → *decision, conceal* → *concealment*), but also derivatives with their bases (e.g., *dark-ness* → *dark, refus-al* → *refuse*). Similarly, Japanese aphasics replaced simple words with compounds containing them (Bisazza & Sasanuma, 1984). These errors presuppose morphological analysis or, at least, analyzability (cf. Miceli & Caramazza, 1987). The same holds for the rare cases of metathesis within compounds, as in German *Blitz-licht* (flash-light) → *Licht-bli[k]tz,* (Dressler, 1979b). For a discussion of Stachowiak's (1978,1979) results see the section on morphosemantic transparency in this chapter. For a case of a bilingual aphasic substituting English with German affixes see Paradis (1978, p. 170).

A Brief History of Research

No comprehensive study on word formation in aphasia has been done to date. There are anecdotal reports on omissions, additions, and substitutions, or on morphological neologisms (e.g., Kleist, 1934, pp. 873, 890ff, 901; Schnitzer, 1972). Word formation has been mentioned as an annex of inflectional morphology in studies of agrammatism (e.g., Kean, 1977; Lapointe, 1983; Stemberger, 1984; Tissot, Mounin, & Lhermitte, 1973). Some studies on specific WFRs are those by Whitaker (1972) on nominalizations, Strachalska (1978) on Polish agent nouns, and Stachowiak (1979) on descriptivity. The study of Glozman (1974) is discussed in the section on a Russian test.

Patients

The tests (established by one of us [W.U.D.]) were administered by the other (G.D.) and by students of the logopedic school of Padua, Italy (supervised by Professor Emanuela Magno Caldognetto).[4] All patients were born and lived in or around Padua and thus spoke a Venetian regional dialect or variant of Standard Italian. These varieties do not differ in the morphological makeup of the test words used.

The patients were placed into two groups. First, six Wernicke's and three Broca's were tested, but since they were not well classified their productions are used here only as supplementary evidence (called "pretest").

The second, main group of patients can be described as follows: A total of 11 aphasic patients participated in the study, including relatively clear cases of Broca's and Wernicke's aphasia. Assessment of aphasia was made on a clinical basis supplemented in all cases by the administration of an Italian version of the Boston Diagnostic Examination test (Goodglass & Kaplan, 1972). The patients had all suffered unilateral left brain damage of cerebrovascular or traumatic origin, as assessed by clinical examination supplemented in most cases by computer tomography (CT) scan.

The patients were all righthanded. They were tested when their aphasic disorder had reached a relatively stable stage. No patient had a peripheral hearing disorder as assessed on a clinical basis.

At the time of this investigation the patients were not hospitalized but attended or had attended the Speech Therapy Department at Padua or Vicenza Hospitals previously. All patients were fully alert and were willing and able to cooperate.

Broca's Aphasics

The group consisted of three men and one woman with a mean age of 37 years (range 23–57). Mean educational level was 7.5 years of school (range 5–13).

CT scan indicated pathological involvement of the left frontoparietal region. The etiology of the lesion was vascular in two cases and traumatic in the other two.

Wernicke's Aphasics

The group consisted of five men and two women with a mean age of 57 years (range 30–73). Mean educational level was 8.5 years of school (range 3–17). CT scan indicated pathological involvement of the left temporoparietal region. The etiology of the lesion was vascular in six cases and traumatic in one case.

Difference Between the Groups

The most obvious difference between the two groups, apart from numerical discrepancy, was their mean age; those in the Broca's group were significantly younger. This is in agreement with a number of studies focusing on the relationship between type of aphasia and age, and suggesting a possibly changing pattern of location of linguistic functions according to age.

Procedure

Patients were tested in a quiet but not soundproof room. The testing sessions, lasting on the average 2 hours, were tape recorded and then transcribed according to International Phonetic Alphabet rules. The test was repeated a few days later.

Syntagmatic Disturbances

A Russian Test

There exists a simplistic preconception that word formation is essentially a method of concatenation, that is, of chaining stems and affixes (as if there did not exist nonconcatenative WFRs such as *to cut* → *a cut, a house* → *to house*). In structuralist terms, concatenation operates on Jakobson's (1964) syntagmatic axis of language.

According to Jakobson, posterior aphasics present an impairment of the paradigmatic axis of language (with selection errors as a consequence), whereas anterior aphasics present an impairment of the syntagmatic axis (with combination/concatenation errors). This dichotomy was taken over by A. R. Luria's Moscow school of aphasiology. Following this framework and the above-mentioned simplistic view of word formation, Glozman (1974) derived the following assumptions on how compounds and derivatives should be affected in Broca's and Wernicke's aphasia: Due to impairment of the syntagmatic axis, Broca's should have difficulties in analyzing complex words into their morphological parts and in deriving the composite meaning of a complex word from the meaning of its parts (e.g., a *writ-er* is an agent [affix *-er*] *who writes*), whereas lexicalized complex meaning should be at their disposal (*e.g., a writ-er* is not anyone who is writing something, but is synonymous with *author*). This relation of synonymy is a paradigmatic relation that should not be impaired in Broca's aphasia.

On the other hand, Wernicke's aphasics, due to impairment of the paradigmatic axis, should have difficulties with lexicalized meanings, but should be able to analyze complex words into their morphological parts and to derive composite meanings from the meanings of the parts.

To test these predictions, Glozman (1974) devised a paradigmatic classification test: There were 15 cards with one word on each of them, and patients had to group the cards (i.e., words) in such a way that they formed word families, such as *inform, inform-ant, inform-ation,* that is, into words with a common derivational base. Her Russian Broca' and Wernicke's behaved as expected.

A Paradigmatic Classification Test in Padua

Since this test was never repeated, we constructed an Italian equivalent as one subtest of our test battery. Again patients had to group triplets of words that belonged to the same word family (each word presented on a separate card). The training example was *fiore* (flower), *fior-eria* (florist's shop), *fior-aio* (florist).

The test, consisting of 24 words, contained only two correct triplets:

1. *bianco* (white), *bianch-eria* (underwear) (usually white), *im-bianc-are* (to whiten, to wash underwear).
2. *grande* (great), *grand-ezza* (greatness), *in-grand-ire* (to enlarge).

The remaining 18 words consisted of six assonant (similar sounding) word triplets, for example, *odio* (hate), *odierno* (of today) (adjective), *odore* (smell). That is, they had no common derivational basis and could not be derived from each other by WFRs.

Patients' responses were classified according to six categories.

1. Correct establishment of a word family (either of the whole triplet or a correct pair—a partial success).
2. Assonance (phonetic similarity) errors (triplets or pairs such as *odio, odierno*).
3. Semantic errors (e.g., when establishing an antonymic pair *odio* [hate], *amore* [love]).
4. Pragmatic errors (i.e, establishing triplets according to pragmatic affinities: two Broca's grouped *sole* (sun) with *biancheria* (white underwear), which may reflect the common practice of Venice and the Venetian to dry the white wash in the sun).
5. Other groupings.
6. No groupings (correct for the 18 words that did not belong to a word family).

Results

Only six Wernicke's but all four Broca's of the main test and four Wernicke's and two Broca's of the pretest were able to do the test. In the main test, the Wernicke's performed 19 groupings (correct or incorrect ones), the Broca's 9. A statistical comparison with the nongrouped word proved to be insignificant. However, by adding the pretest patients, the figures rose to 40 groupings (Wernicke) versus 15 (Broca). Here we found a significant preference of Broca's in refraining from grouping (chi square = 4.3 at the 0.05 significance level).

Table 5.1 presents (completely or partially) correct responses, assonance errors, and semantic errors for Wernicke's and Broca' patients of the main test and the pretest.

Clearly the Broca's performed worse in the correct assignment of the six words to the two word families. But this result was statistically significant only when confidence intervals were evaluated[5] for all patients of the main test and the pretest. This interval for all correct triplets and pairs lay between 0.29 and 0.47; the quotient for correct responses of B and W was 3/12 or about 0.09; 0.09 lies far outside this confidence interval. This result seems to confirm Glozman's (1974) assumption that Broca's have more difficulties with WFRs.

However, the difference between Wernicke's and Broca's aphasics is still bigger for assonance groupings. If Wernicke's have no impairment of word formation, they should never mistake assonant words for members of the same word family.

They should know that semantic affinities are not equivalent with membership in a word family. Still, they performed more semantic groupings than Broca's, who might be expected to mistake semantic groupings for derivational groupings because these also presuppose semantic affinity. Since Broca's are supposed to have an impairment of the syntagmatic but not of the paradigmatic axis, they should be prone to compensate for impaired derivational grouping by increased nonimpaired semantic grouping. But this is not the case.

Therefore the distributions of assonance and semantic groupings disconfirm Glozman's (1974) assumptions. Thus, according to our results, Jakobson's dichotomy of combination and selection errors proved to be irrelevant for word formation in aphasia, as it did for phonology and syntax (cf. Chapter 1 for phonology).

TABLE 5.1. Results of Paradigmatic Classification Test Given to Wernicke's (W) and Broca's (B) Aphasics

	Correct responses		Assonance errors		Semantic errors	
Test	Triplet	Pair	Triplet	Pair	Triplet	Pair
Main test						
6W	5	3	5	2	—	4
4B	3	—	1	3	—	2
Pretest						
4W	2	2	9	2	1	3
2B	—	—	—	—	—	2

Morphosemantic Transparency

INTRODUCTION

The degree of morphosemantic transparency of a compound or derivative equals the degree of semantic compositionality, that is, the degree to which the meanings of the parts yield the meaning of the whole or how well the parts describe the whole. Thus, morphosemantic transparency (as defined in Natural Morphology, cf. Dressler 1979b, 1985; Dressler et al., 1987; Schaner-Wolles & Dressler, 1985), compositionality of meaning (as used in logics and semantics), and descriptiveness (as defined in the Cologne Project of Universals, cf. Stachowiak, 1978,1979) are largely synonymous. For example, *reader* in the sense of someone who reads is more transparent/compositional/descriptive than *reader* as a position in a British university. The opposite of transparency is called opacity.

Morphosemantically more transparent complex words are easier to analyze by normal adults (cf. Smith & Sterling, 1982) and are learned earlier by children (cf. Clark & Hecht, 1982; Schaner-Wolles & Dressler, 1985). And according to both of these psycholinguistic results as well as to general predictions on markedness in the framework of Natural Morphology, aphasics should handle more transparent complex words better than less transparent ones.

This prediction seems to be contradicted by the results of an experiment devised and reported by Stachowiak (1978,1979) in which aphasics were asked to name colored pictures that depicted words of different degrees of descriptiveness (class I being most descriptive, class IV not descriptive at all):

Class I. Morphosemantically rather transparent compounds such as German *Rasier-messer* (razor; literally, raze-knife).
Class II. Morphosemantically rather opaque compounds such as German *Rosen-kranz* (rosary; literally, rose-garland).
Class III. Derivatives such as German *Box-er* (box-er).
Class IV. Simplex words such as German *Käfer* (beetle).

In this naming test, aphasics produced more errors the more transparent the target word was. This is easily explainable, if we assume that more transparent complex words are easier to analyze; therefore a transparent compound (class I) presents three sources of confusion—the whole complex word and its two parts,—whereas a simplex word (class IV) presents only one comparable source of confusion. Thus, Stachowiak's results confirm rather than disconfirm our assumption.

A Reactive Identification Test with Compounds

To test our hypothesis, we used a list of 28 compounds that consisted of transparent and opaque deverbal agent nouns, for example, *porta-lettere* (mail-man; literally, carry-letters) versus *mangia-preti* (rabid anti-clerical; (literally, eat-priests), as well as of transparent deverbal instrument nouns, for example, *aspira-polvere* (vacuum cleaner; literally, suck-dust), and of opaque nonanimate deverbal compounds, for example, *copri-fuoco* (curfew; literally, cover-fire). Patients had to identify the meanings of these compounds.

Results

Table 5.2 presents the percentages of comprehension and correct identification by the Broca's and Wernicke's aphasics of the main test. The subjects comprehended transparent compounds significantly better than opaque ones, and Broca's comprehended more (chi square = 42) than Wernicke's (chi square = 25.93). In correct identification only Broca's scored significantly better (chi square = 10.2) with transparent compounds. There were, however, fewer Broca's than Wernicke's patients, so that it was more difficult to achieve statistical significance with the former.

In performing, the test subjects used various strategies, two of them described here. One can be called a morphological strategy; it consisted of the patient using either both parts of the compounds questioned (full morphological strategy) or only one part (half morphological strategy). For example, a *porta-lettere* is someone "who carries letters" (full morph.) or "who carries mail" (half morph.), or "who brings me letters" (half morph.). The other strategy is a semantic strategy consisting of giving a synonym (e.g., "postman," "mailman") or a semantic description without morphological connection to any part of the compound (e.g., "employee of the post office"). The incidence of these responses is given in Table 5.3.

Table 5.2. Comprehension and Correct Identification of Transparent and Opaque Compounds by Broca's (B) and Wernicke's (W) Aphasics; Main Test

Type of compound	Comprehension		Correct identification	
	B	W	B	W
Transparent				
Agents	80	63	65	33
Things	78	83	41	25
Opaque				
Agents	56	46	6	25
Things	38	42	13	17

TABLE 5.3. Response Strategies by Wernicke's (W) and Broca's (B) Aphasics in Reactive Identification of Compounds

		Strategies			
Compounds		Full morph.[a]	Half morph.	Semantic	Other
Agents					
Transparent	W	5	5	10	10
	B	5	5	8	2
Opaque	W	2	5	6	11
	B	2	1	9	4
Objects					
Transparent	W	5	16	19	20
	B	3	4	14	19
Opaque	W	0	1	5	6
	B	0	0	6	2

[a]Full-morphological strategy consisted of use of both parts of the compounds in question; half-morphological strategy consisted of use of only one part.

These figures were subjected to analyses of variance by Biomedical Programs,[6] of which the most important results were the following: Four separate ANOVA tests for the four strategies of Table 5.3 showed a very significant effect of full morphological strategy being applied to transparent but not to opaque compounds: $F(1.8) = 5.57$ ($p < 0.05$). Sixteen T tests comparing Wernicke's and Broca's aphasics in each line of Table 5.3 showed strong trends for Broca's to use more semantic strategies with opaque agents than Wernicke's (0.5625% vs. 0.25% T values = 2.11 [$p <$ 0.07]). If the opaque object compounds are left out (because of the small number of items), we get (with an analysis of variance (ANOVA) test) a significant interaction showing that Broca's prefer the semantic strategy with opaque agents whereas Wernicke's prefer the half-morphological strategy: $F(6.48) = 2.32$ ($p < 0.05$).

Discussion

The results of the reactive identification test with compounds support our assumption that aphasics can also handle transparent compounds better than opaque ones, both in comprehension and reactive identification. In both performances Broca's aphasics were better than Wernicke's, which disconfirms again the syntagmatic disturbance hypothesis. The better performance becomes even clearer when we look at the choice of response strategies. The morphologial strategy is adequate for identifying transparent compounds; applied to opaque compounds it can only refer to the literal, not to the real, lexicalized meaning (e.g., "A rabid anticlerical is someone who eats priests"). On the other hand, the morphological strategy is easier in a reactive identification test than the semantic strategy, because elements essential for the response are already presented in the stimulus question.

Obviously, Broca's are able to calibrate the differential use of both strategies better than Wernicke's. This presupposes a fairly well-preserved competence of word formation and some metalinguistic insight into the respective appropriateness of alternative strategies.

Morphotactic Transparency

Introduction

The parameter of morphotactic transparency (cf. Dressler, 1979b, 1985; Dressler et al., 1987; Schaner-Wolles & Dressler, 1985) refers to the level of morphological expression and the presence or absence of interference with the operation of concatenation. Let us compare four English derivatives as to their respective degree of morphotactic transparency:

Class I. *excite$-ment* is very transparent because syllable boundary ($) and morphological boundary coincide. There may be a very slight difference in the pronunciation of word-final /t/ in the base *excite* and of syllable-final /t/ in the derivative, but on the whole nothing changes when the affix *-ment* is added to *excite.*

Class II. *exis$t-ence* is less transparent because syllable and morphological boundary do not coincide, that is, when the affix *-ence* is attached to the base *exist,* phonological resyllabification occurs.

Class III. *conclusion* is much less transparent because the attachment of the affix *-ion* to the base *conclude* triggers a morphophonemic rule that changes /di/ to /z/ and buries the morphological boundary.

Class IV. *decision* is still more opaque (morphotactically) because in addition to the interferring rule of class III, the diphthong /ai/ of *decide* is changed to a short vowel /I/.

Psycholinguistic experiments by MacKay (1978) have proved that the base can be best perceptually isolated in derivatives such as those in class I and worst in those in class IV (with a linear progression from IV through I), and that word formation can be processed best in the circumstances in class I and worst in class IV. Similar results have been achieved by Cutler (1981; 1983, p. 63), Jarvella and Meijers (1983, pp. 86ff), and Smith and Sterling (1982, p. 706). Morphotactically more transparent words are learned earlier in first language acquisition than less transparent ones (e.g., Hooper, 1980; MacWhinney, 1978, p. 65; Schaner-Wolles, 1981).

A Reactive Identification and a Reactive Naming Test with Derivatives

Morphotactically transparent and opaque agent noun derivatives were contrasted in two test lists (20 for the identification test, 12 for the naming test). Transparent nouns were of the type *lavora-tore* (worker) (derived from *lavora-re,* to work), opaque ones of the types *lettore* (reader) (derived from *legg-e-re,* to read) and *disertore* (deserter) (derived from *diserta-re,* to desert, with deletion of the syllable /ta/). Only such agent nouns derived from verbs as bases were compared in statistical analysis, since the 10 denominal agent nouns of the identification test proved too difficult to analyze.

The reactive identification test was administered in the same way as the compound test. The stimulus questions of the reactive naming test were of the type: "What do you call a person who works professionally?"

Results

In the reactive identification test, transparent derivations were significantly better understood than transparent ones (Wernicke's chi square = 4.2; Broca's: chi square = 4.33, although there were only four Broca's but seven Wernicke's). Completely correct production was better with transparent derivatives as well, but only Wernicke's reached statistical significance (chi square = 13.7 vs. 2.5 for the Broca's).

In the reactive naming test, both groups had significantly more correct productions with transparent than opaque derivatives (Wernicke's: chi square = 17.28; Broca's: chi square = 6.76).

Only in the reactive naming test did both groups use the morphological strategy significantly more frequently in forming transparent deverbal agent nouns from verb bases than in forming opaque ones (Wernicke's: chi square = 20.63; Broca's: chi square = 10.10).

In the reactive naming test, the subjects sometimes produced morphological neologisms. The data from all patients (main test and pretest) were: *scriv-e-re* (to write) → opaque *scrittore* (writer), replaced once by transparent (non-existing) *scriv-i-tore* (Wernicke's with the normal WFR, which also gives (existing) *vend-i-tore* from *vend-e-re* [to sell]) and thrice (twice by Broca's, once by a Wernicke's) by *scriv-a-tore* (with the wrong stem vowel *-a-*, probably by analogy to *lavora-tore,* etc.); *distrugg-e-re* (to destroy) → opaque *distruttore,* replaced once by transparent (but marginal) *distrugg-i-tore* (Wernicke's); *diserta-re* (to desert) → opaque *disertore,* replaced once by (marginal) *diserta-tore* (Broca's, without haplology, i.e., deletion of the syllable /ta/ before the similar syllable /to/); *inventa-re* (to invent) → opaque *inventore,* replaced twice by transparent (but nonexisting) *inventa-tore* (Wernicke's).

On the other hand, transparent *fuma-tore* (smoker) *(-fuma-re)* was once replaced by *fum-i-tore* (Wernicke's: presumably in analogy to *vend-i-tore,* etc.).[7]

Discussion

The results show—as expected—that transparent derivatives are better understood than opaque ones. Whereas degree of morphotactic transparency determines the speed of analysis for normals, it conditions the amount of failure in aphasics. As to the use of the morphological strategy and its greater adequacy with transparent derivatives, this preference was much more clearly demonstrated in deriving the deverbal agent noun from its base *(vend-e-re* → *vend-i-tore* vs. *scriv-e-re* → *scrivitore)* than in finding the bases for the stimulus derivative *(vend-i-tore* → *vend-e-re* vs. *scrittore* → *scriv-e-re).* Does this mean that different mechanisms are involved in both tasks and that morphotactic transparency aids derivation from the root more than morphological decomposition of the derivative?

Whereas Broca's calibrated the use of the morphological and semantic strategy significantly better than Wernicke's in the analysis of compounds, results for derivatives seem to show the opposite effect. This may, however, be an artifact of the statistical analysis, because the items of the derivative tests were less numerous than those of the compound test.

As to morphological neologisms, aphasics replaced an opaque derivative with the respective transparent five times, once by using the correct WFR (which is blocked idiosyncratically with the verbs *scrivere, distruggere, disertare, inventare*); twice they formed a neologism more transparent than the correct existing derivative by using the WFR incorrectly *(scrivatore* instead of transparent, nonexisting *scriv-i-tore* for existing opaque *scrittore).*

Incorrect use of a WFR occurred only once with a transparent derivative. But aphasics never replaced a transparent derivative with an opaque one. This differential behavior can be described as unidirectional analogy, that is, replacement of marked with unmarked structures (on the parameter of morphotactic transparency) or as relaxation of a language-specific, idiosyncratic blocking of transparent WFRs (similar to relaxation of blocked natural phonological processes, cf. Chapter 1).

Conclusions

The results of the four tests reported here seem to show that word formation in Broca's and Wernicke's aphasia still serves its two main functions:

1. Lexical enrichment, insofar as aphasics (including Broca's, according to Glozman, 1974) form morphological neologisms by applying normal WFRs.

2. Motivation of complex words, insofar as both morphotactic and morphosemantic transparency of morphologically complex words facilitates comprehension and identification.

This facilitation effect supports assumptions of Natural Morphology about markedness relations on the two parameters of morphosemantic and morphotactic transparency and their consequences.

Contrary to Glozman's (1974) assumptions, Broca's performed better than Wernicke's in most of our tests, particularly in word formation semantics. This agrees with their better performance in other areas of semantics (for text semantics cf. chapter 7). Semantics is often reduced by nonlinguists to the paradigmatic axis of language, but in our tests the rather good performance referred to the syntagmatic axis.

In our tests no effect of agrammatism was visible in word formation performance of Broca's. If we combine this with the conclusion of chapter 7 that text cohesion impairments are secondary effects of syntactic disturbances, then we may claim that agrammatism is primarily an impairment of syntax. Since inflectional morphology (but not word formation morphology) serves syntax in delivering inflected word forms for the expression of syntactic categories, secondary impairments of inflection are to be expected. This functional explanation accounts for the much greater defects of Broca's aphasics in inflectional than in derivational morphology (also observed in our tests).

NOTES

[1]Bases may be simplex words such as *black* or *board* or complex words such as *blackboard* as the basis of *blackboard eraser.*

[2]For a neuropsychological review see Caramazza (1987); for the differentiation of word formation and inflection, Miceli and Caramazza (1987). Despite their title, De Bleser & Bayer (1986) dealt only with inflection. On receptive processing of word formation, see Eling (1986).

[3]The letters *c,g* are pronounced [k,g] before back vowels and consonants, but [č,ǰ] before the front vowels *i,e* (= [i,e]). [k,g] before *i,e* are written *ch, gh.* Double consonant signs (e.g., *gg, ggh*) represent monophonemic long consonants ([g:] in this case).

[4]We want to thank Professor Emanuela Magno Caldognetto and her students for their invaluable assistance.

[5]We would like to thank Professor Wilfried Grossmann (Vienna) for suggesting this simple but effective statistical method.

[6]We would like to thank Professor Csaba Pléh and Dr. Andras Vargha (Budapest) for these statistical analyses.

[7]There was another defective form of *fumatore: fumotore.* But this is not a morphological neologism because there are no Italian verbs with stem-final /o/; *fumotore* rather must be analyzed as a phonological paraphasia with an anticipation of the /o/ of the following syllable (cf. chapter 1; Miceli & Caramazza, 1987, pp. 21f).

6
Syntactic and Semantic Factors of Auditory Sentence Comprehension in Aphasia

JACQUELINE A. STARK and RUDOLF WYTEK

Introduction

A review of the literature on language comprehension in general and on auditory sentence comprehension in particular reveals the complexity of the processing assumed to be involved in understanding of sentences. In psycholinguistic terms (cf. Cairns & Cairns, 1976; Clark & Clark, 1977; Swinney, 1981), comprehension of sentences by normal subjects is considered to be a complex, active, and constructive process in which the listener simultaneously and/or successively[1] makes use of linguistic knowledge (phonological, semantic/lexical, and syntactic information), knowledge of the world (pragmatic information), and, stemming from these knowledge sources, a set of "strategies" to induce the meaning of a particular sentence.

The complexity of the postulated processes is mirrored in the studies published to date. Various aspects of language processing have been singled out for investigation—more or less in isolation—to arrive at the essential components or possible parameters of the processing mechanisms involved in the understanding of sentences. Research on auditory comprehension in aphasia has focused on whether different clinical populations can be differentiated by their performance on comprehension tests, as judged by liability to impairment. Either the overall number of errors (quantitative aspects of the performance) or the distribution of errors according to type (qualitative aspects) has been measured.

In this study we investigated auditory sentence comprehension in 169 aphasic patients (classified clinically into four main groups), and systematically varied syntactic and semantic factors in a sentence–picture matching task. The effects of variation in sentence type on the aphasic's comprehension performance were studied in connection with voice distinctions and semantic aspects to determine the role of all of these in the processing of grammatical relations marked by word order and grammatical markers. Our data will be presented after a review of the literature.[2]

Review of the Aphasia Literature on Auditory Sentence Comprehension

Studies of auditory sentence comprehension have focused on investigating differences between normal adults and children and aphasic subjects, stressing the differential susceptibility of the various factors or parameters in different psycholinguistic tasks or modalities. The studies can be divided into three groups:

1. Those that emphasize distinctions among aphasia types, for example, whether the lexical/syntactic distinction works.
2. Those that emphasize the nature of the syntactic processing deficit.
3. Those that emphasize the relation between comprehension and production.

Goodglass, Gleason, and Hyde (1970) investigated the performance of aphasics (Broca's, Wernicke's, anomic, conduction, and global patients) compared with control subjects (adults and children) on four different tasks of auditory comprehension: word comprehension, sequence pointing span, comprehension of directional prepositions, and recognition of the correct use of prepositions in a metalinguistic judgment task (preposition preference). The comprehension tasks chosen for the study appeared to the authors to parallel the kinds of difficulties in production that clinically characterize the various aphasia types. As an example of parallelism between language production and comprehension difficulties, the authors suggested that the anomics' inability to produce nouns might also be evident in an inability to comprehend them. Goodglass et al. found qualitative differences between the aphasic and control subjects with respect to the tasks investigated. Performance patterns among aphasics of different types displayed significant differences in employed tasks (excluding the most severely impaired global aphasia subjects in these comparison's differentiation among the four other diagnostic groups):

1. In word comprehension (Peabody Picture Vocabulary Test) the anomics were most impaired.
2. On the preposition preference test the Wernicke's were most impaired.
3. Results from the sequence pointing span task distinguished the Broca's as having the most impairment.

The directional preposition was the least discriminating of the four tests.

On the basis of these results three functions were identified as allowing discrimination among the aphasia subgroups. Function I (low pointing span score relative to high preposition preference score) separated the

Broca's and conduction from the Wernicke's aphasics. Function II (low Peabody score relative to high pointing span score) distinguished anomic from Broca's and conduction subgroups. Function III (low directional preposition score in contrast to high preposition preference score) separated conduction from Broca's aphasics.

Although the authors demonstrated dissociations between production and comprehension, and patients had specific deficits in one or another of the areas of language investigated, the claim that the selection of features tested was justified is not convincing. In particular, hypotheses concerning the pattern of performance expected from the aphasic subgroups and the actual pattern are absent. For the anomic and Broca's subgroups, the pattern of performance on a single comprehension task is discussed in relation to their performance on other language tasks not investigated in this study.

Goodglass and colleagues' (1970) conclusion, that "the existence of such differential patterning in the disturbance of comprehension further validates the diagnostic groupings as distinct from one another" (p. 606), is pertinent for the present study.

In a later study, Goodglass et al. (1979) investigated another parallelism between production and comprehension in Broca's, Wernicke's, and conduction aphasics using a sentence–picture matching task (four-picture choice), namely, the contrast between subject-embedded sentences (grammatically encoded, compact) versus sentences with contiguous simple propositions (expanded). Although all aphasics obtained better results on the expanded versions of the embedded sentences, the Broca's group benefited most from the expansion and the conduction group benefited the least. The aphasia types tended to respond differentially to the expansion of grammatically nonembedded forms according to type of construction (e.g., before-after, compounds, etc.). The authors found no main effect or interaction due to real-world plausibility. In summarizing the results, the authors pointed out that the embedding of one proposition within another seemed to be the crucial variable in comprehension performance.

On the syntactic level, Parisi and Pizzamiglio (1970) and Lesser (1974) analyzed auditory sentence comprehension in Italian- and English-speaking aphasics, respectively, using a sentence–picture matching test (two-picture choice). In the first study (Italian-speaking aphasics), the performance of Broca's (mean score = 60.1 correct out of 80), anomic (mean score = 71.8), Wernicke's (mean score = 49.5), and mixed or global aphasics (mean score = 50.8) was compared with that of healthy adults (mean score = 75.2), non-aphasic brain-damaged patients (mean score = 73.9), and children. A rank of difficulty of the items tested is given for the total group of aphasics, for the Broca's subgroup, for the Wernicke's subgroup, and for the children. Comparison of the results in terms of order of difficulty of the grammatical contrasts is made only between the Broca's and Wernicke's groups. Quantitatively speaking (mean score), the Broca's scored higher than the Wernicke's. Although the authors stated that a qualitative comparison might be of greater interest, the only real difference in rank order of difficulty (1 to 20 from most difficult to least difficult) between these two groups was their performance on the relative clause contrast (e.g., The cat jumps on the mouse which is on the chair). This type of construction was the most difficult (Rank 1) for the Wernicke's, whereas it was much easier for the Broca's (Rank 13). The possible reason for this differential difficulty is not discussed. A contrasting ranking was also found for the singular-plural and the on-under contrast. The authors found the order of difficulty to be similar when groups of patients of different degrees of impairment were compared irrespective of aphasia type. The most difficult construction in the syntax test was the direct object-indirect object (e.g., The boy shows the cat to the dog), and the subject/object passive voice construction was next in overall order of difficulty (e.g., The cat is chased by the dog).

In Lesser's (1974) investigation of verbal comprehension, the patients were not classified according to aphasia type. With material comparable to that in the syntax test for Italian-speaking aphasics, the English-speaking aphasics achieved a mean score of 64.9 correct responses out of 80. Those construction types in which the sequencing of the words was critical to their interpretation were the most difficult for the aphasics. The short, simple, active, declarative, reversible sentences (S–V–O) were the most difficult sentences (Rank 1). In contrast, direct/indirect object sentences were most difficult for the controls. Of particular interest is that in both studies, the test sentences requiring the correct processing of word order displayed the most errors.

The importance of other parameters, such as the effect of vocabulary, syntactic complexity, and length of the sentence, was investigated by Shewan and Canter (1971). Their results demonstrated only quantitative differences among the different types of aphasia; qualitative differences, however, were found between the aphasia and control groups. An increase in syntactic complexity resulted in the most errors for the aphasics. The most syntactically complex constructions tested in this investigation were irreversible passive sentences, such as "The letter was mailed by the man."

Caramazza and Zurif (1976) examined the performance of Broca's, conduction, and Wernicke's aphasics and control subjects on an auditory sentence comprehension task, that is, a sentence–picture matching task (two-picture choice) consisting of three types of object-relative center-embedded sentences (semantically constrained, reversible, and improbable). The conduction and Broca's aphasics revealed a similar pattern: They performed well on sentences that could be processed on the basis of semantic and pragmatic information (semantically constrained sentences) and performed poorly on sentences requiring processing of syntactic information, that is, "syntactic-like algorithmic processes" (reversible and improbable sentences). The Wernicke's aphasics showed a very different pattern of performance. Although their level of performance was quite high, their pattern of performance could not be accounted for easily—they appeared to be insensitive to both semantic and syntactic factors; they employed "unstructured" strategies.

Heilman and Scholes (1976) also demonstrated that when comprehension was dependent on the processing of syntactic relationships, Broca's aphasics performed less well than when their comprehension performance depended on the processing of major lexical items. In contrast, Wernicke's aphasics appeared to have great difficulty processing the major lexical items (cf. also Scholes, 1978).

In a study of word order problems in agrammatism in sentence comprehension and production, Schwartz, Saffran, and Marin (1980) concluded that the English-speaking agrammatics in their investigation displayed " ... a syntactic mapping defect such that they are unable to utilize a fixed and principled set of procedures to recover the relational structure of spoken sentences" (p. 261). That is, the subjects were unable to derive underlying syntactic-semantic roles, as marked by surface word order. The disorder in sentence production paralleled the comprehension disorder in that the agrammatics showed difficulty producing sentences in which the semantic relations were expresed by the order of noun phrases around verbs or prepositions. That is, the agrammatics could not " ... reliably map semantic relations onto surface word order" (p. 263).

Caplan (1983b) reconstructed Schwartz and colleagues' (1980) data. He questioned their claim that agrammatics could not map "word order" onto thematic information. On the basis of his reconstructed data, Caplan concluded that the agrammatic does not appear to have "lost" any aspect of the system of mapping semantic representations. The agrammatic "can relate this aspect of the semantic information associated with a word to the position of a word in a sentence or a phrase" (p. 159). The agrammatic has simply "added a set of principles dealing with intrinsic animacy of nouns in establishing the mapping between 'word order' and thematic relations conveyed by a sentence or phrase" (pp. 159–160).

Caplan and Futter (1986) reported on data from a single case study of sentence comprehension in an agrammatic subject, in particular the assignment of thematic roles to nouns, which involved a manipulation task, ("acting out the action"). In a discussion of the results on a wide range of sentence types, the authors pointed out that their subject did not randomly assign thematic roles to noun phrases (NPs) in the sentences tested. Rather, the results were to be interpreted as clear evidence that the subject relied " ... on a linear sequence of categories to structure the sentences she hears" (p. 127). However, Caplan and Futter asserted that a strategy of determining thematic roles based solely on the linear order of nouns in the presented sentence could not account for the subject's performance. They summarized the subject's performance as follows: She did not perform randomly; normal grammar did not totally determine the responses; neither could two nonlinguistic interpretative strategies (use of linear spatial or auditory order of elements) account for the results. The discovered regularities in performance were considered to be dependent on the syntactic structure of the sentences presented, "but . . . [were] not completely determined by the structures themselves in the normal way these structures determine meaning" (p. 127). In an analysis of the subject's performance in terms of structure of the test sentences, structures of the following forms

N_1-V-N_2
N_1-V-N_2-N_3
N_1-V_1-N_2-V_2-N_3

were interpreted by the subject according to an interpretive rule (principle 2) proposed by the authors: "Assign the thematic roles of agent, theme, and goal to N_1-V-N_2-N_3, where N_1 does not already bear a thematic role" (p. 128). The agrammatic subject discussed by the authors systematically assigned structure to the forms listed by means of principle 2, which resulted at times in incorrect interpretations. Other sentence types investigated by Caplan and Futter, uninterpretable by means of principle 2, were inconsistently interpreted by the subject.

In summary, the agrammatic subject investigated by Caplan and Futter ". . . [achieved] an initial appreciation of the syntactic form of sentences. She [seemed] to consider sentences, syntactically, as linear series of nouns and verbs, with prepositions and possibly verbal morphology also being noted" (p. 130). The linear order of strings was then interpreted by means of principle 2 whenever it was applicable, and by other strategies when it did not apply to the whole sentence. The authors asserted that their subject's overall performance was not determined by pragmatic factors.

By means of a sentence–picture matching auditory comprehension task (five-picture choice), Heeschen (1980) investigated actor–object relations in various sentence types in German-speaking aphasics. The Broca's aphasics made overall fewer errors than patients with Wernicke's aphasia. The only difference noted between the two groups was that "Broca-aphasics tended to neglect the syntactic aspect of constituent order if a semantic cue was given, while the Wernicke aphasics continued to take the constituent order into account even in sentences where a semantic cue was present" (p. 19). On the basis of his results, Heeschen questioned the "syntactic deficit hypothesis," namely, that Broca's aphasia is characterized by a selective impairment of syntax that is also manifest in language comprehension, that is, a supramodal blockade of syntax.

In a note, Caramazza (1982) commented that Heeschen's conclusion was not supported by the reported results. To refute the "syntactic deficit hypothesis" as put forward by Caramazza and Berndt (1978), Heeschen would have had to demonstrate that the proportion of syntactic to lexical errors was higher for Broca's than for Wernicke's aphasics. According to Caramazza, since Heeschen reported only on reversal errors, a comparison of qualitative differences between the two types of aphasia was not possible. Heeschen did not provide the relevant information to test the syntactic deficit hypothesis.

In a comparison of performance on metalinguistic grammaticality judgment tasks and auditory comprehension tasks, Linebarger, Schwartz, and Saffran (1983) proposed two possibilities for the varying performances of agrammatics:

1. The difficulties consisted in making use of syntactic representations for semantic interpretation.
2. Good performance could be achieved only in one area, that is, there was a trade-off between syntactic and semantic processing.

The agrammatic's good performance on metalinguistic tasks refutes the claim that a loss of the ability to analyze syntactic structures (i.e. of syntactic knowledge) was the source of the difficulties observed in the agrammatics tested by the authors.

Jones (1984) reported on the effect of verb semantics on the processing of word order in simple active declarative sentences by agrammatic and Wernicke's aphasics. Using a comprehension task (three-picture choice), she investigated three types of verbs: (a) directional motion verbs (e.g., to push), (b) nondirectional motion verbs (e.g., to carry), and (c) nonmotion verbs (e.g., to watch).

Agrammatic aphasics demonstrated a word order deficit in the processing of sentences containing the directional motion verbs; these sentences were significantly more difficult than sentences containing the other verb types. Ninety-nine percent of the errors consisted of the reverse role distractor, that is, reversal of the subject with the direct object. Since the subjects were able to decode some aspects of the meaning of the verbs, "the only explanation remaining for the high number of errors made is failure to process the grammatic relationships pertaining between the verb and the two noun arguments" (p. 167). The results thus point out that although the agrammatics were able to access some aspects of the verb meaning, "they were unable to access that information which maps the predicate/argument structure onto the grammatic structure" (p. 167). Furthermore, a particular problem in accessing the prepositional information inherent in the verb was postulated to account for the difficulty of processing sentences containing a directional motion verb such as pull, push, follow, lift, and so on. Jones attributed this difficulty to a "semantic deficit in relation to these verbs" (p. 179), which can be interpreted only on a lexical semantic basis. This interpretation is open to debate.

For the Wernicke's aphasics, the nondirectional and directional motion verbs were equally difficult to process. Analysis of the overall errors made on the sentences revealed interesting differences between the two aphasia types. In contrast to the minimal percentage of verb distractor errors made by the agrammatic aphasics, the verb distractor errors made up 20.3% of the nondirectional and 57.5% of the directional motion verbs for the Wernicke's aphasics. The Wernicke's aphasics (n=6) made proportionally more errors in processing grammatic relationships marked by word order alone.

Aphasia type	Nonmotion	Nondirectional	Directional
Agrammatic (n = 10)			
Total	41	59	10
Mean	4.1	5.9	10.8
% Reverse	92.6	98.3	99.0
% Distractor	7.4	1.7	1.0
Wernicke's (n = 6)			
Total	24	6	73
Mean	4.0	11.5	12.1
% Reverse	100.0	79.7	42.5
% Distractor	0.0	20.3	57.5

The author held that the errors made by the Wernicke's aphasics stemmed from either a lack of recognition of the verb or failure to process the grammatic relationships. The failure with each verb type is discussed separately. The difficulties found with the nonmotion verbs were attributed to an inability to access that part of the semantic representation that maps semantic and grammatic information. In the sentences consisting of directional motion verbs, the Wernicke's aphasics were considered unable to access any of the semantic representation of the verb, resulting in choice of the verb distractor, that is, in the pictorial depiction of a different action. Sentences with nondirectional motion verbs took on an intermediate position; Wernicke's aphasics "... were able to access that information which codes the grammatic relationships, however, they chose the reverse role picture" (pp. 176–177). In terms of processing load, the attention drawn by the author to the role of the complexity of the different types of verbs investigated deserves particular mention.

In the same volume, Lesser (1984) applied lexical functional grammar to production and comprehension experiments consisting of to-complements to reexamine the distinction between lexical and syntactic impairment in Wernicke's and Broca's aphasics, respectively. The aim of the study was to examine the distinction made in lexical functional grammar between the constituent structure of a sentence (phrase structure) and its functional structure (which refers to the grammatical relations among subject, object, etc). The fluent aphasics were impaired in their comprehension of the functional structures of predicative words. On the other hand, the nonfluent Broca's aphasics did not show particular difficulties processing "at this deep level of syntactic representation" (p. 200). Lesser concluded that the dissociation between syntax and the lexicon is supported: "If the lexicon indeed includes specifications for functional and syntactic structures, as lexical grammar claims, a lexical impairment might legitimately be conceived of as incorporating reduction in the ability to use such predicative functions in comprehending and producing sentences" (p. 200).

Tyler (1985) discussed results from a case study of an agrammatic subject's auditory comprehension and ability to construct structural syntactic and interpretative representations in tasks requiring on-line versus off-line processing, for example, constructing global representations while spanning an entire utterance, or making use of local lexical syntactic and semantic constraints in the process of relating verbs to their arguments. One of the questions addressed by Tyler pertained to the location, "with respect to the sequence of processing events, of the comprehension deficit" (p. 261), that is, whether the deficit was due to difficulties in the processes necessary for constructing "on-line, higher-level representations" or to difficulty using these representations in off-line tasks.

On the basis of her experimental results deriving in particular from reaction times in word monitoring tasks using normal, anomalous, and scrambled prose, Tyler proposed that the agrammatic patient tested "could construct a semantic [i.e. interpretative], but not syntactic representation of an utterance" (p. 259). The subject was found to be much more dependent upon pragmatic information than were normal control subjects. The author noted that this greater reliance might result from the subject's syntactic deficit (i.e., difficulty constructing a syntactic representation), which is not a general breakdown in syntactic parsing routines; the subject could make use of some kinds of syntactic information (e.g., sensitivity to violations of subcategorization restrictions between verbs and their arguments). Tyler postulated this syntactic impairment because the subject's performance deviated from normal in the effects of word position in anomalous prose. Interpreting the word effects in normal listeners "as reflecting the development of a structural representation across an utterance" (p. 266), and then inferring from such an interpretation that the agrammatic patient is unable to develop the same kind of structural representation, is open to discussion. Other conclusions arrived at also allow other interpretations. At the present time it is difficult to determine what implications can be drawn about the structure of the language-processing system from the on-line monitoring tasks discussed in Tyler's study. In general, the data used for drawing inferences about "normal sentence comprehension" are open to debate (cf. Swinney, 1981).

In a recent study of reading comprehension, however, Kolk and Friederici (1985) examined two proposals pertaining to the type of syntactic impairment in Broca's as opposed to Wernicke's aphasia:

1. Whether the syntactic impairment in Broca's aphasia is to be considered in an all-or-none fashion.

2. Whether the syntactic disorder in question is solely characteristic of Broca's aphasia.

In a graphic presentation of a sentence–picture matching task (three-picture choice), various sentence types containing three kinds of prepositional phrases were investigated in German- and Dutch-speaking Broca's and Wernicke's aphasics. The findings of Kolk and Friederici indicated that Wernicke's and Broca's error patterns were very similar. Both groups of aphasics manifested a syntactic comprehension disorder. The authors interpreted the pattern of differences between the various types of sentences tested in two ways. In the first interpretation, "... basic (but different) syntactic abilities" (p. 66) were considered to have been lost. In this case, reversible sentences were processed solely by means of "non-syntactic" strategies. According to the second interpretation, the performance by both aphasic groups was not explained by a loss of syntactic abilities; rather, the more syntactic analysis required, the more errors the subjects made.

In a comprehensive study on auditory sentence comprehension, Caplan, Baker, and Dehaut (1985) closely scrutinized essential issues of "syntactic determinants of sentence comprehension in aphasia" in three groups of aphasic subjects. Since their results are significant for the present study, the five questions raised by the authors in their study merit discussion.

The first question, whether syntactic structures influence the assignment of sentential semantic features in aphasia, was answered affirmatively. The previously discussed results of the Caplan and Futter (1985) investigation also hold for this study, namely, that the aphasics did not assign thematic roles randomly. Rather, the elementary structural features of a sentence, such as word order, hierarchical organization of constituents, verb argument structure, and function word vocabulary, played a role in determining the interpretation of sentences. The complexity of a sentence was, thus, considerably determined by noncanonical word order, a third thematic role, and a second verb, in an additive fashion. Although factors such as pragmatic or task-specific information, memory capacities, and so on influenced the aphasics' performance to a certain extent, the effect of syntactic structure was distinguishable by means of the type of task (object manipulation) employed by the authors.

The second issue addressed was the identifiability of aphasia type or subgroup in terms of ability to process syntactic structures. Further, the third issue pertained to whether the differences were of a quantitative (overall severity of aphasia) or qualitative nature (comprehension impairment in specific structures). Statistical analysis revealed that different patient subgroups were identifiable. Concerning the nature of the differences, mainly the overall severity of aphasia and, to a lesser extent, the sentence type determined the differential performance. Regarding the classical aphasia types and the localization of the aphasia-producing lesions, the fourth and fifth questions, respectively, the authors stated that the patient subgroups tested did not correspond to classical aphasia types and the patients did not have lesions in common.

In an analysis of the pattern of dissociation and co-occurrence of symptoms in agrammatic Broca's aphasia, Caramazza and Berndt (1985) maintained that the comprehension and production disorders are to be attributed to impairment of independent mechanisms at the level of the computation of grammatical features. Thus agrammatism is to be viewed as a multicomponent deficit. Three possible accounts for the "very frequent but nonnecessary co-occurrence of asyntactic comprehension with agrammatism" (p. 60) are discussed. The asyntactic comprehension in agrammatic Broca's aphasia is characterized best as a deficit at the level of the semantic mapping functions. "That is, the patient is able to carry out normal syntactic parsing of a sentence but is unable to interpret the output of this computation, especially information regarding the grammatical roles of major lexical items that is needed to specify the logical roles (e.g., agent, patient, etc.) of the sentence" (p. 60). The authors stressed that their choice of the most suitable account of the comprehension deficit was dependent on whether the previously discussed results of Linebarger et al. (1983), pertaining to the agrammatics' ability to perform grammaticality judgments, could be upheld. Only the semantic mapping deficit account is compatible with the dissociation between impaired sentence comprehension and intact grammaticality judgments.

Although the specific research goals and methods employed by the authors of the previously discussed studies vary, two main types of research methodology can be distinguished. The distinction lies in the analysis of (extensive) data from single cases in contrast to group study analysis of aphasics. In several of the studies, performance of aphasics displaying the various traditional aphasia types on a particular language comprehension task was investigated and the results of the different groups compared (cf. Caramazza & Zurif, 1976; Goodglass et al., 1970, 1979; Heeschen, 1980; Heilman & Scholes, 1976; Jones, 1984; Kolk & Friederici, 1985; Lesser, 1974; Parisi & Pizzamiglio, 1970; Shewan & Canter, 1971; etc). Other studies discussed above demonstrate a different research strategy, namely, an in-depth characterization of the deficits or symptoms present in a single aphasic (or in several aphasics displaying very similar patterns of performance), particularly in terms of impairment to postulated mechanisms (e.g., as postulated in the model of sentence processing discussed by Caramazza & Berndt, 1985). The aphasic's (overall) performance is analyzed either without reference to a particular, traditional aphasia type or is considered representative of a particular type of aphasia (or "aphasia syndrome").

Shortcomings of several of the studies discussed in this review include the following:

1. The auditory sentence comprehension performance of the aphasic population tends to be treated as homogeneous. The number of errors (i.e., quantitative analysis) is attributed to severity of language impairment (e.g., Lesser, 1974; Parisi & Pizzamiglio, 1970).
2. When aphasic groups are classified according to type of aphasia in the analysis of errors, the performance of particular subgroups is discussed, while other subgroups included in the study are either not completely analyzed or not compared with all the subgroups tested (e.g., Goodglass et al., 1970; Parisi & Pizzamiglio, 1970).
3. Performance on tasks tapping various dimensions of language comprehension ability—which could contribute to the complexity of an auditory comprehension task—are compared among aphasia types as evidence for differential susceptibility or as evidence against language comprehension as a unitary phenomenon, in contrast to comparison of all aphasic groups on performance of a single task capable of distinguishing various aspects of language processing.
4. Either the results of the study do not unequivocally support the conclusions arrived at by the authors or the data are questionable in the first place (e.g., Caplan, 1983b; Jones, 1984; Tyler, 1985; cf. also Caramazza, 1982, on Heeschen, 1980).

We shall return to details of particular studies in connection with various questions in the discussion section. For the present, it suffices to state that the highly selective review of the cited studies reveals the difficulty of arriving at a conclusive, comprehensive account of whether there exist qualitative and/or quantitative differences in performance on language comprehension tasks by aphasics displaying clinical, classically defined aphasia types. In-depth treatment of crucial issues discussed in most recent studies exemplify the state of the art in this area of research and set the background for the present study.

Goals of the Present Study

With the above research in mind, a goal of the present study is to describe the nature of the auditory sentence comprehension impairments that are present in the various classical aphasia types. That is, our goal is to arrive at a more differentiated description of the auditory sentence comprehension disorder(s) and to determine whether aphasics are distinguishable in terms of quantitative and/or qualitative differences in performance on an auditory comprehension task. Hypotheses concerning the general nature of the deficits expected to be found in the various aphasia types are discussed; specific hypotheses about aphasics' performance on the auditory sentence comprehension task used in this study are delineated.

Hypotheses on the Nature of Auditory Sentence Comprehension Impairment in Various Aphasia Types

To address the questions regarding the nature of the language comprehension disorder(s) manifest in the particular types of aphasia, hypotheses describing the disorders expected to be found in the particular type of aphasia are essential. These are based on linguistic descriptions of the language disorders, briefly formulated as follows:

Global

In global aphasia, a generalized severe language comprehension disorder is expected, since all language modalities and linguistic levels are impaired to a considerable degree. Global aphasics are thus expected to make a great number of all error types due to their very reduced language-processing system.

Broca's

Parallel to the language production disorder, the language comprehension disorder expected in Broca's aphasia can be described as a disorder in the processing of morphosyntactic information, for example, grammatical markers and word order. The Broca's aphasic is impaired in processing of the case markers of the definite article, which simultaneously signal grammatical relations, propositional semantic information, and to a certain extent pragmatic function of the noun phrases in relation to the verb(s) in discourse. In (auditory) sentence comprehension tasks, the disorder should manifest itself in particular error types (e.g., reversals), in reversible syntactic constructions of increasing syntactic and semantic complexity. In terms of a processing model, the underlying cause of the impairment in morphosyntactic processing has not been resolved. Several accounts have been proposed. Caramazza and Berndt (1985) discussed the following possible sources of the deficit:

1. The deficit is at the level of semantic mapping functions. (This hypothesis was cited in the review of the literature.)
2. The syntactic processing device is disrupted: The mechanism that interprets the syntactic information carried by word order and by the grammatical markers is impaired.
3. An impairment of phonological working memory results in limited, that is, ineffective, computation of the syntactic mapping operations. (Cf. Caramazza & Berndt, 1985, pp. 59–61.)

Wernicke's

Linguistically speaking, a disorder in processing of the semantic and/or phonological information of the main lexical items can be postulated for

Wernicke's aphasics. The comprehension difficulties expected in Wernicke's aphasia depend on the severity of the language impairment as evaluated in the clinical setting. In terms of auditory comprehension difficulties, a severely impaired Wernicke's would be comparable to a global aphasic, that is, would display severe comprehension deficits, whereas a mildly impaired Wernicke's subject would be expected to show much better auditory comprehension performance (i.e., make fewer errors).

Moderately and mildly impaired Wernicke's aphasics demonstrate difficulties in maintaining, retrieving, and juxtaposing the surface order of noun phrases. It is our impression that, due to their difficulties in processing the semantic and/or phonological information of the main lexical items, the whole processing system has broken down in the severely impaired Wernicke's aphasic. For the mildly impaired Wernicke's aphasic, including subjects in recovery after a severe language comprehension disorder has subsided, processing of the semantic information/phonological form of the main lexical items is more efficiently achieved; however, the ability to either maintain/retrieve the order of the nouns in working memory or to juxtapose the surface order to arrive at the S–V–O order (agent–patient, etc.) has broken down.

Several possibilities can account for the processing difficulties. One interpretation is that the mild Wernicke's aphasic cannot attend to two aspects of processing at the same time because of limited processing. Processing of the main lexical items is achieved. However, the processing system is then exhausted and the subject cannot arrive at the correct logical order of the nouns, although the processing of case marking of the definite articles is correct. The simultaneous demands overtax the processing system. At the present time it is not ascertainable whether and/or to what extent the decrease in number of errors made by the moderately/mildly impaired Wernicke's aphasic in recovery reflects a separate and qualitatively different performance/impairment, which is perhaps masked by the overall severity of the comprehension disorder, or reflects a mere quantitative difference in degree of language impairment.

Anomic

Clinically speaking, the anomic aphasic is considered to have the least severe auditory language comprehension disorder (Goodglass and Kaplan, 1972, 1983; Goodglass et al., 1970; Kertesz, 1985; Lesser, 1984). The language comprehension impairment in anomics has been characterized by Lesser (1984) as follows: "Anomic patients who score relatively well on tests of auditory verbal comprehension have also been classed with other patients with posterior lesions as having a fuzziness of lexical semantics as well as difficulty in projecting word meanings onto word sound" (p. 193). The degree of "fuzziness" and the difficulty in projecting word meanings onto sounds are assumed to be dependent on the severity of the impairment. For anomics, as for mildly impaired Wernicke's aphasics, difficulties in processing the semantic information of the main lexical items leads to impairment in maintaining the nouns in working memory/ retrieving/arriving at the correct thematic roles (agent–patient), for the same reasons.

Hypotheses Pertaining to the Aphasic's Performance on an Auditory Sentence Comprehension Task

The following main hypotheses concerning aphasics' performance on an auditory sentence comprehension task have been formulated:

Hypothesis 1.1: Quantity Only. Aphasics of different aphasia types (Broca's, Wernicke's, global, anomic) differ only quantitatively in their auditory sentence comprehension performance. The pattern of errors is similar across the aphasia types; errors differ only in number.

Hypothesis 1.2: Severity. Patients with a severe degree of impairment display greater comprehension difficulties than do patients with a moderate or mild degree of impairment regardless of aphasia type; they make more of the same errors.

Hypotheses 1.1 and 1.2 express the standpoint that different aphasia types are *linguistically* not distinguishable.

Hypothesis 2.0: Quality. The auditory sentence comprehension performance of aphasics of different aphasia types and degrees of severity is *qualitatively different,* that is, errors made by patients of the various aphasia types are systematic errors, a fact that reflects impairment of particular underlying mechanisms.

If a combination of quantitative and qualitative aspects in the sense of hypotheses 1.1, 1.2, and 2.0 explains the measureable impairments best, then Hypothesis 3.0 should hold:

Hypothesis 3.0: Quantity and Quality. The auditory sentence comprehension of aphasics of different types is not only quantitatively but also qualitatively different. A combination of quantitative and qualitative aspects differentiates the aphasia types.

Hypothesis 3.1 pertains to the effect of concomitant variables.

Hypothesis 3.1. Other premorbid aspects, such as years of schooling, profession, and so on, and general linguistic notions must also be taken into account in a comprehensive analysis of auditory sentence comprehension performance.

The aim of the present study is to investigate these hypotheses as well as controversial results in the literature with the ultimate goal of arriving at more specific questions concerning the nature of the underlying mechanisms or processes assumed to be involved in auditory sentence comprehension on the basis of analysis of error patterns.

A group study using a single test was chosen to assess specific syntactic and semantic aspects of auditory sentence comprehension. We performed parallel, in-depth testing of selected subjects to arrive at a better understanding of the subject's overall linguistic performance for comparison with the results obtained on a single test. This study thus serves as the basis for further detailed research on auditory sentence comprehension (and sentence production) in aphasia.

Methods

A sentence–picture matching task (four-picture choice), comparable to others discussed in the literature, was developed. This test was designed to meet the following clinical and theoretical linguistic requirements:

1. Practical length. The test should take a reasonably short time to administer, so as not to overtax the patient. That is, it should be just long enough to allow differentiation of aphasia types quantitatively and/or qualitatively.
2. Items varying from simple to complex. This requirement follows from the goal of using severity as one of the explaining variables. Test items ranging from linguistically simple to complex, capable of demonstrating specific difficulties of syntactic or semanto-syntactic processing, were included.
3. Realistic. Test items should correspond to ordinary situations encountered in daily life. This means use of situations depicting persons, things, and actions that reflect manipulations and knowledge of the real world, to avoid confusing the subject unnecessarily.[3]

A combination of the above-mentioned requirements and language-specific characteristics of German determined the item pool of the test employed. The surface form of a German sentence can differ from the form of another sentence in the following ways (cp. Dik, 1980; Givon, 1984; Stockwell, 1977): (a) the serial order of the words, (b) the morphology of the words (the case endings), (c) the serial order of the words plus morphology, and (d) the intonation.

A test making use of these four possibilities by pairing of syntactic aspects (variation in sentence type: simple declarative transitive, subject relative, topicalized) and voice distinctions (active versus passive) with semantic aspects (reversible versus irreversible, animate versus inanimate) enables investigation of the processing of word order and grammatical markers by aphasics. The following is a brief description of the test material.

Subjects

A total of 169[4] subjects with aphasia predominantly of vascular etiology and with German as their native language were routinely tested one month (at the earliest) after onset of the language impairment. Testing consisted of a standardized aphasia examination in German, such as the Aachen Aphasia Test (AAT) and/or an informal aphasia assessment covering spontaneous speech, picture descriptions, naming of depicted objects, sentence production tasks, repetition of words and sentences, word and sentence comprehension tasks, and retelling of a story and a brief examination of reading and writing. On the basis of the aphasia examination—in particular the spontaneous speech rating—the aphasia type was determined and the language impairment classified into one of four degrees of severity (minimal, mild, moderate, or severe).

All 169 aphasics were included in the present statistical analysis, although 13 displayed types of aphasia that seldom occur. Results from patients displaying the 4 main aphasia types (n = 156) will be discussed in greater detail here and are covered in Tables 6.2 through 6.16. Patient variables and results for the 13 with rare types of aphasia (the "Other" group) are given in Table 6.18 and are referred to at various points in the discussion. Aphasic patients were excluded from this study either on the basis of an upper age limit, or bilingualism, or bilateral lesions or because a "mixed" form of aphasia was determined.[5] In the latter case, one type did not dominate the clinical picture. These cases will be analyzed in a follow-up study.

Hemianoptic signs were not present in any of the subjects. Vision was corrected for in those patients wearing eyeglasses.

A summary of subject variables—including mean age, sex, years of schooling, etiology, mean time since onset of aphasia, aphasia type, and degree of severity—is given in Table 6.1. Exact matching of groups for size according to type and degree of severity and also for within-group characteristics was not possible. In this context, the degree of severity is relative to the type of aphasia: A case of minimal or mild global aphasia is doubtful due to the overall severity of the language impairment.

Other than differences in aphasia type and degree of severity rating, a priori no specific variables could be considered as a cause for significant differences in error patterns in this test. We shall return to these variables in the discussion.

Before the patients were tested, 30 native German speakers with a mean age of 50 years (S.D. = 15 years) were tested to control for the adequacy of the test material. The control subjects were comparable to the aphasics in the subject variables age, sex, and years of education.

Material

In the previous section we briefly discussed the linguistic design of the test, especially as it pertains to the syntactic and semantic parameters inves-

TABLE 6.1. Summary of Variables[a] for 156 Patients with Aphasia

Aphasia type	Mean age (years)	Sex	Years of schooling[b]	Etiology[c]	Months (mean) since onset of aphasia	Degree of severity[d]
Global (n = 27)	57.3 (S.D. = 10.8; med. = 58.7)	M = 17 F = 10	0 = 4 1 = 2 2 = 11 3 = 6	All CVA 4 = 4	24.2 (S.D. = 29.7; med. = 15.2)	Mo = 14 S = 13
Broca's (n = 46)	56.7 (S.D. = 11.1; med. = 57.5)	M = 31 F = 15	1 = 1 2 = 31 3 = 8 4 = 6	CVA = 44 Trauma = 1 Abscess = 1	26.1 (S.D. = 31.6; med. = 14.2)	R = 4 Mi = 9 Mo = 21 S = 12
Wernicke's (n = 44)	61.8 (S.D. = 8.5; med. = 62.1)	M = 19 F = 25	0 = 7 1 = 1 2 = 19 3 = 11 4 = 6	CVA = 38 Tumor = 3 Trauma = 1 Abscess = 2	12.4 (S.D. = 16.0; med. = 5.8)	Mi = 5 Mo = 22 S = 17
Anomic (n = 44)	52.1 (S.D. = 11.9; med. = 54.2)	M = 21 F = 18	0 = 4 1 = 4 2 = 19 3 = 7 4 = 5	CVA = 34 Tumor = 2 Trauma = 1 Abscess = 2	23.0 (S.D. = 49.7; med. = 3.7)	R = 5 Mi = 14 Mo = 8 S = 12

[a]All patients were right-handed.
[b]0 = not known; 1 = grammar school (6–8 years); 2 = vocational school (9–10 years); 3 = high school (12 years); 4 = university degree (at least 16 years).
[c]Left hemisphere lesion.
[d]S = severe, Mo = moderate, Mi = mild, R = minimal (residual language impairment).

tigated. Four sentence types were crossed with reversibility/irreversibility and active/passive to arrive at a total of 32 test items. A summary of the test design is presented in Table 6.2.

In the case of both the bitransitive (subject–indirect object–direct object, or triple noun phrase) construction (with a verb valency of three) and the subject relative clause construction, only reversible sentences were included. The subject relative clause construction was included to investigate the effect of length of utterance in relation to sentence type:

Type	Length
Simple declarative, transitive, active	5–6 words
Subject relative clause	9–10 words
Bitransitive (subject–indirect object–direct object)	7–8 words

A summary of the linguistic variables for the 32 test sentences is given in Table 6.3.

Except for the passive construction "by" phrase, test sentences with prepositional phrases were not included in this study for several reasons. Although prepositions belong to the grammatical class of function words (form class), their semantic role varies according to the sentential context. Therefore, selective aphasic impairment of prepositions can stem from different sources (cp. Friederici, 1982; Kolk & Friederici, 1985; etc.).

In contrast to English, in a German indirect object construction, case markers and the usual word order (S–V–IO–DO) distinguish the noun phrases: "Die Frau zeigt dem Jungen das Mädchen" ("The woman is showing the boy the girl"). In German there is no variant with a prepositional phrase, that is, an outer dative equivalent to the English version: "The woman is showing the girl to the boy," only an inner dative. The indirect object before the direct object is the most common ordering of these noun phrases.

In contrast to the marginal role played by morphological marking of a noun phrase in English, the salient role of morphology as a basic marker of grammatical relations in German (e.g., marking of the noun phrases) is to be stressed. Morphology, that is, the case markers of the articles and other determiners, is determined by and denotes grammatical functions. Word order (i.e., the ordering of the noun phrases around the verb), however, is determined by pragmatic roles (cp. Comrie, 1981; Dik, 1980; Eisenberg, 1986).[6] In German the definite/indefinite articles are marked for case and gender of the nouns they precede. The grammatical relations (e.g., subject, direct object, and indirect object) and semantic roles (e.g., agent, patient, recipient, etc.) of the nouns are determined by the case endings of the articles. In general, the case endings on articles are distinctive markers. However, in some cases the forms coincide. For example, neuter and feminine gender articles have no distinctive case marker in the nominative and accusative.

TABLE 6.2. Linguistic Parameters of the Sentence Types

Sentence type	Voice (no. of sentences)	Semantic aspects	Example (translated into English)
Simple declarative (transitive: subject–verb–indirect object)	Active (4)	Reversible	The mother is looking for the son. (nom.[a]) (acc.)
	Active (4)	Irreversible	The woman is ironing the shirt. (nom.) (acc.)
	Passive (4)	Reversible	The woman is awakened by the man. (nom.) (dat.)
	Passive (4)	Irreversible	The banana is picked up by the boy. (nom.) (dat.)
Topicalized transitive	Active (4)	Reversible	The girl, the boy is carrying her. (G. The girl [acc.] – V – the boy [nom.])
	Active (4)	Irreversible	The ball, the boys are looking for it. (G. The ball [acc.] – V – the boys [nom.])
Bitransitive: subject–verb–indirect object–direct object	Active (4)	Reversible	The woman introduces the girl the boy. (nom.) (dat.) (acc.)
Subject relative	Active (4)	Reversible	The teacher, who is holding a book, greets the girl. (nom.) (nom.) (acc.) (acc.)

[a]nom. = nominative; acc. = accusative; dat. = dative.

TABLE 6.3. Linguistic Characterization of Test Sentences

Item no.	Active	Passive	Reversible Yes	Reversible No	Simple declarative	Topicalized	Subject relative	Dative (DO–IO)	Case marking[a]	Animacy[b]
1	X		X		X				2	A
2	X			X	X				1	M
3		X	X						1	M
4		X		X					1	I
5	X		X			X			2	M
6	X		X					X	3	A
7	X			X		X			2	M
8	X		X				X		1	M
9	X		X		X				3	A
10	X			X	X				0	M
11		X	X						3	I
12		X		X					1	M
13	X		X			X			0	A
14	X		X					X	1	A
15	X			X		X			2	M
16	X		X				X		0	M
17	X		X		X				3	A
18	X			X	X				2	M
19		X	X						3	A
20		X		X					3	M
21	X		X			X			3	I
22	X		X					X	3	A
23	X			X		X			3	M
24	X		X				X		3	M
25	X		X		X				2	A

26	X			X	X				1	M
27		X	X						3	A
28		X		X					3	M
29	X		X			X			1	A
30	X		X					X	3	A
31	X			X		X			0	M
32	X		X				X		3	M

[a]0 = unmarked; 1 = marked; 2 = initial position marked; 3 = final position marked. See text for explanation of case marking.
[b]All noun phrases are animate (A) (e.g., boy, girl), inanimate (I) (e.g., car, bus), or mixed (M) (agent = animate while other objects are inanimate).

For each sentence the case markings of the articles for the total sentence were characterized as follows:

0 = Unmarked. The subject (nominative case) and object (accusative case) noun phrases are not unambiguously marked. For example, the neuter and feminine gender have the same form in the nominative and accusative case, in contrast to the masculine gender.
1 = Marked. All noun phrases are distinctly marked (S, DO, IO).
2 = Initial position marked. The direct object is in the accusative case in a topicalized sentence (O–V–S: e.g., *Den* Sohn sucht die Mutter [It's the son, the mother is looking for]) or the nominative case in a declarative sentence is distinctly marked.
3 = Final position marked. The subject is distinctly marked in the nominative case in a topicalized sentence (O–V–S: e.g., Die Mutter sucht *der* Sohn [nom.] [It's the mother, the son is looking for]) or the direct object is marked in an active declarative or bitransitive sentence.

In connection with case marking, there is a distinct intonation pattern. Table 6.3 gives a summary of the case markings (0, 1, 2, or 3) for the 32 test sentences.

The picture material for the test sentences was constructed to limit the possible error types.[7] For each stimulus sentence, four simple ink drawings on one DIN A4 sheet of paper were presented (refer to Figure 6.1). One of the four drawings depicted the content of the test sentence. Depending on the sentence type, the other drawings consisted of three of the following distractors:

1. Verb. The verb differed from the required one. This distractor was used for all test sentences. Wherever possible, the verb distractor was a semantically related verb, such as an opposite, for example, push versus pull.
2. Direct object. The grammatical direct object of the sentence differed. For example, a girl was depicted instead of a boy.
3. Subject. The grammatical subject of the sentence differed.
4. Subject–direct object reversal (S–DO). A reversal of the grammatical subject with the grammatical direct object was made.
5. Direct object–indirect object reversal (DO–IO). A reversal of the indirect with the direct object was made. This type of error was possible on the subject–indirect object–direct object (i.e., triple noun phrase) sentences.

An example of the test material used is given in Figure 6.1: "Der Bub stösst/schiebt das Maedchen" ("The boy is pushing the girl"). The position of the correct drawing was randomly selected for all sentences.[8]

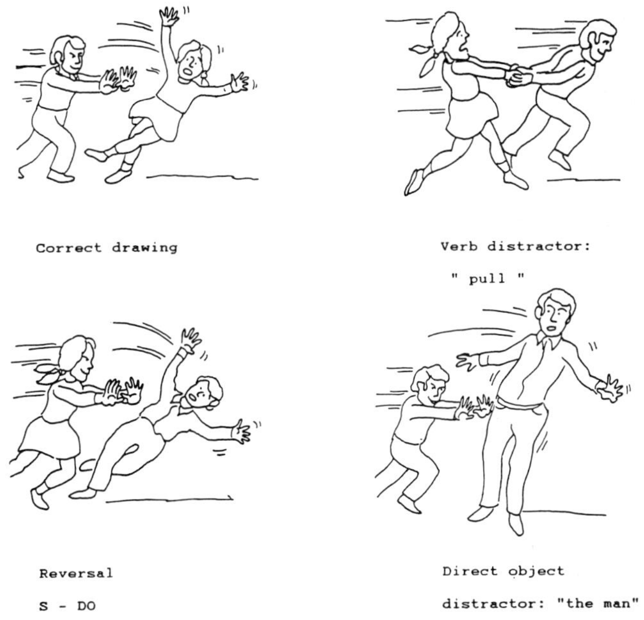
Correct drawing
Verb distractor:
" pull "
Reversal
S - DO
Direct object
distractor: "the man"

FIGURE 6.1 An Example of the Picture Material for a Test Sentence
Test Sentence: The boy is pushing the girl. (German: Der Bub stoesst/schiebt das Maedchen.) (Drawings by James W. Warren.)

PROCEDURES

The test was administered to all subjects individually—not as the first task in the session and also not as the last one. Each sentence was read aloud by the examiner with the proper intonation, and the subject was then requested to choose from the set of four pictures the one that best represented the meaning of the sentence. A repetition of the test sentence was given on the subject's request or following a pause during which no reaction occurred. The number of repetitions was noted for analysis of certainty of response. The first response was used for analysis unless the subject was uncertain in pointing and immediately changed the response without a repetition of the test sentence. If the patient responded to the test sentence without hesitation and only later became uncertain and changed the response, the test sentence was repeated. In this case, however, the initial response was considered in the analysis. The test was completed in one session; its administration took between 20 and 40 minutes, depending on the severity of aphasia of the subject.

Statistical Analysis

In recent publications the merits and limitations of case versus group study methods in neuropsychological research have been assessed, for example by Caramazza (1986). Caramazza concluded that only from extensive single case studies can one infer (processing) mechanisms that are assumed to function in healthy subjects, "since patient group study methodology does not allow valid inferences about the structure of cognitive systems" (p. 33). We agree with the main tenor of Caramazza's argument. However, a combination of both group and single case study research methodology seems to be the best strategy for neurolinguistic research at the present stage of development in the field. That is, parallels in intact and impaired mechanisma/processes investigated in group studies can be closely scrutinized in a large number of case studies. In other words, each form of investigation complements the other. By means of group studies, information relevant for basic research and for developing specific questions regarding the nature of the impaired performance(s) can be attained. Subsequently, these and additional data can be subjected to comprehensive analysis in extensive case studies to arrive at a broad perspective of the aphasic subject's total performance. The results of data analyses from both methods of investigations should be considered in developing hypotheses on the structure of cognitive systems. For example, the question of severity of aphasia in reference to performance in auditory sentence comprehension is surely best answered by longitudinal research. In a group study, statistically significant results among groups underline the relevance of relationships of the linguistic variables investigated and are an expression of specific trends.

The statistical tests included analysis of variance of ranks (Kruskal-Wallis H test [K-W]), group comparisons by Mann-Whitney U test (M-W), and cross-tabulations with appropriate measures of associations and frequency tabulations in unconditional and conditional form.[9] For assessment of differences in location of linguistic variables, the Kruskal-Wallis test was used. For clarification of pairwise differences, the Mann-Whitney test was also used with the independent variables degree of severity of language impairment, years of schooling, and a combination of these. Cross-tabulations were done for all linguistic variables crossed with the group variables (4 and 5 group classification, which will be defined in short) and with the variables degree of severity and certainty of response, always for the complete test of 32 sentences as well as for each sentence separately. Simple frequency tabulations were computed for the linguistic variables for the whole sample and for each type of aphasia separately.

Table 6.4 shows the assignment of numbers to level of severity and type of aphasia. The 169 patients were classified into the 17 groups and results from these groups were then put together and analyzed according to a set of independent medical and linguistic variables, as follows:

TABLE 6.4. Aphasia Type Groupings

Level of severity grouping (1–17)	Aphasia type grouping (0–4)
1 = Severely impaired global 2 = Moderately impaired global	1 = Global
3 = Severely impaired Broca's 4 = Moderately impaired Broca's 5 = Mildly impaired Broca's 6 = Minimally impaired Broca's	2 = Broca's
7 = Severely impaired Wernicke's 8 = Moderately impaired Wernicke's 9 = Mildly impaired Wernicke's	3 = Wernicke's
10 = Severely impaired anomic 11 = Moderately impaired anomic 12 = Mildly impaired anomic 13 = Minimally impaired anomic	4 = Anomic
14 = Transcortical motor 15 = Transcortical sensory 16 = Semantic 17 = Conduction	0 = Other aphasia types

1. Classical. The aphasia type grouping 1–4 refers to the four main aphasia types: Broca's (=B), anomic (=A), global (=G), and Wernicke's (=W), irrespective of level of severity.
2. Classical plus. The aphasia type grouping 0–4 includes the four main types of aphasia and the "Other" (=O) category. This category consists of single patients displaying less frequently occurring types of aphasia such as transcortical motor, conduction, or semantic aphasia (Head, 1926).
3. Classical–severity. The grouping 1–13 is a finer division of the 1–4 grouping, taking into account the levels of severity (e.g., 1 = global, severe, . . . , 13= anomic, minimal).
4. Classical plus–severity. The grouping 1–17 includes the less frequently occurring aphasia types in addition to the 1–13 grouping.
5. Severity only. The groupings referred to in the Kruskal-Wallis H test and the Mann-Whitney U test according to degree of severity are: 1 = minimal, 2 = mild, 3 = moderate, and 4 = severe.

In the present study, analysis of the results will be discussed mainly with respect to the above groupings 1 and 5.

Results

The control subjects ($n=30$), tested primarily to check for the adequacy of the picture material, made on the average one error or indicated uncertainty in one instance, predominantly on the subject–indirect object–direct object construction. However, with repetition of the test sentences the errors/uncertainties were corrected.

For 156 aphasics, the total number of correct responses amounted to 3,578, or 71.7% of the total possible responses (n=4,992). (For n=169 aphasics, 3,717, or 68.7%, of the total possible responses (n=5,408) were correct.) From the total possible responses,[10] 1,414, or 28.3%, were entered into the main error analyses. Two-hundred-fourteen, or 4%, of the responses were unanalyzable either because they could not be unambiguously evaluated according to one type of error (i.e., two responses), or there was no response. Of the 3,578 correct responses, 144 (4%) were evaluated as correct following an immediate self-correction. The variable "subjective certainty of response" displayed the following distribution:

1. Certain: 4,351 responses (80.5%)—single presentation of test sentence, response without hesitation.
2. Uncertain: 1,057 responses (19%), further differentiated as follows: (a) one to two repetitions necessary before responding, 763 responses (14.1%); (b) three or more repetitions needed, 119 responses (2.2%); (c) first response incorrect, then corrected, 144 (2.7%).
3. No response: 31 cases (0.6%).

A detailed analysis planned for a future follow-up study of the distribution for the variable "subjective certainty of response" in connection with the linguistic variables, that is, sentence type(s), will shed light on the relation between processing strategies and syntactic structure.

Analysis of Errors by Aphasia Type

The distribution of errors by aphasia type is presented in Table 6.5 and Figure 6.2. The Broca's aphasics made the fewest errors overall (n=221) but made the most reversal DO–IO errors (n=83), 45% of the total for this error type. The Wernicke's group made the most errors overall; the anomic and global groups, which were composed of fewer patients, were in between in terms of total number of errors. Since the groups varied in size, an averaging of the errors was required. The average number of errors for each aphasia type is given in Table 6.6. (An example of group total errors averaged for group size is: Broca's aphasics [n=46] made 34 verb errors resulting in an average of 0.7 verb errors per Broca's subject.) The data presented in Tables 6.5 and 6.6 and in Figure 6.2 demonstrate the differential susceptibility of patients of the various aphasia types to certain kinds of errors; this susceptibility is particularly striking when the percentage of possibilities to make the error is considered.

The Broca's aphasics made few verb (mean = 0.7), subject (mean = 0.2), or direct object (mean = 0.3) errors. The number of S–DO reversal errors and, to a greater extent, the DO–IO reversal errors were striking (mean =

TABLE 6.5. Distribution of Errors by Aphasia Type

Error type	Broca's (n = 46)	Anomic (n = 39)	Wernicke's (n = 44)	Global (n = 27)	Total number of errors	Significance of statistical tests[a]
Verb (4,992[b])						
Number of errors	34	78	158	127	397	K-W 1–4, K-W 0–4:**
% of aphasia type errors	15.4	30.7	28.8	32.5		M-W:AB**; AG**; BG**; BW**; GW*; AW*
% of possibilities[c]	2.3	6.2	11.2	14.7	7.9	
% of total errors	0.2	5.5	11.2	9.0	28.1	M-W: 8–17; (11–17)
Subject (2,496)						
Number of errors	11	16	51	46	124	K-W 1–4, K-W 0–4:**
% of aphasia type errors	5.0	6.3	9.3	11.8		M-W:AG**; AW**; BG**; BW**
% of possibilities	1.5	2.6	7.2	10.6	8.8	
% of total errors	0.1	.1	3.6	3.2	5.0	M-W: 9–17
Direct object (4,368)						
Number of errors	14	16	111	80	221	K-W 1–4, K-W 0–4:**
% of aphasia type errors	6.3	6.3	20.2	20.5		M-W:AG**; AW**; BG**; BW**
% of possibilities	1.1	2.6	16.8	10.6	15.6	
% of total errors	0.1	.1	7.8	5.6	5.1	M-W: 4–16; 5–16
Reversal S-DO (2,340)[d]						
Number of errors	79	92	160	101	432	K-W 1–4, K-W 0–4:**
% of aphasia type errors	35.7	36.2	29.2	25.8		M-W:AG**; AW**; BG**; BW**
% of possibilities	11.4	15.7	24.2	25.0	30.6	
% of total errors	5.6	6.5	11.3	7.1	18.5	M-W: 8–17; 11–17
Reversal DO-IO (624)						
Number of errors	83	52	68	37	240	K-W 1–4, K-W 0–4:*
% of aphasia type errors	37.6	20.5	12.4	9.5		M-W:AB*; BG*
% of possibilities	45.1	33.3	38.6	34.3	17.0	
% of total errors	5.7	3.7	4.8	2.6	38.5	M-W: 4–15; 8–15
Group total number of errors	221	254	548	391	1,414	
% of total errors	15.6	18.0	38.8	27.7		M-W:AB, $p < 0.087$; AG**; AW**; BG**; BW**; GW*
% of total responses	4.4	5.1	11.0	7.8	28.3	

[a]Refer to the text and Table 6.4 for an explanation of the groupings and abbreviations; ** = $p < 0.01$; * = $p < 0.05$.
[b]Total number of examples.
[c]The possibility to make a particular error depends on the sentence type.
[d]The S–DO reversal error of sentence 13 is not included in this analysis (cf. note 12).

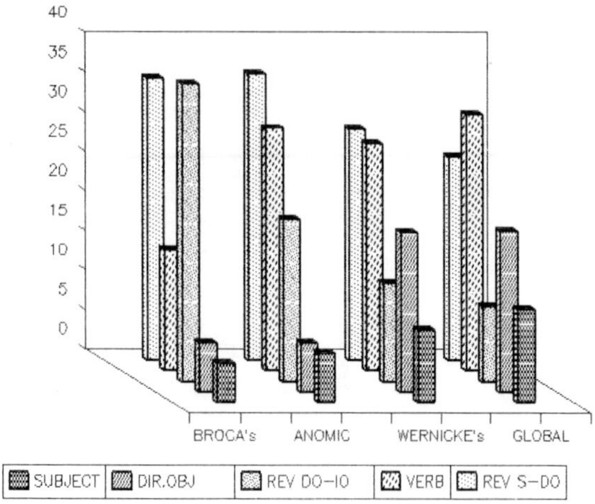

FIGURE 6.2 Distribution of Errors by Aphasia Type

1.7 and 1.8, respectively). The following statistically significant differences ($p < 0.01$) in error distributions were found for the Broca's group in paired comparisons with the other aphasia types:[10]

Verb. Anomic, global, Wernicke's.
Subject. Global, Wernicke's (anomics and Broca's patients made too few errors).
Direct Object. Global, Wernicke's (anomics and Broca's patients made too few errors).
S–DO Reversal. Global, Wernicke's.
DO–IO Reversal. Anomic, Global ($p < 0.05$).

TABLE 6.6. Distribution of Errors by Aphasia Type Averaged for Group Size; Mean Number of Errors per Subject

Error type	Broca's (n = 46)	Anomic (n = 39)	Wernicke's (n = 44)	Global (n = 27)	Average Total
Verb	0.7	2.0	3.6	4.7	2.5
Subject	0.2	0.4	1.2	1.7	1.3
Direct object	0.3	0.4	2.5	3.0	1.4
Reversal S–DO	1.7	2.4	3.6	3.7	2.8
Reversal DO–IO	1.8	1.3	1.5	1.4	1.5
Average total number	4.8	6.5	12.4	14.5	8.8
Mean lexical errors[a]	1.2	2.8	9.4	7.3	5.2
Mean syntactic errors[b]	3.5	3.7	5.1	5.1	4.3

[a]Verb, subject, and direct object are considered lexical errors.
[b]Reversal S–DO and reversal DO–IO make up the syntactic errors.

In terms of error distribution, the anomics were similar to the Broca's aphasics. The two differed, however, with reference to the verb ($p < 0.004$), DO–IO reversal ($p < 0.019$), and to a lesser extent S–DO reversal (mean Broca's = 1.7 versus mean anomic = 2.4) errors. The anomics made highly significantly more verb ($p = <0.01$), and significantly fewer DO–IO reversal errors than the Broca's aphasics. In terms of the average number of overall errors, the anomics made more errors (mean = 6.5) than the Broca's aphasics (mean = 4.8); however, the two groups did not differ significantly in terms of the sum of errors ($p < 0.087$). (Refer to Tables 6.5 and 6.6 for a summary of significance with respect to total number of errors).

The Wernicke's aphasics had a mean of 12.4 errors, with verb (mean = 3.6), direct object (mean = 2.5), and S–DO reversal (mean = 3.6) errors predominating. The Wernicke's aphasics differed statistically significantly from the Broca's in the verb ($p < 0.0001$), subject ($p < 0.0001$), direct object ($p <0.0004$), and S–DO reversal ($p < 0.000$) errors. The error types verb ($p < 0.02$), subject ($p < 0.002$), direct object ($p < 0.0003$), and S–DO reversal ($p < 0.005$) differentiate the Wernicke's from the anomic aphasics.

The global aphasics displayed the greatest mean error score (mean = 14.5), that is, they made errors on 45% of the test sentences. The mean number of errors for all error types did not significantly differ from that for the Wernicke's group, except for the verb error ($p < 0.04$). In regard to statistically significant differences between the other aphasia types, the global aphasics differed significantly from the Broca's in all error types and from the anomics in all error types except the DO–IO reversal error.

The "Other" group consisted of the following moderately impaired aphasics: (a) two conduction, (b) three transcortical motor, (c) three transcortical sensory, and (d) one initially moderately impaired aphasic tested over a period of 3 years at intervals of 6 months (who recovered to a mild degree of impairment). This subject could be best described as fitting the description of semantic aphasia, as put forward by Head (1926). The Classical Plus–Severity grouping included these less commonly occurring aphasia types separately (refer to Table 6.4). When these aphasia types were grouped together and compared with the four main aphasia types (K-W with the 1–17 grouping), all the aphasia types differed highly significantly in the verb, subject, direct object, and S–DO reversal errors ($p < 0.0001$) and significantly in the DO–IO reversal error ($p < 0.04$).

In pairwise analysis (1–17 grouping) only the following groups differed significantly:

1. The conduction aphasics differed significantly from the moderately impaired Wernicke's in the verb and S–DO reversal errors and from the mildly impaired Wernicke's in the subject error type.

2. The moderately impaired Wernicke's and the moderately impaired Broca's differed significantly from the transcortical sensory aphasics in the DO–IO reversal error.
3. The moderately and mildly impaired Broca's aphasics differed significantly from the semantic aphasic in the direct object error.
4. The moderately impaired anomics differed from the conduction aphasics in the verb and S–DO reversal error types.

These significances must be interpreted with great reservation. The results for the "Other" group are included only to allow comparisons between specific aphasia types and also as an indication of susceptibility to particular linguistic error types. The overall role of the "Other" group is minimal in terms of the number of errors ($n=63$) and percentages (4.3% of total errors); thus, its inclusion does not affect the overall analysis to a great extent. (Results for the "Other" group are summarized in Table 6.18 in the appendix.)

The mean number of errors by aphasia type for the "Other" group was:

Type of aphasia	Mean number of errors	% Reversal errors
Transcortical motor	6.7	95.0
Transcortical sensory	8.0	58.3
Semantic	3.2	81.1
Conduction	1.5	100.0

The most errors made by the "Other" group were S–DO and DO–IO reversals. With respect to the DO–IO reversal error type, when considering the possibilities to make such an error, the percentage of this error type was below chance (51.9%).

In summary, the results of analysis by aphasia type point to quantitative and qualitative differences among the aphasia types with regard to overall distribution of different error types. The differences are statistically significant among the aphasia types (K-W 1–4, 0–4, and 1–17 groupings) and in pairwise comparisons of the aphasia types (M-W U tests).

With regard to the frequency of each error type, the question arises as to the context in which the errors were made, that is, the error frequency and distribution in terms of sentence type. Analysis of the data according to the different sentence types is presented in the following sections.

Analysis of Errors by Sentence Type

Reversible Versus Irreversible Sentences

Starting with the dichotomy reversible versus irreversible, classified according to a priori knowledge, a summary of the frequency of errors (and percentages) by aphasia type is given in Table 6.7, both results—absolute and relative counts—being informative. For irreversible sentences, 87% of the total responses were correct (n = 242 errors), whereas 62.4% of the reversible sentences were correct (n = 1,172 errors), considered with respect to the possibility of making an error. The Broca's aphasics differed significantly from the other aphasia types in their good comprehension performance with irreversible sentences. For the Broca's aphasics, the direct object errors (n = 5) were the only errors made on the irreversible sentences; these amounted to 2% of the total errors made on irreversible sentences. In the reversible sentences, the Broca's errors amounted to 18.4% of the total reversible errors. This discrepancy between performance on irreversible versus reversible holds for all aphasia types when the mean number of errors (mean for group size) is considered. This is also the case when the percentages of errors for each type are examined for the Broca's and anomics, albeit to a varying extent. The opposite holds for global and Wernicke's aphasia, that is, the percentage of the errors made by subjects with these two aphasia types is greater for the irreversible than for the reversible types[11]:

	Irreversible		Reversible	
Type of aphasia	% Total irreversible errors	Mean no. of errors/subject	% Total reversible errors	Mean no. of errors/subject
Broca's	2.0	0.1	17.5	4.7
Anomic	11.8	0.7	18.3	5.8
Wernicke's	46.5	2.6	35.0	9.9
Global	38.4	3.5	24.0	11.0

Considering the group total possibilities to make an error (expressed in percent), the ratios for the aphasia types in the irreversible versus reversible sentences are:

Type of aphasia	Ratio	Irreversible:Reversible (% total errors:% total errors)
Broca's	23.5	1.0:23.5
Anomic	4.8	6.0:28.8
Wernicke's	2.3	21.6:49.3
Global	1.8	29.0:55.0

These results indicate that quantitative differences exist between irreversible and reversible sentences over all sentence types. However, the pattern and/or error frequencies vary according to the type of aphasia. These dif-

TABLE 6.7. Distribution of Errors According to Reversible/Irreversible Dichotomy

	Error type					
Aphasia type[a]	Verb	Subject	Direct object	S–DO Reversal	DO–IO Reversal	Errors sentences/ total errors
Reversible sentences (n = 3,120)[b]						
B	34 (15.7%)[c]	11 (5.1%)	9 (4.2%)	79 (36.6%)	83 (38.4%)	216/221
A	57 (25.3%)	13 (5.8%)	11 (4.9%)	92 (40.9%)	52 (16.4%)	225/254
W	105 (24.2%)	23 (5.3%)	78 (18.0%)	160 (36.9%)	68 (15.7%)	434/548
G	87 (29.3%)[c]	19 (6.4%)	53 (17.8%)	101 (34.0%)	37 (12.4%)	297/391
K-W 1–4[d]:	**	**	**	*	*	
M-W:	AB*; AG**; AW*; BG**; BW**; GW*	BG**; BW*	AG**; AW**; BG**; BW*	AG**; AW**; BG**; BW*	AB*; BG**	
Irreversible sentences (n = 1,872)						
B	0	0	5 (100%)			5/221
A	21 (72.4%)	3 (10.3%)	5 (17.2%)			29/254
W	53 (46.5%)	28 (23.7%)	33 (28.9%)			114/548
G	40 (42.5%)	27 (28.7%)	27 (28.7%)			94/391
K-W 1–4:	**	**	**			
M-W:	AB**; AG**; BG**; BW**	AB*; AG**; AW**; BG**; BW**	AG**; AW**; BG**; BW**			

[a]B = Broca's, A = anomic, G = global, W = Wernicke's.
[b]The S–DO reversal error was possible only in 2,340 sentences and the DO–IO reversal error in 624 sentences.
[c]Number of errors; in parentheses the percentage of that error type.
[d]Refer to the text and to Table 6.4 for a listing of the groupings and tests; ** = $p < 0.01$; * = $p < 0.05$.

ferences can, for example, be expressed in terms of odds ratios, as given in the above case.

A comparison of the verb and direct object errors of Broca's aphasics for the reversible versus irreversible sentences, for example, illustrates far better performance with irreversible sentences compared with reversible ones: The Broca's aphasics made no verb errors and about half as many direct object errors in the irreversible sentences (cf. Jones, 1984). The subject errors also confirm this. In this context it must, however, be stressed that the linguistic complexity of the reversible sentences allowing a subject error is greater than that of their irreversible counterparts. In general, similar tendencies are found with the error frequencies of the other aphasia types, although the odds ratios between reversible and irreversible sentences are much smaller. When one looks at the increase in errors made on reversible sentences, it is not just a question of finding "syntax" errors—reversals. There is also an increase in "lexical" errors—verb, direct object. If these lexical processing problems exist, why do they not show up in the irreversible sentences? Possibly because the additional difficulty of the reversibility makes overall processing harder, which makes the entire system more error prone.

The aphasia types differed highly significantly (K-W grouping 1–4, $p < 0.01$) for the verb, subject, and direct object errors in both the reversible and irreversible sentences and in the subject–direct object reversal error, and significantly ($p < 0.05$) in the direct object–indirect object reversal error, an error type possible only in the reversible sentences. A summary of the significances obtained in pairwise comparisons (Mann-Whitney) is listed under the respective error type in Table 6.7.

Simple Declarative Transitive Active

Data on the simple declarative transitive active sentences—total, reversible, and irreversible—are given in Table 6.8. Statistically significant ($p < 0.05$) and highly significant ($p < 0.01$) differences were found among the aphasia types (B, A, G, W) as well as between particular aphasia types for all of the error types.

The mean total number of errors for each aphasia type corrected for group size was:

	Reversible	Irreversible	Total	Total no. of errors	% S–DO rev. errors
Broca's	0.3	0.04	0.35	16	56
Anomic	0.4	0.1	0.5	17	41
Wernicke's	1.4	0.6	2.0	89	22
Global	1.7	0.9	2.6	71	29

TABLE 6.8. Distribution of Errors for Simple Declarative Transitive Active Sentences

Aphasia type[a]	Error type: Verb	Subject	Direct object	S–DO reversal	Total errors
Simple Declarative Active					
B	2 (12.5%)[b]	0	5 (31.2%)	9 (56.2%)	16
A	6 (35.3%)	1 (6.2%)	3 (17.6%)	7 (41.2%)	17
W	25 (28.1%)	6 (6.7%)	32 (36.0%)	26 (29.2%)	89
G	23 (32.4%)	8 (11.3%)	24 (33.8%)	16 (22.5%)	71
K-W 1–4[c]:	**	**	**	*	
M-W:	AB*; AG**; AW, $p = 0.056$; BG**; BW**	AG**; BG**; BW*	AG**; AW**; BG**; BW*	AG**; AW*; BG**; BW*	
Simple Active Reversible (SAR)					
B	2 (14.3%)		3 (21.4%)	9 (64.3%)	14/16[d]
A	6 (40.0%)		2 (13.3%)	7 (46.7%)	15/17
W	17 (27.0%)		20 (31.7%)	26 (41.3%)	63/89
G	16 (34.8%)		14 (30.4%)	16 (34.8%)	46/71
K-W 1–4:	**		*	**	
M-W:	AG**; BG**; BW**		AG**; AW**; BG**; BW**	AG**; AW*; BG**; BW*	
Simple Active Irreversible (SAI)					
B	0	0	2 (100%)[b]		2/16[d]
A	3 (60.0%)	1 (20.0%)	1 (20.0%)		5/17
W	8 (30.8%)	6 (23.1%)	12 (46.1%)		26/89
G	7 (28.0%)	8 (32.0%)	10 (40.0%)		25/71
K-W 1–4[c]:	*	**	**		
M-W:	AB*; BG**; BW**	AG**; BG**; BW*; GW $p < 0.07$	AG**; AW*; BG*		

[a]B = Broca's, A = anomic, W = Wernicke's, G = global.
[b]Number of errors for the aphasia type; in parentheses the percentage of that error type for the specific aphasia type.
[c]Refer to the text and to Table 6.4 for a listing of the groupings and tests; ** = $p < 0.01$; * = $p < 0.05$.
[d]Ratio of particular error type to total number of errors.

Subject Relative Sentences

The frequency distribution of errors for the subject relative sentences are presented in Table 6.9. Statistically significant differences were found among the aphasia types for all error types and between aphasia groups particularly for the direct object and the S–DO reversal errors.

A comparison of the simple declarative active reversible with the subject relative active reversible shows that almost the same number of errors were made on the shorter simple reversible sentences ($n = 138$) as on the

TABLE 6.9. Distribution of Errors for Subject Relative Sentences

Aphasia type[a]	Error type: Verb	Direct object	S–DO reversal	Total errors
B	5 (83.3%)[b]	1 (16.7%)	0	6
A	12 (52.2%)	2 (8.7%)	9 (39.1%)	23
W	22 (31.4%)	22 (31.4%)	26 (37.1%)	70
G	16 (34.8%)	16 (34.8%)	14 (30.4%)	46
K-W 1–4[c]:	*	**	**	
M-W:	BG*; BW*	AG**; AW**; BG**; BW**	AB**; AW $p < 0.057$; BG*; BW**	

[a]B = Broca's, A = anomic, W = Wernicke's, G = global.
[b]Number of errors for the aphasia type; in parentheses the percentage of that error type for the specific aphasia type.
[c]Refer to the text and Table 6.4 for a listing of the groupings and tests; ** = $p < 0.01$; * = $p < 0.05$.

longer relative sentences (n = 145). It must be noted that in this restrictive relative clause construction the reversal role distractor remains on the subject noun phrase. The frequency distribution of error types reveals interesting differences between the two construction types. A striking difference between the two is that Broca's aphasics made no reversal errors, twice as many verb errors (however, n = 5), and fewer direct object errors in the subject relative sentences. The Broca's verb errors on the subject relative sentences made up 83.3% of their total errors for that construction, as opposed to 12.5% on the reversible simple active sentences. The anomics and the Wernicke's also made more verb errors in the subject relative sentences. The error type frequencies for the global aphasics was similar for both types of sentences.

Topicalized Sentences

A total of 345 errors[12] was made on the topicalized sentences—reversible and irreversible—in comparison with 193 total errors for the simple active sentences. That is, 44% more errors were noted for the topicalized sentences. The frequency distribution of errors and the statistically significant differences among the aphasia types are given in Table 6.10. In terms of the total topicalized sentences, highly significant differences were found among the aphasia types (B,A,G,W) for all error types. The aphasia types did not differ significantly only for the direct object error types in the irreversible topicalized sentences. (Refer to Table 6.10 for a listing of the statistically significant differences between aphasia types.)

The subject–direct object reversal error for one of the reversible topicalized test sentences (see note 12) was excluded from the error analysis

TABLE 6.10. Distribution of Errors for Topicalized Sentences

Aphasia type[a]	Error type: Verb	Subject	Direct object	S–DO reversal	Total errors
Total Topicalized Sentences					
B	3 (7.3%)[b]	0	4 (9.8%)	34 (82.9%)	41
A	21 (31.3%)	2 (3.0%)	5 (7.5%)	39 (58.2%)	67
W	41 (30.8%)	13 (9.8%)	27 (20.3%)	52 (39.1%)	133
G	36 (34.6%)	12 (11.5%)	17 (16.3%)	39 (37.5%)	104
K-W 1–4[c]:	**	**	**	**	
M-W:	AB**; AG**; AW $p < 0.06$; BG**; BW**	AG**; AW**; BG**; BW**	AG*; AW**; BG*; BW*	AG*; AW*; BG**; BW**	
Topicalized Reversible (Sentence 13 Not Included)					
B	3 (7.7%)		2 (5.1%)	34 (87.2%)	39/41[d]
A	10 (19.6%)		2 (3.9%)	39 (76.5%)	51/67
W	15 (18.3%)		15 (18.3%)	52 (63.4%)	82/133
G	20 (29.8%)		8 (11.9%)	39 (58.2%)	67/104
K-W 1–4:	**		n.s.	**	
M-W:	AG**; BG**; BW*		BG*	AG*; AW*; BG**; BW**	
Total S–DO Reversal (Sentence 13 Included)					
B				70 (93.3%)	75/77[d]
A				67 (84.8%)	79/95
W				80 (72.7%)	110/161
G				51 (64.5%)	79/116
K-W 1–4:				**	
M-W:				AG**; AW**; BG**; BW**	
Topicalized Irreversible					
B	0	0	2 (100%)		2/41[d]
A	11 (68.8%)	2 (12.5%)	3 (18.7%)		16/67
W	26 (51.0%)	13 (25.5%)	12 (23.5%)		51/133
G	16 (43.2%)	12 (32.4%)	9 (24.3%)		37/104
K-W 1–4:	**	**	*		
M-W:	AB**; AG**; AW $p < 0.06$; BG**; BW**	AG**; AW*; BG**; BW**	AG*; AW*; BG $p < 0.06$; BW $p < 0.06$		

[a]B = Broca's, A = anomic, W = Wernicke's, G = global.
[b]Number of errors; in parentheses the percentage of that error type for the specific aphasia type.
[c]Refer to the text and to Table 6.4 for a listing of the groupings and tests; ** = $p < 0.01$; * = $p < 0.05$.
[d]Ratio of particular error type to total number of errors.

because this test sentence was not unambiguously marked for case endings, and reliance only on intonation proved to be insufficient. Test sentence 13 read[13]:

Die Mutter schreit das Mädchen an.
Intonation pattern: 3 2 1

The intended English equivalent:

It's the mother the girl is yelling at.

not

The mother is yelling at the girl.

In comparison with the simple declarative transitive (SAR), even if the S–DO reversal error for test sequence 13 is not counted as an error, a 50% increase of S–DO reversal errors (averaged over all aphasia types) is noted for the reversible topicalized (TR) construction:

Aphasia type	Ratio TR:SAR	TR:SAR (no. of errors)	% Reversal errors TR:SAR
Broca's	3.8	34:9	87:56
Anomic	5.6	39:7	76:35
Wernicke's	2.0	52:26	63:29
Global	2.4	39:16	58:22

For the Broca's group, apart from an increase in subject–direct object reversal errors, minimal differences were found between the simple active and topicalized constructions. For the global, anomic, and Wernicke's aphasics, not only were there more reversal errors, there was also an increase in the number of verb errors. Ninety-five percent of the Broca's errors made on topicalized constructions were on the reversible topicalized sentences, compared with 76% for the anomic, 64% for the global, and 62% for the Wernicke's aphasics.

Passive Sentences

The passive sentences reveal an error pattern similar to that of the topicalized sentences. The total number of errors in the passive sentences amounted to 347. In Table 6.11 the frequency distribution of errors and the statistical significance for the passive sentences are given.

For total passive sentences, the aphasia types differed highly significantly in all error types. The Broca's aphasics differed highly significantly from the Wernicke's in all error types for the total, reversible, and irreversible passives. In comparison with the topicalized sentences, the Broca's made three times as many verb errors on the passive sentences. This result is being further analyzed in terms of verb semantics (cp. Jones, 1984).

TABLE 6.11. Distribution of Errors for Passive Sentences

Aphasia type[a]	Error type				
	Verb	Subject	Direct object	S–DO reversal	Total errors
Total Passive Sentences					
B	11 (21.6%)[b]	0	4 (7.8%)	36 (70.6%)	51
A	21 (32.8%)	0	6 (9.4%)	37 (57.8%)	64
W	45 (32.1%)	9 (6.4%)	30 (21.4%)	56 (40.0%)	140
G	30 (32.6%)	7 (7.6%)	23 (25.0%)	32 (34.8%)	92
K-W 1–4[c]:	**	**	**	**	
M-W:	AB*; AG $p < 0.06$; BW**	AG**; AW**; BW**	AG**; AW*; BW**	AW*; BW**	
Passive Reversible					
B	11 (22.0%)		3 (6.0%)	36 (72.0%)	50/51[d]
A	14 (25.0%)		5 (8.9%)	37 (66.1%)	56/64
W	26 (25.2%)		21 (20.4%)	56 (54.4%)	103/140
G	13 (21.7%)		15 (25.0%)	32 (53.3%)	60/92
K-W 1–4:	*		**	*	
M-W:	BG $p < 0.06$; BW**		AG*; AW*: BG**; BW*	AW*; BG*; BW**	
Passive Irreversible					
B	0	0	1 (100%)		1/51[d]
A	7 (87.5%)	0	1 (12.5%)		8/64
W	19 (51.4%)	9 (24.3%)	9 (24.3%)		37/140
G	17 (53.1%)	7 (21.9%)	8 (25.0%)		32/92
K-W 1–4:	*	**	*		
M-W:	AB*; AG**; BG**; BW**	AG**; AW*; BG**; BW**	AG**; AW**; BG**; BW*		

[a]B = Broca's, A = anomic, W = Wernicke's, G = global.
[b]Number of errors; in parentheses the percentage of that error type for the specific aphasia type.
[c]Refer to the text and to Table 6.4 for a listing of the groupings and tests; ** = $p < 0.01$; * = $p < 0.05$.
[d]Ratio of particular error type to total number of errors.

Table 6.11 shows significant differences in error frequencies between the other aphasia types for the reversible and irreversible passive sentences as well.

The mean number of errors corrected for group size was:

Aphasia type	Reversible	Irreversible	Total passive	% S–DO rev. errors
Broca's	1.1	0.02	1.1	72
Anomic	1.4	0.2	1.2	66
Wernicke's	2.3	0.8	3.2	54
Global	2.2	1.2	3.4	53

Performance on Active Versus Passive Sentences

In the discussion of errors made on reversible versus irreversible sentences, the data were collapsed across active and passive sentences. Since in the analyses presented for the various sentence types active and passive sentences were considered separately, a comparison of the relations between these types of sentences (leaving all other aspects equal) is warranted. The data are summarized in Table 6.12.

Although all aphasics made more errors on the more difficult passive construction, interesting differences in the ratio passive/active were found. The Wernicke's and globals were similar in performance and contrasted with the Broca's and anomics, who also showed similar performance. The fact that the Broca's and anomics had a higher ratio of number of errors on the passive sentences to number on the active sentences can be interpreted in two ways. Either these subjects are more sensitive to the distinction "active" versus "passive" in terms of syntactic complexity or the ratio shows a less severe impairment of auditory comprehension, in contrast to the Wernicke's and global aphasics.

Bitransitive Subject–Indirect Object–Direct Object (Triple Noun Phrase) Sentences

The frequency distribution of errors and the statistically significant differences for the bitransitive/three argument dative (or triple noun phrase) constructions are summarized in Table 6.13.

Expressed in terms of the total number of errors, with the mean corrected for group size and the percentage of IO–DO reversal errors, the pattern for this construction is:

Aphasia type	Total number of errors	Total corrected for group size (mean no./subject)	% IO–DO rev. errors
Broca's	107	2.3	72
Anomic	80	2.0	65
Wernicke's	116	2.6	59
Global	70	2.8	47

In this construction type, subject, verb, and indirect–direct object reversal errors are possible. The subject errors made by the Broca's aphasics made up the total number of subject errors for this aphasia type ($n = 13$).[14] In contrast, the subject errors on this construction for the anomics amounted to 81% of their total subject errors, 48% for the globals, and 54% for the Wernicke's patients. In comparison with other single construction types, the number of verb errors made by the Broca's patients in this construction was 38% of the Broca's total verb errors, whereas the number of verb errors made on reversible passive constructions amounted to 32.4%,

TABLE 6.12. Comparison of Simple Active Declarative Sentences ($n = 1{,}248$) and Passive Sentences ($n = 1{,}248$)[a]

Aphasia type	Total errors (%)		Ratio of passive/active
	Active	Passive	
Broca's	16 (23.9)	51 (76.1)	3.2
Anomic	17 (21.0)	64 (79.0)	3.8
Wernicke's	89 (38.9)	140 (61.1)	1.6
Global	71 (43.5)	92 (56.4)	1.3

[a]The total number of errors is presented in this table. The data are collapsed across reversible/irreversible sentences. Refer to Tables 6.8 and 6.11 for the breakdown according to reversible and irreversible and for the distribution according to error type.

14.7% for the subject relative sentences, and 9.0% for simple declarative active reversible sentences.

The ratio of the simple active declarative reversible construction (SAR) to the three-argument dative construction (S–IO–DO), based on the mean number of errors corrected for group size, was:

	SAR:S–IO–DO
Broca's	0.3:2.3
Anomic	0.4:2.0
Wernicke's	1.4:2.6
Global	1.7:2.8

TABLE 6.13. Distribution of Errors for Bitransitive Subject–Indirect Object–Direct Object (Triple Noun Phrase) Sentences

Aphasia type[a]	Error type			Total errors
	Verb	Subject	DO–IO reversal	
B	13 (12.1%)	11 (10.3%)[b]	83 (77.6%)	107
A	15 (18.8%)	13 (16.2%)	52 (65.0%)	80
W	25 (21.5%)	23 (19.8%)	68 (58.6%)	116
G	22 (28.2%)	19 (24.4%)	37 (47.4%)	78
K-W 1–4[c]:	$p < 0.06$	*	*	
M-W:	AG*; BG*	AG $p < 0.06$; BG**; BW*	AB*; BG**	

[a]B = Broca's, A = anomic, W = Wernicke's, G = global.
[b]Number of errors; in parentheses the percentage of that error type for the specific aphasia type.
[c]Refer to the text and to Table 6.4 for a listing of the groupings and tests; ** = $p < 0.01$; * = $p < 0.05$.

The number of errors made by the Broca's aphasics on this single construction type accounted for over 48% of their errors. In contrast, the percentages of total errors on this construction type, in comparison with the overall group average number of errors, accounted for 31.5% of the anomics, 20% of the globals, and 21% of the Wernicke's errors.

Analysis of Error Frequency by Degree of Severity

The same error analysis—overall frequencies and frequencies by sentence type—was done according to degree of severity. Table 6.14 presents the overall frequency distribution of errors for the minimal, mild, moderate, and severe aphasics in general (i.e., irrespective of the type of aphasia). The significance of the statistical tests is given for each error type.

Four group divisions were attended to in the statistical analyses:

1. Kruskal-Wallis H test for differences across the four degrees of severity.
2. Mann-Whitney U test for pairwise analysis of degrees of severity, for example, moderate with severe.
3. Kruskal-Wallis H test for each aphasia type separately according to severity degree, to determine the effect of severity.
4. Mann-Whitney U test for pairwise analysis of aphasia types holding degree of severity constant.

(The groupings used in the analyses are discussed in the section on statistical analysis and shown in Table 6.4.)

Correction of the number of errors in the degree of severity analyses was necessary to an even greater extent than in the analyses according to aphasia type because of the unequal group sizes. Since mild or minimally impaired global aphasics are by definition very questionable, and since minimally impaired Wernicke's aphasics were not included in this study, the size of the severity groups mild and minimal was necessarily small.

For almost all individual error types—exempting the direct object-indirect object reversal—there is an increase in the average number of errors from the residual to the severe degree of aphasia. The overall mean number of errors shows an increase of at least 55% across the severity scale. The largest difference in mean number of errors is between the subjects with moderate and severe degrees of impairment (+5.8 errors). The difference is highly significant for the verb, subject, direct object, and S–DO reversal errors, and is significant ($p < 0.05$) for the DO–IO reversal. Although an increase in the mean number of errors is found for all error types with the exception of the DO–IO reversal, the absolute values vary according to error type/mean number of errors.

A subject or direct object error is indicative of severe impairment. In contrast, verb errors and to a greater extent S–DO reversal errors are present in a mild or moderate degree of severity.

TABLE 6.14. Distribution of Errors by Degree of Severity

Error type	Severity of aphasia: Residual ($n = 9$)	Mild ($n = 33$)	Moderate ($n = 73$)	Severe ($n = 54$)	Total	Significance of statistical tests[a]
Verb (4,992[b])						K-W R–S**
No. of errors	4	31	141	221	397	M-W degrees: Mi-Mo**; Mi-S**; Mo-S**
% respective degree	17.4	22.0	27.2	30.2		R,Mi:K-W n.s.; Mo:K-W 1–4**
% total errors	—	2.2	10.0	15.6	28.1	M-W:AB**; AW**; BG*; BW**; GW**
						S:K-W 1–4**
						M-W:AB**; AW**; BG**; BW**
Subject (2,496)						K-W R-S**
No. of errors	1	7	30	86	124	M-W degrees: Mi-S**; Mo-S**
% respective degree	4.3	5.0	5.8	11.7		R:K-W n.s.; Mi:K-W 1–4**; Mo:K-W*
% total errors	—	—	2.1	6.1	8.8	M-W:BG*; BW*
						S:K-W 1–4**
						M-W:AB*; AG*; BG**; BW**
Direct object (4,368)						K-W R-S**
No. of errors	0	6	50	165	221	M-W degrees: Mi-Mo**; Mi-S**; Mo-S**
% respective degree	—	4.2	9.7	22.5		R:K-W n.s.
% total errors	—	—	3.5	11.7	15.6	Mi:M-W:AB*
						Mo:K-W 1–4**
						M-W:AG**; AW; BG**
						S:K-W 1–4**
						M-W:AG*; AW**; BG**; BW**
						K-W R-S**
Reversal S-DO	6	55	186	185	432	M-W degrees: Mi-Mo**; Mi-S**; Mo-S*
(2,340)[c]	26.1	39.0	35.9	25.3		R,Mi:K-W 1–4 n.s.
	—	3.9	13.1	13.1	30.5	Mo:M-W:AB $p < 0.06$**; AW*; BG**; BW**

						K-W R-S n.s.
Reversal DO-IO (624)	12	42	111	75	240	M-W degrees: Mo-S*
	52.2	29.8	21.4	10.2		R,Mi,Mo:K-W 1–4 n.s.; S:K-W 1–4*
	1.0	2.9	7.8	5.3	17.0	M-W: AB**; BG*; BW*
Degree total number	23	141	518	732	1,414	
% total errors	1.6	10.0	36.6	51.8		

[a]Refer to the text and to Table 6.4 for a listing of the groupings and tests; ** = $p < 0.01$; * = $p < 0.05$. R = minimal (residual language impairment), S = severe, Mo = moderate, Mi = mild.
[b]Total number of examples.
[c]Sentence 13 is not included in analysis (cf. note 12).

Pairwise analyses of the degree of severity for the verb and direct object errors using the Mann-Whitney U test are highly significant for the mild-moderate, mild-severe, and moderate-severe degrees, that is, for all possible groupings by severity. This is true also for the S–DO reversal error type, except for the moderate-severe degree, which is significant only at the 0.05 level. The Kruskal-Wallis H test over the four degrees of severity is highly significant ($p < 0.01$) for the verb, subject, direct object, and S–DO reversal error but not for the DO–IO reversal error.

For the verb error, in patients with a moderate degree of severity pairwise analyses of aphasia types yielded significant differences between anomics and Broca's, anomics and Wernicke's, Broca's and globals, and Broca's and Wernicke's. For severe degreee of impairment the following aphasia types differed significantly: anomic and Broca's, anomic and Wernicke's, Broca's and global, and Broca's and Wernicke's with respect to the verb error. Significant differences between the anomic and Broca's aphasics with mild severity were found for the direct object errors, although most of the significances for the error types pertained to the moderate and to an even greater extent to the severe level of impairment.

The DO–IO reversal error was more equally distributed throughout the degrees of severity. Significant differences ($p < 0.05$) were found only between the moderate and severe degrees of impairment for this error type. For the DO–IO reversal error, highly significant ($p < 0.01$) differences were found in pairwise comparisons of anomic and Broca's subjects with a severe degree of impairment, and significant differences ($p < 0.05$) were found between the Broca's and global and between Broca's and Wernicke's types of aphasia.

Cross-Tabulation of Overall Errors by Aphasia Type According to Degree of Severity

The mean number of errors increased with progressing degree of severity within each aphasia type. The only exception was the minimal difference between the Broca's mild (mean = 4.3 errors) and the Broca's moderate (mean = 4.2 errors) groups. The mean number of errors for each aphasia type are given in Table 6.15.

Within each aphasia type, significant differences were found among the degrees of severity for particular error types.

1. Broca's: Showed a trend ($p < 0.06$) for the S–DO reversal error type.
2. Anomics: All error types showed highly significant differences except for the DO–IO reversal error.
3. Globals: For the S–DO error type, highly significant differences were noted between the moderately and severely affected subjects.
4. Wernicke's: Highly significant differences were noted for the verb, subject, and direct object error types, whereas only a trend ($p < 0.07$) for

TABLE 6.15. Distribution of Errors by Aphasia Type According to Degree of Severity

Aphasia type	Severity degree[a]	Error type					Total errors (mean[c])
		Verb	Subject	Direct object	S–DO reversal	DO–IO reversal	
	R (n = 4)	2 (18.2%)[b]	0	0	4 (36.4%)	5 (45.4%)	11 (2.8)
Broca's	Mi (n = 9)	11 (28.2%)	2 (5.1%)	3 (7.7%)	9 (23.1%)	14 (35.9%)	39 (4.3)
(n = 46)	Mo (n = 21)	11 (12.5%)	5 (5.7%)	3 (3.4%)	31 (35.2%)	38 (43.2%)	88 (4.2)
	S (n = 12)	10 (12.1%)	4 (4.8%)	8 (9.6%)	35 (42.2%)	26 (31.3%)	83 (6.9)
K-W R-S[d]					$p < 0.06$		
	R (n = 5)	2 (16.6%)	1 (8.3%)	0	2 (16.6%)	7 (58.3%)	12 (2.4)
Anomic	Mi (n = 14)	13 (18.3%)	3 (4.2%)	1 (1.4%)	36 (50.7%)	18 (25.3%)	71 (5.1)
(n = 39)	Mo (n = 8)	25 (37.9%)	2 (3.0%)	2 (3.0%)	21 (31.8%)	16 (24.2%)	66 (8.3)
	S (n = 12)	38 (36.2%)	10 (9.5%)	13 (12.4%)	33 (31.4%)	11 (10.5%)	105 (8.8)
K-W R-S		**	**	**	**		
	Mi (n = 5)	7 (22.6%)	2 (6.4%)	2 (6.4%)	10 (32.2%)	10 (32.2%)	31 (6.2)
Wernicke's	Mo (n = 22)	49 (23.6%)	13 (6.2%)	21 (10.1%)	89 (42.8%)	36 (17.3%)	208 (9.5)
(n = 44)	S (n = 17)	102 (33.0%)	36 (11.6%)	88 (28.5%)	61 (19.7%)	22 (7.1%)	309 (18.2)
K-W Mi-S		**	**	**	$p < 0.07$		
	Mo (n = 14)	56 (35.9%)	10 (6.4%)	24 (15.4%)	45 (28.8%)	21 (13.5%)	156 (11.1)
Global	S (n = 13)	71 (30.2%)	36 (15.3%)	56 (23.8%)	56 (23.8%)	16 (6.8%)	235 (18.1)
(n = 27)							
K-W Mo-S			**	**			

[a]R = residual minimal, Mi = mild, Mo = moderate, and S = severe degree of impairment.
[b]Number of errors (percentage) for each error type.
[c]Mean number of errors per aphasic is given in parentheses.
[d]K-W = Kruskal-Wallis H test; ** = $p < 0.01$; * = $p < 0.05$.

the S–DO reversal error among the three degrees of severity could be found.

The other error types were either uniformly distributed in frequency among the severity degrees or the number of errors was too few for analysis.

Discussion

The issues to be addressed in the discussion of the present results are the quantitative and/or qualitative differences among the aphasia types—within-group versus between-group variation. Do the results obtained in this study provide support for any of the general statements delineated in the section on hypotheses? Moreover, do the results reveal anything about the impairment of underlying processing mechanisms or the structure of processing components? The results do support to a considerable degree the given descriptions of the expected impairment in a particular type of aphasia. However, further elaboration of the above general statements is required.

Quantitatively speaking, that is, taking the sum of errors, most of the aphasia types differed from one another either highly significantly ($p < 0.01$) or significantly ($p < 0.05$). The mean number of overall errors presented in Table 6.6 confirms the differences, as do results of the Mann-Whitney pairwise analyses by aphasia type in terms of the total number of errors. The aphasia types that differed significantly from one another and their levels of significance are:

	Broca's	Anomic	Global	Wernicke's
Broca's	-----------	$p < 0.087$	$p < 0.01$	$p < 0.01$
Anomic	-----------	-----------	$p < 0.01$	$p < 0.01$
Global	-----------	-----------	-----------	$p < 0.05$

If the S–DO reversal error in sentence 13 is counted as an error, minimal changes in significance arise for the global-Wernicke's comparison: $p < 0.057$ instead of $p = <0.05$.

Differences in frequencies in individual errors and the distribution of the errors with regard to the various sentence types support the hypothesis that the aphasia types are not only quantitatively but also qualitatively distinguishable. The pattern of error frequencies is thus more complex. Therefore, the frequency of an error must be analyzed with reference to the sentence type on which it is made. These distinctions make up the qualitative differences to be accounted for when addressing questions pertaining to the impaired mechanisms. For example, all of the subject errors of the Broca's aphasics were made on the bi-transitive triple noun phrase sentence type, that is, on sentences requiring the processing of the highest degree of morphosyntactic information. Consideration of the pattern of error frequency according to aphasia type demonstrates the qualitative differences.

Global Aphasia

The global aphasics not only made the most errors but also showed no preference for a particular type of error. Except for the DO–IO reversal error, the mean number of errors for each error type exceeded that of all the other types of aphasias. The overall range of the mean number of errors for each error type exemplifies the scope of the comprehension impairment in global aphasia compared with the other aphasia types. For example, the mean number of errors per subject for the direct object error for the Broca's aphasic was 0.3, in contrast to 3.0 for the global aphasics. The number of errors was more uniformly distributed among the various syntactic constructions. The percentage of errors of the total number of errors made on a single syntactic construction ranged from 6.4 to 20%:

Sentence	% of group's total errors
Active irreversible	6.4
Passive irreversible	8.2
Topicalized active irreversible	9.5
Active reversible	11.8
Subject relative active reversible	11.8
Passive reversible	15.3
Topicalized active reversible	17.1
Subject–indirect object–direct object active reversible	20.0

Thus, an increase in syntactic and semantic complexity plays a role whether or not an error is made, even for the global aphasics. This role is, however, much less accentuated in global aphasia than in the other aphasia types. The mean number of errors made on the reversible sentences was greater than on the irreversible ones; this also held true for the other aphasia types.

The mean number of errors of the global aphasics was, however, above chance level; only 55% of their responses were correct. Because of this high percentage of errors, and since the globals had a mean onset of aphasia at the time of testing of 24.2 months, the global aphasics included in this study probably have chronic global aphasia. It is rather improbable that they represent a transition from global to Broca's aphasia, as is sometimes observed in global aphasia with onset up to approximately 12 months previously. That is, in some cases of global aphasia, after the initial severe overall language impairment affecting all modalities and all linguistic levels has subsided, a pattern of language performance remains that is characteristic of severe Broca's aphasia. (Cp. "Syndromenwandel," Leischner, 1979; or Kertesz, 1979.)

A comparison of moderately impaired and severely impaired globals reveals that for the subject and direct object error types, the two levels of severity differed highly significantly. The degree of severity of the aphasia appears to be the determining factor. For the other error types, the differences between the two degrees of severity were not significant. Except for the DO–IO reversal error, the severely impaired globals made more errors than the moderately impaired ones.

In terms of interpreting the pattern of errors, global aphasics appear to perform on a hit or miss basis. Which test item or sentence type they understand is—to a great extent—determined by the momentary, transitory efficiency of a very impaired language-processing system. The type of error the global aphasic makes depends on which part of the sentence—if not the complete sentence—he or she (correctly) processes. The global aphasic's overall limited performance can be described in terms of the "shutter principle" (Cf. Wepman, 1972, p. 208) or with the analogy of a bottleneck effect. (". . . There is a (brief) moment when, like the opening of a shutter of a camera, the child is amenable to direct stimulus . . . During the period of rehearsal he seems to be closed off from other external stimuli; his shutter appears to be closed." Wepman, 1972, p. 208.) In this context, the far-reaching effect of perseveration should not be underestimated, nor can it be exactly determined in auditory comprehension tasks requiring a nonverbal pointing response.[15] One example of perseveration would be a subject's retaining the lexical item "boy" and thus pointing to a boy on the following test item instead of a girl, not because the subject has not correctly understood the test sentence but because he or she is perseverating the lexical/semantic item "boy."

Broca's Aphasia

Although they were the largest group in this study, the Broca's aphasics made the least total number of errors (n = 221). Only 15% of their responses were incorrect. However, the frequency of mean errors per subject—corrected for group size—indicates differential susceptibility of both error and sentence types. For example, the reversal errors made up 73% of the total errors, or 3.5 of the 4.8 mean number of errors made by each Broca's aphasic over all sentence types in which such an error could be made.

The Broca's aphasics displayed the greatest range in error frequency among the sentence types: 0 to 48%, depending on sentence type. The percentage of total group errors for the various sentence types was as follows:

Sentence type	% of Broca's group's total errors
Active irreversible	0
Passive irreversible	0
Topicalized active irreversible	0
Subject relative active reversible	2.7
Active reversible	6.3
Topicalized active reversible	17.6
Passive reversible	22.6
Subject–indirect object–direct object active reversible	48.4

The increase in complexity of the sentence types under investigation in terms of the processing of morphosyntactic information (case marking, word order, etc.) is mirrored by a strictly concordant rise in the number of errors. Those sentences requiring exact processing of, for example, grammatical case markers (i.e., the case of the definite articles) to arrive at a correct interpretation of the semantic roles of the noun phrases, are more liable to call forth incorrect responses. The error type is predominantly reversal of subject and direct object, or of indirect object and direct object. However, in the latter case, that is, in the sentence type consisting of three noun phrases, the subject noun phrase also contributed to processing difficulties, and subject errors were noted in this case. (Refer to note 14.) The compactness of the sentence (i.e. of the three noun phrases, each requiring processing of the definite article) presented the greatest processing difficulties for the Broca's aphasics. Verb errors were also made on the more difficult reversible sentence types. The significance of verb semantics should not be overlooked (cf. Jones, 1984).

It is interesting to note that the subject relative clause construction, although longer than the reversible simple active declarative, was easier for the Broca's aphasics to process. An explanation for this could be that the added length had a facilitative effect, in that the subject and object noun phrases were separated by additional information, which, however, clarified only the subject noun phrase. The patient thereby gained time to process the subject noun phrase case markers, that is, they acquired part of the morphosyntactic information necessary to process the complete sentence, before they heard the second noun phrase.

In the case of the reversible passive sentences, the need for processing of the passive markers (the preposition "by," i.e., "von," a conjugated form of the verb "werden," and the past participle) contributed to the difficulty in processing the case markers. Another possible interpretation is that, since the structure of the sentence was similar to that of an active counterpart (future tense) until the "by" phrase was heard, the Broca's aphasic was so involved with syntactic processing that his or her initial assumption (that the subject noun phrase is the agent) was maintained. The difficulties of processing the "by" phrase and the past participle morphemes ("ge," "t") did not counteract the initial assumption; rather the added complexity made the whole processing system more prone to error. The patient adhered to his or her initial processing strategy (the first noun phrase is the agent). Possibly the Broca's aphasic recognized some difference, for example, that another sentence type was presented for processing, but the processing continued according to the initial assumption.

In terms of the homogeneity of the Broca's group performance, the four degrees of severity just reach the significance level ($p < 0.049$) with regard to the total number of errors. In general, the frequency of errors increased with increase in severity with the exception of mean errors between the mildly and moderately impaired patients—4.3 errors per patient as opposed to 4.2, respectively. The overall error pattern across the four degrees of severity indicates that as a group Broca's aphasics are very similar in terms of the difficulties encountered in processing sentences presented orally.

Wernicke's Aphasia

In terms of mean number of errors, the severe Wernicke's were comparable to the severe Globals: 18.1 versus 18.2 mean errors per aphasic. In all of the error types except reversal errors (S–DO, IO–DO), the differences between the degrees of severity were statistically significant, that is, the Wernicke's aphasics of the three severity degrees investigated showed different patterns of errors. The greatest increase in the number of errors was found between the moderately and severely impaired patients for the verb, subject, and direct object errors.

A sensitivity to syntactic and semantic aspects was found for the various sentence types tested. The error frequency expressed in terms of the percent of errors according to sentence type is:

Sentence type	% of Wernicke group's total errors
Active irreversible	4.7
Passive irreversible	6.7
Topicalized active irreversible	9.3
Active reversible	11.5
Subject relative active reversible	12.7
Topicalized active reversible	15.0
Passive reversible	18.8
Subject–indirect object–direct object active reversible	21.2

The range of the error percentages (4.7–21.2%) for the Wernicke's group was less than that for the Broca's and the anomic groups, but greater than that for the globals. Reversibility, as well as sentence length, played an important role in the performance of the Wernicke's group. The reversal errors made up 27% of the errors of the severe aphasics, 59% of the errors of the moderately affected aphasics, and 64% of the errors of the aphasics displaying a mild degree of impairment. The percentage increase in this type of error went in the opposite direction to degree of severity: The mildly impaired Wernicke's made more reversal errors than the moderately and severely impaired Wernicke's, although the average number of errors decreased from severely to mildly impaired. This reversal of pattern supports the assumption that especially the severely impaired and to a lesser degree the moderately impaired Wernicke's aphasics display a different pattern of errors, which is either an indication of a more severe impairment of the same processing mechanism(s) or of an impairment of different processing mechanisms. In other words, the auditory comprehension disorder of the mildly and moderately impaired aphasics becomes more specific as the severe overall (or multicomponent) difficulties in the processing of lexical and phonological information subside. The more severe general or overall impairment seems to be either a semantically or phonologically based difficulty in the processing of lexical items.

A specific, less severe difficulty is manifest in the processing of the order of the noun phrases in reversible constructions. On the basis of data obtained in this study (and from personal experience), in contrast to the situation with Broca's aphasics the difficulty does not appear to stem from inability to process the case markers of the definite articles, but rather from inability to correctly process the *position* of the nouns around the verb, in particular to mentally change the order of the noun phrases in a reversible construction such as in the passive or topicalized construction, to arrive at the correct interpretation. In responding to a passive construction, for example, several Wernicke's aphasics reported that "it belongs the other way around or in another order"; however, they were unable to perform the reversal of the noun phrases to arrive at the correct interpretation of the sentence. The longer a sentence is, the more information must be retained before the second or third noun phrase is processed. This overburdens the processing system due to limitations in semantic/lexical or phonological processing of the main lexical items, and the Wernicke's aphasic displays great difficulty arriving at, retrieving, or maintaining the correct order of the noun phrases. The poorer performance on the subject relative sentences supports this assumption. In contrast, the interruption between the subject and the direct object noun phrase in the subject relative sentence type had a facilitative effect for the Broca's aphasics in that they gained time to process the morphosyntactic information (i.e., the case markers). The morphology of the noun phrases appears to be correctly interpreted by the Wernicke's patients. This conclusion is again based on indirect evidence from testing: On many occasions the less impaired Wernicke's aphasic repeated the test sentence aloud, as did the Broca's aphasic. The difference between their repetition performance was that the Wernicke's patient correctly repeated the case markings, while the Broca's transformed the accusative case, for example, into a nominative in a topicalized sentence. We are assuming that even though the Wernicke's had case markings to figure out the thematic roles, the difficulties they encountered in processing word order overrode the correct interpretation of these markings. Therefore, the same type of error in Wernicke's and Broca's aphasia may stem from different sources of difficulty or impairment to different mechanisms or processes. This issue is presently being investigated further.

Anomic Aphasia

The performance of the anomic aphasics was interesting for several reasons:

1. In clinical descriptions, anomic aphasics are usually described as having mild auditory language comprehension impairment (Goodglass & Kaplan 1983; Kertesz, 1985).
2. The frequency of errors for the four degrees of severity differed significantly in the verb, subject, direct object, and subject–direct object reversal error types (comparable to the Wernicke's group).

These within-group differences, in association with varying degrees of severity of aphasia, point to qualitative differences among anomics with regard to their performance on auditory comprehension tasks. That is, on the basis of results for the anomic group on the task used in this study, classification of a subject as displaying anomic aphasia without consideration of the degree of severity would not be adequate. The anomics, as well as the Wernicke's group, were not homogeneous with reference to their auditory comprehension difficulties: Within each group the four degrees of severity showed differences in terms of the total number of errors (K-W $p < 0.000$). This, however, is only a quantitative difference—the *pattern* of the errors is of significance in determining whether qualitative differences exist. For severely and moderately impaired anomic aphasics, verb errors made up 20% more of their errors (36.2 and 37.9%, respectively) compared with verb errors of the minimally and mildly impaired subjects (16.6 and 18.3%, respectively). The verb errors of severely impaired anomics appeared to be a trade-off for IO–DO reversal errors (mean number per anomic):

Verb: 3.2
Reversal IO–DO: 0.9

All the other error types showed an increase in mean number of errors in correlation with an increase in severity of impairment.

The anomics were sensitive to the reversible/irreversible dichotomy: 88.6% of their errors were made on reversible constructions. Since a verb error is possible in every sentence, the percent of verb errors in the reversible sentences (73%) in contrast to those in the irreversible sentences (27%) demonstrates the effect of this factor in the processing of sentences.

The influence of the syntactic complexity of the sentence type in combination with sentence length is manifest in the error frequency as expressed in percentage of errors (of the total number) according to sentence type:

Sentence type	% of anomic group's total errors
Active irreversible	2.0
Passive irreversible	3.1
Active reversible	5.9
Topicalized active irreversible	6.3
Subject relative active reversible	9.0
Topicalized active reversible	20.0
Passive reversible	22.0
Subject–indirect object–direct object active reversible	31.0

The anomics displayed the second largest range in terms of sensitivity to syntactic constructions: 2 to 31% (the Broca's ranked highest: 0–48.4%).

In contrast to the Broca's performance on the subject relative clause construction (2.7% errors), the added length and complexity of this construction resulted in greater processing difficulty for the anomic (9% errors) as well as for the Wernicke's aphasics (12.7% errors). Furthermore, the anomics made errors on the first three sentence types, although these were a small percentage of the total errors, which contrasts with the Broca's aphasics' performance.

To account for the anomic's error pattern in terms of processing difficulties, it appears that the aforementioned lexical/semantic fuzziness postulated by Lesser (1984) could account for the verb errors in particular, that is, for the performance of the severely impaired anomics. Processing of the semantic aspects of the verb breaks down with increase in sentence length and with need for syntactic and semantic processing. The range of the percentage of errors made on the various syntactic constructions lends support to this assumption. In addition to or in combination with that processing deficit, difficulties in lexical processing or the processing of the order of the nouns (subject and direct object noun phrases, also the subject–indirect object–direct object noun phrases) in reversible sentence constructions were manifest in the error patterns of the anomic aphasics. This processing difficulty was consistent for the anomic group as a whole, with the exception of the reversal direct object–indirect object error type for the severe anomic aphasics. The hypothesis put forward for the mild Wernicke's aphasics also holds for the anomics: On the basis of the data, processing of the case marking of the definite articles does not appear to be impaired. Rather, overall lexical processing of the nouns and/or processing of the order of the nouns around the verb, in particular arrangement or rearrangement of noun phrases in the syntactic framework to arrive at the correct interpretation of the sentence, seems to be the cause of the difficulty.

Other Aphasia Types

The aphasics in the "other" group have been briefly discussed. The reason for including these subjects in the study was to allow a comparison, for example, of anterior versus posterior aphasics, and consideration of the linguistic variables investigated as well as the aphasics' pattern of performance in a broader context. The grouping 1–17 allowed such a pairwise comparison of these small groups (single cases) with single cases of the main aphasia types or with the aphasia type groups. For example, the transcortical motor aphasics (mean number of errors = 6.7) did not differ from the severely impaired Broca's (mean number of errors = 6.9). One interpretation of the significance of the similar performance pattern (same errors) is that the sentence comprehension deficit of anterior aphasics may reflect the same underlying impairment in the processing of grammatical markers. Comparisons of aphasics studied in extensive case studies can elucidate this and other similarities and also differences in the processing of aurally presented sentences.

General Discussion

The unresolved issues cited in the introductory review of the literature on auditory sentence comprehension and the results of this study reflect the complexity of the factors involved. Aspects of the nature of the comprehension difficulties in the various clinically defined types of aphasia—quantitative versus qualitative differences—were discussed in relation to the level of severity and the linguistic factors for each aphasia type in the preceding sections. The influence of other intervening variables, such as years of schooling and interactions among the variables, must be considered. An attempt to separate out the influence of these factors follows.

With respect to the hypotheses proposed regarding the nature of the comprehension disorder, Hypothesis 3.0, Quantity and Quality, best describes the aphasics' performance on the sentence-picture matching test employed in this study. Hypothesis 2.0, Quality, accounts for the data with the exception of the Broca's group in comparison with the anomic group. In terms of the following error types, the two groups differ qualitatively: verb and DO–IO reversal (refer to Table 6.6). The overall quantitative difference between these two aphasia types is only a trend ($p < 0.087$): The Broca's aphasics (n = 46) made a total of 221 errors (mean errors per subject = 4.8) and the anomic aphasics (n = 39) made a total of 254 errors (mean per subject = 6.5). When aphasia types of various degrees of severity with approximately the same mean number of errors are compared, the distribution of error types also differs in several cases. For example, a comparison of the distribution of errors of the moderately impaired Wernicke's (mean number of errors = 9.5) with the severely impaired anomics (mean = 8.8), or of the severely impaired Broca's (mean = 6.9) with the mildly impaired Wernicke's aphasics (mean = 6.2), illustrates that the quantity of errors does not solely explain the aphasics' error pattern differences. Hypothesis 1.2, Severity, also does not explain the overall distribution of errors. However, the severity of the language impairment—initially determined primarily on the basis of results from production tasks—also has considerable influence on comprehension performance. The performance of aphasics with the most severe overall comprehension disorder, that is, the severely impaired globals (mean number of errors 18.1) and the severely impaired Wernicke's (mean number of errors 18.2), supports the qualitative hypothesis for the subject and direct object error types.

These comments show how difficult it is to sift out qualitative from quantitative aspects, as they are both expressed numerically as errors. Nevertheless, quantity alone does not account for the overall error distribution. The overall error distribution and the patterns for the various sentence types were used to determine the nature of the comprehension disorder in terms of the hypotheses proposed for each aphasia type. The analysis by sentence types yielded distinct patterns of errors for different aphasia types; these have been discussed in the previous sections for each aphasia type. The differences between Broca's and Wernicke's aphasics is important in this context. For example, can the performance patterns associated with these two aphasia types be taken as evidence for impairment of different underlying mechanisms? What do these mechanisms or processes consist of? Do any of the error types included in the test shed light on aspects that should be incorporated into hypothetical accounts of these processing mechanisms? At least three aspects can be derived from the distractor types (i.e., possible errors):

1. Processing of grammatical relations in a language (with rather free word order), that is, parsing of the structure of noun phrases, especially in reversible sentences.
2. Processing of grammatical markers (e.g., number, gender) as an expression of the grammatical relationships of subject and object, and also of the preposition "by" in passive sentences, and so on.
3. Processing aspects (semantic and phonological) of the major lexical entries, especially of the nouns and verbs in the sentences.

In Broca's aphasia, the difficulties in processing sentences appear to stem from impairment of the second aspect of processing. In comprehending reversible sentences, the Broca's aphasic falls back onto the less marked form (S–V–O) or onto the "agent-before-patient strategy" and other strategies (discussed in Caplan et al. [1985] and by other authors cited in the review of the aphasia studies). When the articles are not distinctly marked, word order is crucial in determining the grammatical roles. However, in German, grammatical roles are determined predominantly by case marking on the articles when these articles are distinctly marked, followed by word order and intonation. If only the sentence-processing deficit is considered, it is difficult to decide between the semantic mapping and the syntactic deficit hypotheses. The crucial issue is whether or how these two hypotheses can be differentiated on the basis of the results obtained in this study, since the error types cannot differentiate the two hypotheses. The information that denotes grammatical roles corresponds to the syntactic information carried by word order and grammatical markers in German. In both cases the interpretation or use of this information is impaired. On the basis of our results on only auditory sentence comprehension it is not possible to choose among the hypotheses discussed by Caramazza and Berndt (1985). With reference to impairment of the syntactic processing device, grammaticality judgments are problematic for this account of the agrammatic Broca's aphasics' comprehension deficit. However, the mapping deficit can take care of our findings.

The Broca's aphasic's processing of word order is thus secondarily impaired, that is, is limited to a basic ("psycholinguistic universal") structure due to his or her inability to use the structural information expressed by grammatical markers/morphemes (cf. Zurif, 1980). It is exactly these markers that denote the grammatical roles—thematic/semantic and pragmatic/discourse roles in reversible sentences in German. Since the irreversible, that is, semantically constrained, sentences are processed correctly, the third aspect—semantic processing of the major lexical items—can be assumed to be intact. It could be that the need for simultaneity in processing of the grammatical marker and the (role of the) first noun in real time exceeds processing ability.

In Wernicke's aphasia, the difficulties in auditory processing of input can be attributed to impairment of the second and third aspects. The word order difficulty is due to inability to maintain, to retrieve, or to arrive at the correct ordering of the nouns. It has not been resolved whether the underlying sources of this processing difficulty are of a lexical/semantic nature or have a syntactic basis (cf. Lesser's (1984) distinction between functional and constituent structures). It is also not certain whether the comprehension disorder in Wernicke's aphasia results from impairment of two separate mechanisms. These possibilities were previously commented on and are based on the differences in error patterns among the three degrees of severity in Wernicke's aphasics. The question remains how initial severe processing difficulties subside in recovery. The initial severity of these difficulties prevents differentiating which specific process or processes are impaired. In recovery, do the deficits become more specific, or does one impaired process improve while other processing difficulties remain?

On the basis of the previous discussions, it is assumed that what in certain cases appears to be a similar deficit is, however, a reflection of impairment of different aspects of language processing or differential impairment of the same process. The differences in overall errors and in the distribution of these errors lend support to the view that the Broca's and Wernicke's aphasics' performance in auditory sentence comprehension is qualitatively different. The finding that the lexical to syntactic errors is so much greater for Wernicke's in comparison with Broca's aphasics. Considering all sentences together, the Broca's made almost three times more syntactic errors than lexical errors (ratio of 2.7), whereas the Wernicke's made approximately twice as many lexical errors as syntactic errors (ratio of 1.8). The ratio of syntactic to lexical errors simultaneously expresses the susceptibility of a particular error type (e.g., Broca's vs. Wernicke's) and the overall degree of impairment (e.g., Global, Wernicke's). It is important to stress that analysis showed that the Broca's lexical errors were made only on the sentences of greater syntactic complexity. This can be interpreted as follows: Due to greater syntactic processing demands, the whole processing system is overtaxed. Thus, even lexical/semantic errors are made. In contrast, when the syntactic demands are within limits, that is, do not overburden the Broca's aphasic, lexical errors are not made, only syntactic errors. For the Wernicke's aphasic, the opposite holds true. The performance of the Broca's and Wernicke's aphasics was compared because these two types have been the topic of investigation in many recent studies (cf. Kolk & Friederici, 1985; Scholes, 1978). The ratio of syntactic to lexical errors is given for all aphasia types in Table 6.16. (Refer to note 14.)

In a broader context, a distinction between anterior and posterior aphasics in terms of the qualitative differences in performance seems valid (cf. Scholes, 1978). Left anterior brain damage results in difficulties in processing the grammatical markers necessary for interpreting the various roles of the nouns in sentences (cf. Zurif, 1980). Left posterior brain damage gives rise to overall lexical processing difficulties of the

TABLE 6.16. Lexical/Semantic Versus Syntactic Errors in Four Types of Aphasia

	Total errors (%)		
Aphasia type	Lexical/semantic (verb, subject, direct object)	Syntactic[a] (reversal S–DO, reversal IO–DO)	Ratio syntactic/ lexical
Broca's	59 (26.7)	162 (73.3)	2.7
Anomic	110 (43.3)	144 (56.7)	1.3
Wernicke's	320 (58.4)	228 (41.6)	0.7
Global	253 (64.7)	138 (35.3)	0.5

[a]Errors on sentence 13 not included in analysis (refer to footnote 12).

main lexical items and thereby reduces the efficiency of the processing, that is, of maintaining or constructing the correct order of nouns in reversible sentences. One possible description of the processing deficits is that lexical/semantic difficulties in processing the structure (semantic and/or phonological) of the major lexical items are of such magnitude that the result is very limited processing of the order of the nouns around the verbs. Further experiments are necessary to test this specifically.

In addition to the influence of severity and aphasia type on the aphasic's auditory sentence comprehension performance, the role of concomitant variables must be considered. In this context an interesting aspect to consider is the influence of years of schooling on the significances for each error type. (Years of schooling are given in Table 6.1 according to aphasia type.) The finer differentiation of four levels was collapsed into two levels: (a) grammar school and vocational school, and (b) high school graduation and university graduation.

With aphasia type as the grouping variable, the errors were analyzed by Kruskal-Wallis analysis of variance of ranks and chi square according to these two levels of schooling. Table 6.17 shows significances for the error types according to level of schooling. The level 2 aphasics made fewer subject and direct object errors, and these errors were more evenly distributed among the aphasia types, which resulted in fewer significant results for these error types. Since with level 2 schooling all results show lesser significance (except for the DO–IO reversal error), a possible interpretation could be that a higher level of schooling allows for a leveling of specific aphasia type effects. For the DO–IO reversal error type, a different pattern is observed. Aphasics with level 1 schooling made more DO–IO reversal errors (n = 154; mean = 1.7), however, no significant differences were found among the aphasia types for this error type. Although aphasics with level 2 schooling made fewer DO–IO reversal errors (n = 91; mean = 1.4), highly significant differences among the aphasia types were found. The same interpretation as that for the subject and direct object errors in-

TABLE 6.17. Effect of Years of Schooling on Possible Type

Error type	Total aphasics		Schooling[a] Level 1		Schooling[a] Level 2	
	K-W	x^2	K-W	x^2	K-W	x^2
Verb	$p < 0.000$	0.000	0.000	0.000	0.001	0.000
Subject	$p < 0.000$	0.000	0.000	0.000	0.047	0.018
Direct object	$p < 0.000$	0.0	0.000	0.000	0.371	0.016
S–DO reversal	$p < 0.000$	0.0004	0.000	0.0002	0.014	0.021
DO–IO reversal	$p < 0.040$	0.168	0.831	0.8239	0.003	0.011

[a]Level 1 = grammar and vocational school; level 2 = high school graduation and university graduation.

dicates that this error type—which is only possible in the most complex sentences tested—is much more probable with education level 1 aphasics. The difficulty is not due solely to aphasia-specific processing difficulties, but also to the overall linguistic complexity of the sentences. The influence of years of schooling on this error type could be interpreted as indicating that aphasics with level 1 schooling have greater difficulty processing this bitransitive sentence type correctly. Aphasics with level 2 schooling can handle this sentence type more adequately. The aphasia type-specific processing deficits show up more clearly with aphasics at the higher educational level. Although the role of educational level should not be overlooked, the aphasia-type-specific deficits are still the overall determining factors. In particular, results from the Broca's aphasics are striking for both schooling levels for the DO–IO reversal error type. These results show the importance of taking into consideration not only the variables aphasia type, severity of impairment, and syntactic complexity, but also educational level.[16] The last is surely a determining factor of the test but cannot be used as an independent variable in all analyses due to sample size.

Another issue to be addressed is the often stated differentiation between real-time linguistic processing in on-line tasks and the use of strategies in off-line tasks. The term "strategy" has the connotation of something persistently and consciously employed. This is not the case. Rather, a "strategy" here is a reflection of unconscious processing of particular linguistic units/segments/structures that has become increasingly automatized with constant use. A dividing line between real linguistic processing and the use of quicker, more strategic processing based on linguistic principles is difficult to draw in an across-the-board fashion, due to several factors such as fatigue, nonlinguistic memory aspects, and so on. The impact of such factors is difficult to measure. The errors made by the aphasics in this study can thus be ascribed to real processing difficulties dependent on the aphasia type. All processing was probably more automatized before onset of aphasia. After onset, certain aspects of linguistic processing (i.e, strategies) become even more important or basic. These so-called strategies become the principal means of processing language, for example by Broca's aphasics. Caplan et al. (1985) and Caplan and Futter (1986) have stressed that adhering to such strategies results in errors when the sentences to be processed have a different linguistic structure. The crucial aspect that seems to get lost in discussions of strategies is that the use of strategies is an expression of the aphasic's impairment: Strategies are applied by aphasics because of inability to process the necessary linguistic information (cp. Kolk & Friederici, 1985). One indication that the difficulties are real and systematic and not due to linguistic memory factors is confirmed by the fact that repetitions of the test sentences failed to improve performance in most instances.

The overall distinction between on-line and off-line tasks as reflecting different types of linguistic processing is rather more closely related to a distinction among possible types of tasks that can be employed to investigate particular research questions. The demands involved in comprehending/interpreting "normal" sentences using the sentence-picture matching paradigm are different from those necessary, for example, in fast reaction time monitoring tasks, in which a button must be pressed as soon as a target word in a test sentence is heard. The ways in which these tasks differ in terms of computational processes have not been fully specified, since the computational processes for each task have not been stated in detail. The instructions given to the subject definitely play a role in how the subject goes about solving the task (i.e., test items). If similar results for both types of tasks are found, the same hypothetical process might be postulated as being the shared processing aspect. However, if the results diverge, this is not a guarantee that the on-line task tapped more "real" linguistic processing than the sentence-picture matching task. Rather, it is more probable that various aspects of processing—which are in turn investigated by means of different tasks—are probed. To arrive at the shared processing components, results from the tasks mentioned must be interpreted and other investigations must be designed to address specific research questions (cf. Frazier, 1982; Garrett, 1982).

An understanding of how psycholinguistic processes operate over time is important when analyzing an aphasic's performance on any task. Pertaining to the aphasic's processing of aurally presented sentences (cf. Marslen-Wilson & Tyler, 1981), however, the whole sentence must be heard before the aphasic can respond. This does not mean that the aphasic waits until the examiner has completed the sentence before beginning to process it. On the basis of the response pattern, processing seems to begin as soon as the examiner has produced the first noun phrase.[17]

Reduction in processing abilities with reliance on more basic structures or processes (i.e., strategies) results in characteristic error patterns for the Broca's, Wernicke's, anomic, and other aphasia types. The overall error distribution shows that in all cases, no matter how the underlying difficulties are to be described, aphasic subjects do not perform in an all-or-nothing fashion. Linguistic factors such as syntactic complexity, frequency of use, and concomitant variables determine the varying levels of performance. The notion of syntactic complexity, although difficult to define, is based on sentence type, number of arguments a verb takes, semantic aspects such as reversibility/irreversibiltiy, and animacy/inanimacy, compactness, redundancy, and length of utterance. This notion of syntactic complexity has a considerable effect on normal language processing. Therefore its influence on aphasic language processing should not be underestimated. The aphasics' performance supports the assumption that it is not the result of "de novo organization of unimpaired mechanisms" (cf. Caramazza & Berndt, 1985, p. 8; Saffran, & Schwartz & Marin, 1980; Zurif, 1980). Rather, the aphasics' performance reflects prevailing linguistic structure (with minor variations that may be due to chance) in spite of their specific processing difficulties. The distribution of the errors among the sentence types illustrates that the aphasics are sensitive to overall variations in structure in spite of their processing difficulties. The sensitivity to specific linguistic factors mirrors the aphasia type's disorders, which have already been discussed. With reference to syntactic complexity, no aphasic found the bitransitive sentences easier to process than simple active declarative irreversible sentences, and so on. For the sentence types investigated, the following ranking of syntactic complexity was derived for the aphasia types (based on the number of errors made on each sentence type)[18]:

Assumed sentence complexity	Ranking of sentence by aphasia type			
	Broca's	Anomic	Wernicke's	Global
1 Active irreversible	2	1	1	1
2 Topicalized active irreversible	2	3	3	3
3 Passive irreversible	1	2	2	2
4 Active reversible	5	3	4	4
5 Subject relative active reversible	4	5	5	4
6 Topicalized active reversible	6	6	6	7
7 Passive reversible	7	7	7	6
8 Subject-direct object-indirect object active reversible	8	8	8	8

The Wernicke's aphasics have a ranking most similar to the assumed order of difficulty. The question arises why this assumed order should demonstrate differences in the other direction, that is, should be completely different for the aphasics in the first place. If this assumed ranking were completely different for all aphasia types, the possibility of de novo organization of syntactic structure based on concepts other than syntactic complexity or other semantosyntactic aspects could be considered. It is not at all clear how such a severe generalized breakdown of syntactic and semantic processing of sentences could be characterized. The ranking of the sentences does not confirm such a breakdown; rather the types of errors made by the various aphasia types within this ranking make up the qualitative differences and the amount of these errors the quantitative differences among the aphasia types. The aphasics' overall performance is a result of differential sensitivity to syntactic and semantic factors due to particular difficulties in processing sentences. The aphasics' better processing of irreversible compared with reversible sentences reflects prevailing linguistic structure, that is, notions of sentence complexity: Reversible sentences are more difficult to process than irreversible ones for both aphasics and control subjects (cf. Heeschen, 1980; Jones, 1984; Kolk & Friederici, 1985; Lesser, 1984; etc.).

The aphasics' overall error distribution can also be interpreted in terms of universal linguistic principles or constraints. These are expressed, for example, in the relational hierarchy postulated by Perlmutter and Postal, or Ross's primacy constraint (cf. Pullum, 1977), or Keenan and Comrie's (1977) accessibility hierarchy. Although these principles have not been applied to aphasia data in this context, and they are derived from different linguistic considerations, their application to the results of this study seems warranted.

The relational hierarchy is interpreted by Perlmutter and Postal (discussed in Pullum, 1977) in the following way:

Relational hierarchy

S < DO < IO < OO

where S (=subject) "has precedence over" or "outranks" the DO (=direct object), and so on (cf. Johnson, 1977). With reference to the application of linguistic rules, Ross's primacy constraint states that subjects have primacy over objects. The accessibility hierarchy proposed by Keenan and Comrie (1977) relates to the relative accessibility to relativization of noun phrase position in simple main clauses in universal grammar:

S	<	DO	<	IO	<	OBL	<	GEN	<	OCOMP
(subject)		(direct object)		(indirect object)		(oblique)		(genitive)		(object of comparative)

where subject (S) is more accessible than direct object (DO), and so on.[19]

These diverse hierarchies can be applied to aphasia data with respect to the intactness/impairment of particular aspects/categories, and so on, that is, relative ordering of error type as an indication of severity of impairment or specific deficits according to aphasia type. Since these hierarchies were formulated in terms of linguistic universal properties, how these hierarchies are incorporated into a model of language processing has not been delineated. "In each case it has been found that the GR (grammatical relations) hierarchy can be applied to predict the degree of activeness,' accessibility to the operation of various processes, extent of particular participation in grammatical operations, etc." (Pullum, 1977, p. 272). Pullum further asserted that the fundamental principle of linearization depends on the GR hierarchy.[20] Although the linguistic characterization of word order is theoretical, any sentence-processing model must account for the computation of the ordering of words, in particular of noun phrases in relation to each other and in relation to the verbs.

The results of this study coincide with these hierarchies in that the aphasics made fewer subject errors than direct object errors on irreversible sentences and fewer subject errors than indirect object errors on triple noun phrase sentences (in relation to the possibility to make these errors). Therefore, it can be hypothesized that the aphasics had greater access to the dominating elements of this hierarchy (i.e, subject and direct object).

With reference to the results of the present study, what can be derived from these diverse hierarchies is that the subject of a sentence is first in order and importance. One of the reasons for this primary role is that the subject is grammatically most marked by means of case marking of the article (or pronoun), by verb congruence and in terms of position. For irreversible sentences, therefore, it can be stated that the noun phrase that is grammatically most strongly coded remains intact. (This holds irrespective of word order variations in the irreversible topicalized sentences.) The semantic constraints are decisive in this case and with reference to irreversible passive sentences.

In reversible sentences, however, reversals of the subject and direct object are not considered as separate errors, but rather as the reversal of the two noun phrases (S–DO reversal). The incorrect processing of reversible topicalized and passive sentences, in particular of the subject (= agent) and direct object (=patient), *paradoxically* points to the prominent role of the subject, that is, to the relative ordering of subject (=agent) in sentence-initial position to verb-second position in main clauses: Regardless of sentence type, the first noun is processed as the agent. The verb-second position in the main clause is the only really fixed position in German (and the verb-final position in subordinate clauses). The S–V–O strategy does in part derive from the prominence of the subject (i.e, agent) in sentence-initial position.

The frequency of the direct object–indirect object reversal error type can also be accounted for on the basis of these hierarchies. The best possibility to demonstrate the prominence of the subject over the direct object and the direct object over the indirect object is a comparison of the error frequency of these noun phrase types in bitransitive sentences. The ratio of DO–IO reversal to subject errors is 4.6. The meaning of the DO–IO reversal error is that the indirect object, which is the second noun phrase of the sentence, is incorrectly processed as the direct object. With reference to the above discussed hierarchies, it can be hypothesized that due to the greater availability of the direct object over the indirect object, the indirect object is processed as the direct object. The real goal, the indirect object, is left over and processed by default.

Concerning the results of this study, in particular the possible error types, caution must be taken in considering what is going on in terms of grammatical relations when particular errors are made. The reversal errors are rather unequivocal: When an aphasic points to the drawing depicting the reversal distractor, we can reasonably assume that the grammatical relations of these noun phrases have been incorrectly processed and therefore reversed grammatical relations have been derived (i.e., arrived at). However, with regard to grammatical relations, it is not clear what is going on with the subject and direct object errors. When an aphasic points to the direct object distractor, it is not possible to claim that the patient does not know, for example, what a direct object is. Rather the

TABLE 6.18. Summary of Patient Variables and Data for the "Other" Group (n = 13)

Patient variables[a]

Mean age (years)	Sex	Handedness	Schooling	Etiology	Mean time since onset of aphasia	Degree of severity
47.0 (SD = 12.0)	11 men 2 women	Right	2 years = 3 3 years = 10	Cerebrovascular accident	8.7 months SD = 5.2	Mild = 5 Moderate = 8

Distribution of Errors

Category	Verb	Subject	Direct object	S–DO reversal	DO–IO reversal	Total
Overall	11	1	2	22	27	63
Mean no. of errors/subject	0.8	0.1	0.1	1.7	2.1	4.8
According to degree of severity						
Mi (n = 5)	2	0	0	4	8	14
Mo (n = 8)	9	1	2	18	19	49
According to Sentence Type						
Simple active declarative, total	2	0	1	4	—	7
Simple active declarative reversible	0	—	1	4	—	
Simple active declarative irreversible	2	0	0	—	—	—
Subject relative active reversible	1	—	0	0	—	1
Topicalized active, total	3	0	0	6 (+15)[b]	—	9 (+15)
Topicalized active, reversible	2	—	0	6 (+15)	—	
Topicalized active irreversible	1	0	0	—	—	
Passive, total	1	0	1	12	—	14
Passive reversible	1	—	1	12	—	
Passive irreversible	0	0	0	—	—	
Subject–indirect object–direct object active reversible	4	1	—	—	27	32

[a]Due to the size of the aphasia groups, the "Other" group is considered altogether.
[b]Refer to Table 6.10 and note 12; the number of errors in parentheses is for sentence 13.

error indicates that the specific information about a person or thing has not been correctly processed, perhaps due to incorrect semantic/lexical processing of specific features (male/female, etc.). For this reason these error types are considered to be of a semantic or lexical nature. This also pertains to the verb distractor. The role of the verb is presently being analyzed according to verb types discussed in Jones (1984). In this study, the verb distractors were often semantically similar to the target verb; the target and the distractor verb sometimes differed in one or a few features, for example, push versus pull. The processing of semantic information of the verb is thus very important not only in consideration of the verb as a major lexical item, but also in terms of verb semantics in relation to the syntactic structure (e.g., how many arguments a verb obligatorily requires and can optionally take). In spite of these reservations, all the error types do point to specific difficulties in the processing of sentences. The weight of the errors is differential. Considering the errors in terms of these hierarchies supports the assumption that the aphasics' performance reflects prevailing linguistic structures, such as the hierarchy of syntactic complexity or the accessbility of noun phrases, that is, the relative intactness of a noun phrase type over others according to the grammatical roles in a sentence.

Summary

The role of several syntactic and semantic factors in the processing of grammatical relations marked by word order and grammatical markers, as well as interactions among them, was investigated by means of a sentence-picture matching task. The results from 169 aphasics were analyzed in terms of the effect of variation in sentence type in connection with voice distinctions and semantic aspects on the aphasic's comprehension performance. Analysis of the pattern of errors revealed qualitative and quantitative differences within and among the aphasia types on the various sentence types. These differences demonstrated the necessity of taking into consideration not only aphasia type but also degree of severity of the language impairment and other variables. A group study using a single test allowed for the sifting out of the influence of various linguistic factors, that is, syntactic and semantic aspects, which were found to be particularly important in determining the nature of auditory sentence comprehension deficits. Additional follow-up investigations of either single cases or group studies are necessary to address specific issues.

Notes

[1]Research on normal subjects has focused on whether the processes are serial and noninteractive or parallel and interactive (Tyler & Marslen-Wilson, 1980, 1981). Although this distinction is an important one, it does not constitute the main emphasis of our paper.

[2]Linguistic analyses of performance on the Token Test are not discussed in this review of studies on auditory sentence comprehension, for several reasons. We acknowledge the discriminatory power of this test for distinguishing aphasic from nonaphasic patients, as well as for detecting very mild receptive deficits. However, due to the test material and test design, exactly what the Token Test measures is not entirely clear (cf. Cohen, Kelter, & Schäfer, 1977; Naumann, Kelter, & Cohen, 1980). Lesser (1976) commented that "the difficulties some aphasic patients experience with the Token Test may not be entirely in the understanding of spoken language" (p. 246). She further suggested that "Token Test results from aphasics do not provide material suitable for linguistic analysis" (Lesser, 1976, p. 79). A linguistic analysis of qualitative differences is in our opinion not purposeful, because the response variables are so limited (correct/incorrect). Length of utterance and amount of redundancy are two aspects out of several that influence the aphasic's response in the various sections of the Token Test. On the other hand, the authors of the Token Test (De Renzi & Vignolo, 1962) and other authors (e.g., Whitaker & Selnes, 1978) have stressed the linguistic nature of the test and also its useful application in the measurement of child language acquisition.

Survey articles dealing with general factors involved in language comprehension with particular emphasis on treatment of comprehension deficits are also not discussed in this survey of the literature. Both Brookshire (1978) and Marshall (1981) have given comprehensive accounts of the multiple factors that affect the aphasic's auditory comprehension performance and are to be considered in the treatment of comprehension difficulties. The importance of such variables cannot be overlooked. An understanding of the interaction of variables such as linguistic, timing, and contextual variables, and of factors including supplemental inputs, manner of presentation, task requirements, and so on, is essential for optimal therapeutic intervention and theoretical descriptions of the deficits (cf. Marshall (1981) and Brookshire (1978) Blumstein et al. 1985.

[3]The test items used in this study were constructed to reflect possible everyday situations. This is one reason why the Token Test is not considered the most appropriate test to measure auditory sentence comprehension, although the original aim of this test was to detect subtle receptive disorders in the processing of spoken language. The aphasics tested with the Token Test differed greatly in their overall reaction to the test situation and material (i.e., pointing to and manipulating different colored tokens in the form of circles and rectangles).

[4]Over 300 aphasics have been tested during the past 9 years to date. These subjects will be considered in future analyses of the data, including data from the "mixed" aphasics.

[5]The age limit was set at 75 years, although the overall general health of each patient was also considered. All patients in this study had a left hemisphere lesion. CT scans were available for many of the patients; localization of the lesion was not among the subject variables listed in Table 6.1.

[6]Although German has a relatively free word order, the usual or basic word order in main clauses is S–V–(IO)–DO and in subordinate clauses is subordinate conjunction–S–(IO)–DO–V.

[7]The types of possible errors depend on the sentence type. The number of drawings to choose from was limited to four, allowing three distractors per sentence. The distractor types were systematic in that the types remained constant for the sentence types in which they were possible. For example, for the irreversible sentences, verb, subject, and direct object distractors were used; for reversible sentences, a verb, direct object, and S–DO reversal distractor; and for bitransitive sentences, a verb, subject, and DO–IO reversal distractor. A verb distractor was used for each test sentence. The use of only one distractor, that is, a two-picture choice, does not allow adequate differentiation of the types of processing difficulties. Moreover, with only two drawings for the subject to choose from, good perform-

ance has a much higher probability of being due to chance. An upper limit for drawings to be presented at once for each test sentence seems to be five with four distractors (cf. Heeschen, 1980; Kolk & Friederici, 1985). The objection that in sentence–picture matching tasks the choice of distractors limits the aphasic's possible errors does not appear to be satisfactory, when the error types are properly chosen. We believe that an object manipulation (acting out) task is more restrictive, especially in the analysis of errors, because of inherent difficulty in unambiguously demonstrating the activity, that is, the verb, of the sentence.

[8]The distribution for position of correct drawing was:

DIN A4 (top)

Position 1: 10 sentences (31.3%)	Position 2: 11 sentences (34.4%)
Position 3: 6 sentences (18.8%)	Position 4: 5 Sentences (15.6%)

For example, in 10 (31.3%) of the test sentences (not consecutive ones) the correct drawing was in the upper left frame of the sheet.

[9]In the choice of appropriate statistical methods, the scale of measurement and the distribution type of each of the dependent (most linguistic) variables stemming from the auditory comprehension test are important. The patient variables are mostly of a nominal type, with some of them having an ordinal scale. However, linguistic variables are all measurements of errors made in answer to a visual stimulus. Therefore, the linguistic variables are expected to be characterized best by a Poisson distribution and subsequently possibly by a normal distribution. This is confirmed by computing the Kolmogorov–Smirnov test of goodness of fit, first for the normal distribution as parent distribution and second for the Poisson distribution. Most error-type variables of this study were in very good agreement with the assumption of a Poisson distribution. Irrespective of the type of distribution, each variable can be considered an ordinal variable usable in nonparametric tests, the loss of information that occurs with the use of nonparametric statistics being of no importance. Therefore, the main statistical computations were done under the assumption that all variables were ordinally or nominally scaled.

[10]The four main aphasia types are the ones primarily discussed in the text; the results (error frequencies and significances) for the "Other" group of aphasics are listed in Table 6.18.

[11]For one of the reversible topicalized sentences, the S–DO reversal was not counted as an error (sentence 13). Refer to notes 12 and 13.

[12]Test sentence 13 was unmarked in terms of case marking. As a topicalized sentence, the only disinguishing aspect was intonation. Therefore, the results for the topicalized sentences are given with the S–DO reversal error of sentence 13 not counted as an error and also counted as an error. In Tables 6.5, 6.6, 6.7, 6.13, and 6.14 the S–DO reversal error is not considered as an error in the analyses. In Table 6.10 both possibilities are listed.

[13]Analysis of the results for the picture chosen for sentence 13 reveals the following:

Variable	Verb	Direct object	Topicalized	S–V–O
Choice of picture no.	3	1	2[a]	4[b]
Broca's	0	0	9	37
Anomic	2	0	7	28
Wernicke's	4	3	6	29
Global	7	0	7	12

[a]Correct as topicalized O–V–S.

[b]Incorrect as topicalized reversible S–DO (correct as S–V–O).

[14]In three of the four triple noun phrase sentences, the subject distractor was lexical in character; for the other sentence it represented a syntactic foil. Analysis by sentence revealed that 95% of the Broca's subject errors were made on that one sentence with a syntactic distractor: "*The boy* shows the baby to the mother," instead of *the girl* or *the man* as sentence subject, which would be a lexical distractor (target sentence: "*The mother* shows the baby to the boy"). This can be taken as further substantiation that the Broca's difficulties stem from limitations in syntactic processing.

[15]Very few aphasics perseverated the position of a drawing. This type of response pattern was observed in six severely impaired aphasics, but results from these patients were not considered for analysis, since the testing was not completed due to the perseveratory tendency. These patients did not scan the four drawings in response to each sentence; they consistently pointed to the drawing in a certain position for one test sentence after another.

[16]Although these results are interesting only for the DO–IO reversal error, the selection of sentence types to be investigated in aphasia should be made with extreme caution. Some of the sentence types used by Caplan et al. (1985) are especially difficult and in addition are not often used in everyday conversation.

[17]Incorrect initial processing was corrected in only a small percentage (2.7%) of the responses.

[18]The notion of linguistic complexity, in particular of syntactic complexity, is based on the interaction of several factors which include those listed in the text. The ranking of the syntactic complexity of the sentence types used in this study was determined by pairing reversibility with sentence type, length of utterance, compactness, and redundancy (e.g., markedness of the case endings).

[19]Johnson (1977) stated that: "... the '<' of the Postal & Perlmutter RH is not logically equivalent to the '>' of the Keenan-Comrie AH. The symbol < of the RH is a theoretical term which has no direct interpretation such as "as accessible to" (p. 158).

[20]In this context Hawkins' (1983) suggestion can be cited "... that there is every reason for extending the rigor of Keenan and Comrie's relativization implications to suitably reformulated universals of word order" (p. 63).

7
On Text Disturbances in Aphasia

WOLFGANG U. DRESSLER and CSABA PLÉH[1]

Introduction and History of Research

Contributions characterizing specific disturbances of discourse or text organization have been rather late and few (for the 1970s see Dressler & Stark, 1976; Engel, 1977; Stachowiak, Huber, Poeck, & Kerschensteiner, 1977; for the 1980s see below). Our use of the term "discourse" refers to the American tradition of discourse analysis, and of the term (written or oral) "text" to the German tradition of text linguistics (see Beaugrande & Dressler, 1981; Dijk, 1977a,b; Halliday & Hasan, 1976; for narratives, the main text type studied here, see Reinhart, 1984). The word "specific" relates to the issue of whether there are disturbances of discourse at a higher level than, and beyond, the organization of individual sentences. Particularly we mean by "specific textual disturbances" the:

1. Written or oral disturbances
   a. Disturbances of various linguistic levels (with possible consequences for the textual level) or
   b. General cognitive disturbances
2. Specific aphasic disturbances in general or specific aphasia types in particular

The existence or absence of such specific text-related organizational disturbances—also in the area of nonaphasic disturbances (cf. Dressler & Wodak, 1984, 1986; Lavorel, 1986; Rochester & Martin, 1979)—can be used as an argument in linguistics and text theory (whether discourse analysis or text linguistics) concerning the issue whether text organization is a specific level of linguistic organization above and beyond the sentence level and whether it belongs to the domain of linguistic capacities, that is, to human language faculty (Saussurean faculté du langage) in its broadest sense, or instead to more general cognitive and psychosocial skills.

One important distinction in text linguistics (cf. Beaugrande & Dressler, 1981) is the differentiation of "coherence" and "cohesion": Coherence refers to the semantic and pragmatic connectedness of a text, that is, to its content level, whereas cohesion refers to the syntactic, morphological, and lexical means of connecting sentences to paragraphs or other textual chunks and to whole texts. Another important differentiation refers to text types, two of which will be studied here: narratives (for aphasics cf. Freedman-Stern, Ulatowska, & Baker, 1984, pp. 189ff; Koll-Stobbe, 1984, 1985a; for normal but elderly people cf. Obler, 1980) and picture stories, in which spatially organized units have to be transformed into temporally organized narratives (cf. Koll-Stobbe, 1985a,b, for aphasics).

One typical approach to investigating textual disturbances is represented by A. R. Luria's Moscow school of aphasiology (cf. Luria, 1976). These investigators try to connect textual disturbances to more general cognitive deficits or to hypothetical inner stages of text planning. For example, Cvetkova (1966), on the basis of an analysis of text recall by patients with prefrontal or parieto-occipital lesions, concluded that in prefrontal lesions individual sentences remain intact but that the patient is unable to unfold the macrostructure of the text, that is, to maintain the topic and to return to the topic.

In his general outline of the neuropsychology of memory, Luria (1974, pp. 145–180) traced this type of aphasic disturbance in text recall to the general disturbances of goal-directed activities in these patients.

In her 1975 monograph on dynamic aphasia, Ahutina, as well as Luria (1976), attributed a primary disturbance of the inner programming of speech to this particular kind of lesion of the anterior speech centers and pointed out that the slightest symptoms consist of disturbances of suprasentential organization, which result in patients' inability to relate propositions to each other spontaneously during speech planning. More severely disturbed patients are unable to initiate spontaneous speech and are restricted to reactive utterances. This can be characterized as a disturbance of intentional activity in general (including speech activity; Dressler, 1983, p. 19). Although individual grammatical patterns are available to these patients, the patients are said to be unable to relate the cognitive semantic matrix of inner speech to the syntactic matrix of actually produced discourse.

However, reduction of textual capacities to cognitive ones must not be generalized to all aphasic syndromes. For example, Huber and Gleber (1982) have demonstrated that ordering of pictures and ordering of sentences (of a connected discourse) are not disturbed in the same way in different aphasia types.

Although Luria's approach may have increased our insight into hypothetical stages of speech planning, it has contributed relatively little to our understanding of the actual linguistic symptoms of aphasic text disturbances.

Ulatowska, Weiss-Doyel, Freedman-Stern, and Macaluso-Haynes (1983) and Ulatowska, Freedman-Stern, Weiss-Doyel, Macaluso-Haynes, and North, (1983) reported that the production of narrative and/or procedural discourse by anterior and posterior aphasics showed neither specific textual disturbances nor cognitive ones (in less severe cases). The details investigated only rarely (e.g., co-reference of pronouns) went beyond the sentence domain. For example, the mean length of sentence/clause or frequency of sentence embedding investigated by Ulatowska et al. are not central problems of textual structure but rather of sentence syntax.

Recently, however, in the more linguistically oriented approach to aphasia, some works have appeared in which disturbances in the "surface" organization of text are analyzed (for an overview see Dressler, 1983, 1984a). For our present purposes, the work by Berko Gleason et al. (1980) is the most relevant one among these studies. These investigators studied textual organization in fluent (Wernicke's) and nonfluent (Broca's) patients. They found that posterior lesion (Wernicke's-type) patients used relatively more verbs and deictic elements than either normal controls or Broca's patients. The texts produced by both groups of aphasics were characterized by looser criteria in the use of anaphoric pronouns, that is, on the surface organization their speech was characterized by less explicit cohesion.

Work by Koll-Stobbe (1985a, 1986) contains, in addition to general text linguistic reflections, a report on the aphasic's capacity to transcode picture series into a narrative. Relevant results will be cited where they apply to the present study.

Kaczmarek (1984a [different groups of patients, different aims and methods than in Kaczmarek, 1984b]) gathered many data on cohesive devices and disturbances in narrative recall and picture stories (without, however, any text linguistic analysis).[2] He concluded (p. 90) that, also in discourse, anterior lesion aphasics show more disturbances on the syntagmatic axis (i.e., errors in connecting units) and posterior lesion aphasics more errors on the paradigmatic axis (i.e., selection errors). This supports the Jakobson (1964) and Luria (1973) model.

Freedman-Stern et al. (1984) studied the written production of a Wernicke's aphasic in three different text types and concluded that discourse structure was preserved (particularly coherence and thematic organization) despite "severe disruption of sentences" (p. 198) leading, secondarily, to impairment of cohesion (pp. 194, 199). (On dialogues cf. De Bleser, 1987; for the reduction of content produced by aphasics cf. Joanette, Goulet, Ska, & Nespoulous, 1986.)

Goals of the Present Study

The study reported here had similar concerns. We were also primarily interested in possible difficulties in the surface marking of cohesion in aphasic speech. However, we used two text types in order to see whether some discourse characteristics of aphasic speech vary according to requirements of text type. Both samples were of narrative speech; one was based on picture stories (cf. Koll-Stobbe, 1985a), the other on story recall (cf. Freedman-Stern et al. 1984, p. 189). Thus we used the same text types as Kaczmarek (1984a), who unfortunately did not contrast the results of the two types with one another.

Procedure

Speech Samples

In this study (from our Viennese aphasia project[3]) we analyzed text productions of 16 moderately disturbed patients: five Wernicke's, four anomics, four Broca's, and three global (nonfluent, simultaneously anterior and posterior lesions) aphasics.[4] All patients came from Vienna or from the vicinity; some characteristics are given in Table 7.1.

Eight texts were obtained from each patient. Four were recorded before intensive speech therapy, and four after therapy. The four texts belonged to three types. The patients had to produce two picture story texts, on the basis of the picture series shown in Figures 7.1 and 7.2. The first picture story will be referred to as the *Cat* story (Fig. 7.1), the other as the *Rain* story (Fig. 7.2). Patients also had to recall two short stories, presented here in their English translation. An analysis into story constituents according to Labov and Waletzky (1967) is given in Tables 7.2 and 7.3. The first story recall will be referred to as the *Donkey* story, the other as the *Rails* story. Thus, our sample consists of 128 texts (32 for each of the four tasks).

Scheme of Analysis

The eight texts of each patient were tape recorded and then transcribed (in narrow transcription) by a native speaker of German (H. K. Stark). The

TABLE 7.1. Characteristics of 16 Patients Studied

Aphasia type	Number of patients	Sex (male:female)	Age (years)	Education[a]
Wernicke's	5	3:2	40–62	2 Pflichtschule, 3 Mittelschule
Broca's	4	2:2	53–66	3 Pflichtschule, 1 Mittelschule
Anomic	4	2:2	44–56	2 Pflichtschule, 2 Mittelschule
Global	3	2:1	46–55	1 Volksschule, 2 Mittelschule

[a]Pflichtschule corresponds to elementary and grammar/junior high school, Mittelschule to high school, and Volksschule to elementary school.

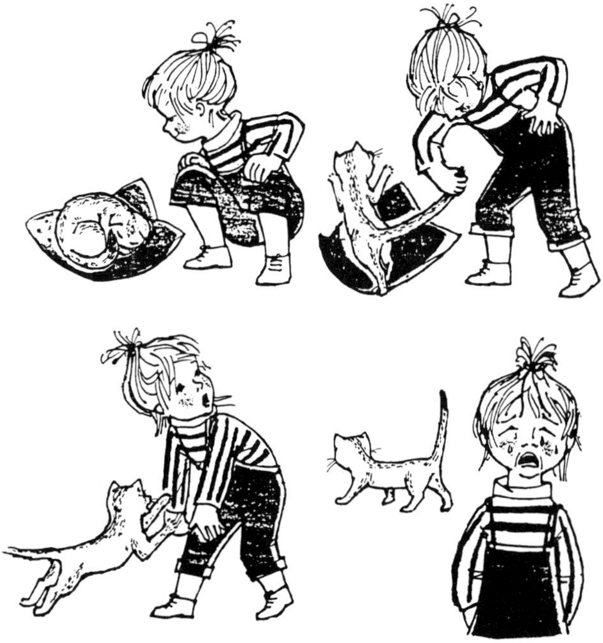

FIGURE 7.1 Picture material used for the cat story. Reprinted with permission © Jugend und Volk Verlagsgesellschaft m.b.H., 1975.

transcription was then transformed into standard orthography by E. Lindner, indicating the standard meaning of dialect expressions and noting in parentheses the intended sentence or word (in case of incomplete constructions and nonexisting word forms). This transliteration was compared again with the tapes. Neologisms and pauses were marked as well.

The normalized texts were then segmented and coded in all but three cases by a Hungarian psychologist (J. Frater) who speaks German fluently. The codings were checked by Austrian students who were unaware of the exact purposes of the research. Finally, the suggested corrections were again double-checked by one of us (C.P.) and only then was the coding accepted as "final." In the three remaining cases, native German speakers did the first steps of coding.

These text editing and coding matters are not as trivial in the case of aphasic speech as one usually imagines. As Dressler (1983, 1984a) has argued, linguists who treat aphasic texts should not forget all of their expertise in treating other mutilated texts (e.g., those studied by a philologist), their task being, especially when they are attempting to analyze larger speech segments, that of text reconstruction to a large extent.

The very coding procedure used revealed some problems of reliability (such problems are usually found in psychology). The main divergences

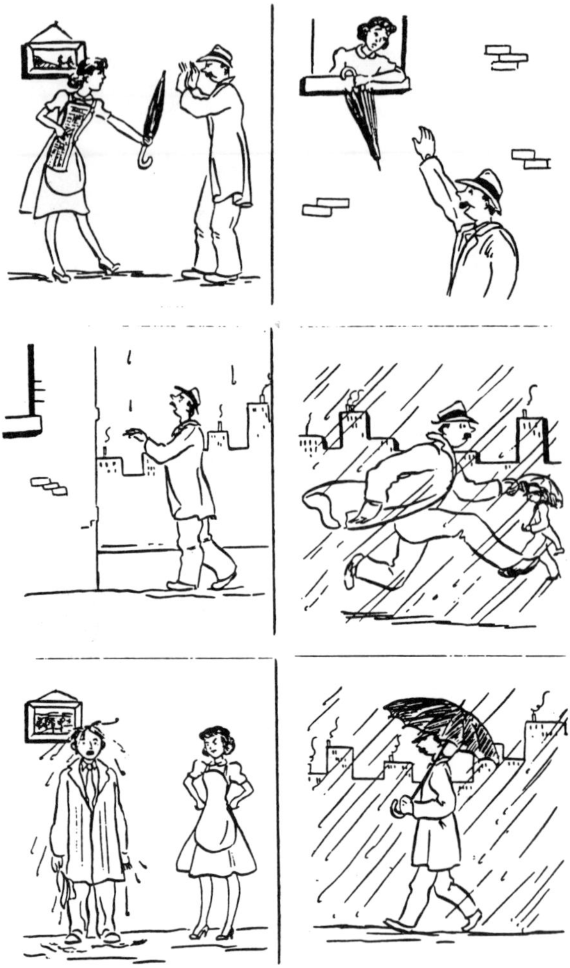

FIGURE 7.2 Picture material used for the rain story. Reprinted with permission © The Psychological Corporation, 1981.

between the codings of native and nonnative speakers, for example, were connected with the problem of anaphora usage: Native speakers were much more liberal in accepting a proform as anaphoric, while nonnative speakers required more explicit textual cohesion.

This side result of our study suggests that the problem of textual coherence and cohesion in aphasia could be studied by systematically varying the linguistic and situational knowledge of the unintended receivers of aphasic communication.

Each text produced by a patient was analyzed according to eight different aspects, using altogether 39 coding categories. Table 7.4 presents the

TABLE 7.2. Original for Story Recall: Donkey

Orientation	1. Ein geiziger Müller hatte einen Esel.	1. A stingy miller had a donkey.
Complication	2. Um diesen Esel billig zu ernähren,	2. In order to feed this donkey cheaply,
	3. bedeckte er ihn mit einem Bärenfell	3. he covered him with a bear's hide
	4. und trieb ihn jeden Abend auf den Acker eines Bauern im nächsten Dorf.	4. and drove him every evening to the field of a peasant of the nearest village.
	5. Der Esel ließ sich dort das Korn nach Herzenslust schmecke,	5. There the donkey ate the grain with relish,
	6. denn kein Mensch wagte es, ihn zu verjagen.	6. for nobody dared to drive him away.
	7. Jeder hielt den Esel für einen Bären.	7. Everybody mistook the donkey for a bear.
Solution I	8. Endlich aber faβte der Bauer, dem das Feld gehörte, Mut	8. Finally the peasant to whom the field belonged took heart
	9. und lauerte dem Tier auf.	9. and lay in wait for him.
	10. Er hatte seinen grauen Mantel angezogen	10. He had put on his gray coat
	11. und sein Gewehr mitgenommen,	11. and had taken his gun,
	12. um das Tier zu töten.	12. in order to kill the beast.
Solution II	13. Als der Esel den Bauern kommen sah,	13. When the donkey saw the peasant coming,
	14. hielt er ihn für eine Eselin	14. he took him for a she-ass
	15. und begann vor Freude zu schreien.	15. and began to cry for joy.
	16. Der Bauer erkannte nun den Esel an seiner Stimme,	16. Now the peasant recognized the donkey by his voice,
	17. fing ihn ein,	17. seized him,
	18. und führte ihn in seinen Stall.	18. and drove him into his stable.
Coda	19. So kam der Geizhals um seinen Esel.	19. Thus the miser lost his donkey.

categories and shows their grouping into three columns of analysis as they were actually used on the coding sheets. Table 7.5 gives an example of an actually coded text.

With the *Donkey* and *Rails* stories, a different analysis was also performed. The originally presented stories were segmented, as shown in Tables 7.2 and 7.3, and in each protocol the clear presence or absence of each unit was coded, the "uncertain" category also being used. Additions, that is, propositions not present in the original story, were also coded (including their place in the linear sequence).

TABLE 7.3. Original for Story Recall: Rails

Orientation:	1. Zwei Meter vor einem 18 Monate alten Kind konnte unlängst ein Lokomotivführer den Zug anhalten.	1. Recently an engine driver was able to stop a train 2 meters away from an 18-month-old child.
	2. Das Kind war in einem unbeaufsichtigten Augenblick auf die Gleise geklettert.	2. The child had been playing on the rails in an unobserved moment.
Complication:	3. Der Bub hat im Garten des Hauses, an dem die Bahntrasse vorbeiführt, gespielt.	3. The boy was playing in the garden of the house the train embankment passes.
	4. Als die Mutter, die im Haus arbeitete,	4. When the mother, who was working in the house,
	5. die Pfiffe des herankommenden Triebwagenzuges hörte,	5. heard the whistles of the approaching train,
	6. eilte sie hinaus	6. she ran out
	7. und sah den Buben	7. and saw the boy
	8. zwischen den Schienen laufen, stolpern und stürzen.	8. running, stumbling, and falling between the rails.
	9. In diesem Augenblick war der Zug noch dreihundert Meter von dem Kind entfernt.	9. At this moment the train still was 300 meters from the child.
	10. Die Frau konnte ihr Kind nicht mehr erreichen,	10. The woman was no longer able to reach her child,
Evaluation:	11. Vor Schreck schien ihr das Herz im Leibe stillzustehen.	11. her heart seemed to stand still in terror.
Solution:	12. Doch zwei Meter vor dem zwischen den Schienen liegenden Kind blieb die Lokomotive stehen.	12. However, 2 meters in front of the child, who was lying between the rails, the engine came to a stop.
	13. Mit der sofort eingeschalteten Schnellbremsung	13. Because of the immediately applied instant brake
	14. war es dem geistesgegenwärtigen Lokomotivführer gelungen, den Zug eben noch rechtzeitig anzuhalten.	14. the vigilant engine driver had succeeded in stopping the train just in time.
	15. Ein Schaffner stieg aus	15. A conductor got out
	16. und legte den Kleinen in die Arme der Mutter.	16. and put the small (boy) into his mother's arms.
Coda	17. Bevor die Mutter noch richtig danken konnte,	17. Before the mother was able to thank him properly
	18. war der Zug schon wieder fort.	18. the train was already away.

TABLE 7.4. Scheme of Analysis

Sentential features	Textual features	Disturbances
1. *Units:* number of sentences or sentoids 2. *Functions:* a rough characterization of the function of the unit Act: event or action Desc: descriptive sentence Dir: direct speech Crit: critic of what was said earlier Gen: generalization of earlier speech Subj: reactions to the task, complaints, etc. *WoDi:* word-finding difficulties 3. Compound sentences: conjunction, disjunction, that, relative and temporal clauses distinguished 4. Lexical statistics Noun tokens (NTOKEN) Noun types (NTYPE) Verb tokens (VTOKEN) Verb types (VTYPE) (Aux not included)	1. *Tense of the verb:* present (pre), perfect (perf), past, future (fut) 2. *Situationality* NP: full noun phrases ProAn: clearly anaphoric pronouns ProEx: nonanaphoric 3rd person pronoun *Elli:* nongrammatical ellipsis 3. *Deixis* Place: here, there, etc. Time: now Obj: this, that, etc. 4. Intersentential relations: expressed connectives AND DISJ: but, or, etc. THEN CAUSE: all causal connectives	Pauses (pau) Repetitions (rep) Incomplete constructions (Inc) WroWo: nonexisting words CorrGr: grammatical corrections, including gender change in the article CorrLex: changes of word or of part of a word Addi(tions)

STATISTICAL ANALYSIS

The 39 coding categories used in the "formal coding" were analyzed by analysis of variance (hence, ANOVA) using several "quasi-experimental" designs. Besides the original raw indices, derived scores were also used.

First, each indicator was analyzed in a 4 × 2 × 4 design according to the type of aphasia, therapy (before or afterward), and text (*Cat, Rain, Donkey, Rails*) as (a) between-subjects and (b) within-subjects factors. Four-way ANOVAs were used when different categories within a class of categories were also compared, for example, when the relative number of verbs and nouns was compared along the three other dimensions. One-way ANOVAs were also performed to clarify the interactions found in the more complex models. In this case, one category within a given text was compared among the four groups of patients.

Memory coding was also analyzed with ANOVAs. All the analysis was

TABLE 7.5. Picture Story Produced by a Broca's Aphasic: Child and Cat

Picture 1:	Das ist Butzika (=Mutzikatze) - ah - (das) Mädchen ist sie (?) Katze oder Mädchen. (1)[a] Th: Was tut das Mädchen? Pat: Aufwecken. (2)	This is a pussy-cat - ah - girl is she (?) cat or girl. (1) Th: What is the girl doing? Pat: Wake (inf.) up. (2)
Picture 2:	Die ist ein ganz . . . hm, hineinzwicken in (den) Schwanz. (3) Th: Zwicken oder . . . Pat: eine reissen Nase (an der Nase reissen?) (4)	This (she) is a completely . . . hm, pinch into (the) tail. (3) Th: Pinch or . . . Pat: a tear (inf.) nose (tear on the nose?) (4)
Picture 3:	und das ist ge-gibt ihm tegt (geht) auf li (sie) los. (5) Th: Wer? Pat: *Ge* (=die) *K*atze. (6) Th: Auf wen? Pat: auf e(in) . . . Mädchen. (7) Th: Was wird die Katze tun? Pat: her-hinhauen. (8) Th: Warum?	and this is - gives him goes against her. (5) Th: Who? Pat: The cat.(6) Th: Against whom? Pat: against a . . . girl. (7) Th: What will the cat do? Pat: strike here there. (8) Th: Why?
Picture 4:	Reinst - reizt - raunzt die Kleine, weil sie aufikrieg hat eine (9) (=dial.: weil sie eine raufgekriegt hat, weil sie gekratzt worden ist).	Cleans (neologism) - irritates - nags the small (one) because she has got one (9) (dial.: has been slapped).

Th = therapist; Pat = patient.
[a]Numbers in parentheses used for coding of sentences. See Table 7.4 for explanation of coding symbols.

Sentences	Text	Disturbances
1. Desc	2 Elli, 3 NP, ProEx	
2. Act	Pre, Elli	CorrGr
3. Act	ProEx, Pre, Elli	Inc, Pau
4. Act	NP, Pre	Inc
5. Act	2 ProEx, Pre	WroWo
WoDi	ProAn	CorrGr
6. Desc	NP	
7. Desc	NP	WroWo, Pau
8. Act	Pre, Elli	CorrGr
9. Act	NP, CAUSE, Pre	CorrLex, Inc
WoDi	Perf, ProAn	
Analysis		
Units = 9	Pre = 6	Pau = 2
NTOKEN = 9	NP = 7	Inc = 3
NTYPE = 5	ProEx = 4	WroWo = 2
VTOKEN = 4	ProAn = 2	CorrGr = 3
VTYPE = 4	Elli = 5	CorrLex = 1
Art = 6	CAUSE = 1	
Desc = 3	Perf = 1	
WoDi = 2		

done with programs 2V and 7D of the Biomedical Programs (BMDP) program package (Dixon & Brown, 1979).

From the several hundred statistical tests performed, only the ones giving clearly significant results are reported here. Thus the omission from consideration of a seemingly important feature implies that this category does not differentiate either between patients or between texts. Results are presented in meaningful groups. Sometimes nonsignificant differences are discussed when they make sense in relation to significant ones. This chapter thus concentrates on quantitative analyses.

Results

General Fluency[5]

Aphasias are commonly divided into nonfluent (global, Broca's, etc.) and fluent ones (Wernicke's, anomic, etc.). Nonfluent aphasics are much more fluent in automatisms and formulaic speech. These differentiations are made according to quantitative criteria taken over from psychology (in final analysis), such as mean length of utterance (measured in words, etc.) per time unit, and so on.

However, this is also a problem of text linguistics, as has been noted in error analysis of second language acquisition. For example, Gutstein (1982) demonstrated that the increase in fluency of Japanese learners of English depends heavily on the communicative functions of the respective text types and chunks. Before Fillmore's research (e.g., Fillmore, Kempler & Wong, 1979; cf. Quasthoff, 1978, 1983) text linguists/discourse analysts were hardly interested in problems of fluency, presumably because fluency seems to be merely a problem of performance and because linguists are often supposed to deal with competence only, competence usually being neatly separated from performance (cf. here chapter 1). Our procedural approach[6] tries to overcome this cleavage.

Verbs

As Figure 7.3 shows for verbs and nouns together and Table 7.6 for verbs and nouns separately, not surprisingly Wernicke's patients were more fluent when talking about pictures, while anomic patients were more fluent in recall. At the same time, the generally poor performance of Broca's and global patients did not vary according to the task. The text-by-aphasia type interaction in noun plus verb tokens was $F_{3,36} = 2.71$, $p < 0.02$, while in types it was statistically even clearer ($F = 3.62, p < 0.005$). As Table 7.6 shows, the interaction appeared both in verbs and in nouns.

Another way to interpret these interactions is to say—on the basis of the first columns of F values in Table 7.6—that while the types of aphasia had

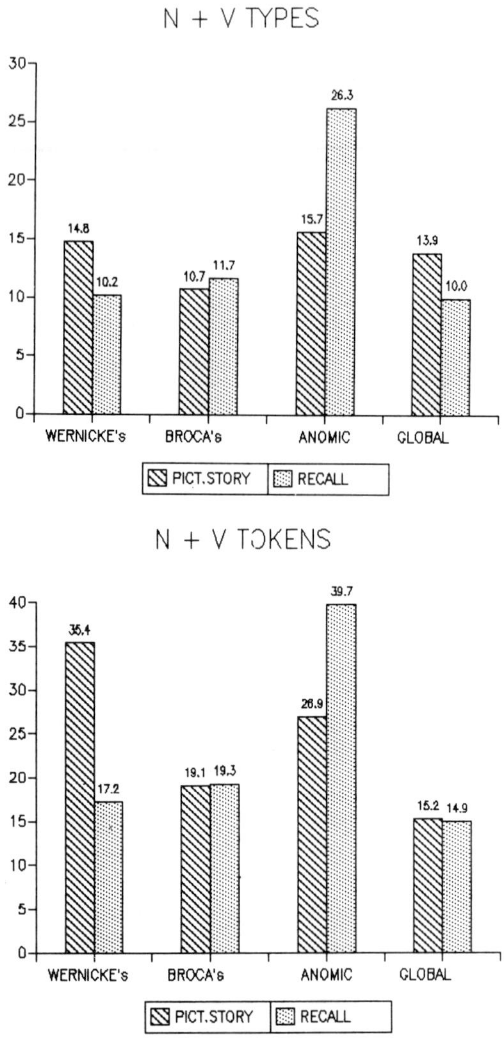

FIGURE 7.3 Noun and verb types and tokens in picture story and story recall.

no effect on fluency in picture stories, it had clear effects on fluency—always favoring the anomic group—in story recall.

These results support the view that anomics have no considerable deficit either in comprehension or memory but rather a word-finding problem, which emerges particularly in nomination tasks (cf. Buhr, 1976; Goodglass, 1983; Lesser, 1978, pp. 75, 104f; Luria, 1976, pp. 355ff; Stachowiak, 1979, pp. 10, 163, 165; Weigl, 1979). In the production of picture stories, nomination of picture content is constitutive all the more so as patients tend to reduce picture stories to picture nominations (cf. Dressler,

TABLE 7.6. Mean Number of Noun and Verb Tokens and Types for Different Text Types According to Aphasia Type

Indicator	Wernicke's	Broca's	Anomic	Global	F (3,12)	F (9,36) Disc × Text	
N Token							
Picture	17.4	10.6	12.9	6.4	1.95	n.s.	2.45
Recall	8.8	12.2	19.8	8.0	7.20	0.005	0.05
N Type							
Picture	6.0	4.5	5.7	4.7	1.0	n.s.	2.58
Recall	5.3	6.4	10.7	4.8	6.10	0.01	0.05
V Token							
Picture	18.0	8.5	14.0	8.8	1.67	n.s.	2.33
Recall	8.4	7.2	19.9	6.9	2.72	0.10	0.05
V Type							
Picture	8.8	6.2	10.0	9.2	1.0	n.s.	2.94
Recall	4.9	5.3	15.6	5.2	5.77	0.01	0.01

Wodak & Pléh, 1984). Thus, anomics have problems with picture stories, whereas story recall is easier because the lexical material to be used (particularly relevant content words) has been presented when the original story was read aloud (priming), that is, lexical access is easier.

However, Wernicke's patients have a verbal comprehension deficit that interferes when stories are read aloud to them for recall, but not when pictures are presented to them visually. This difference between text types is due to the nature of the disturbance outside the text level. This goes beyond fluency.

Type/token ratios computed for nouns and verbs separately did not vary according to the type of aphasia or text. Verb type/token ratios (mean = 0.75) were, however, higher than noun type/tokens ($F_{1,10}$ = 4.12, $p < 0.07$).

Sentence Embedding

There was one more positive result concerning the categories in the first column of Table 7.4. Although compound (and therefore embedded) sentences were naturally very rare (cf. Ulatowska et al., 1981, p. 353) (e.g., only one in the picture story of Table 7.5), the increased fluency of anomic patients in recall was evident in the use of compound constructions, too. The means for pictures and recalls in the sum of compound sentences was respectively as follows: Wernicke's: 0.7, 1.2; Broca's: 0.4, 0.2; anomics: 0.7, 3.2; globals: 0.3, 0.7. The aphasia × text interaction gave $F_{3,36} = 2.10$, $p < 0.05$.

Kaczmarek (1984a, p. 71, Table 14 row 4) obtained similar results (percentages of all words used by the respective group: anomics, 19.2; Wernicke's 8.1; Broca's, 1.6). The extreme reduction of sentence embedding in Broca's aphasics is a feature of agrammatism, that is, of a deficit in sentence grammar (syntax).

Syntactic cohesion and semantic coherence are higher within a sentence than between two adjacent sentences. When more embeddings have to be controlled for coherence and cohesion, the planning of a sentence represents a more difficult task. This also strains memory capacity (which may be subnormal in aphasia). Thus, if anomics are capable of planning more complex (compounded, embedded) sentences in story recall than in picture stories, this may be traced to the same factor as fluency discussed in our scheme of analysis.

Wernicke's Versus Broca's Aphasics

One negative fact should be mentioned in connection with the categories of the first column of Table 7.6. In contrast to Berko Gleason et al. (1980), we found no differences between Wernicke's and Broca's aphasics in their verb and noun fluency. While Berko Gleason et al. found a higher verb fluency in Wernicke's and a higher nominal fluency in Broca's patients (as a comparison of the upper and lower parts of Table 7.6 show), there were no such divergencies in our samples. The number of verbs and nouns was roughly equal in all groups, both in types and tokens. The only possible source of this difference might be that Berko Gleason et al. omitted "general" nouns (e.g., thing) (cf. Buckingham, 1979, pp. 278ff) in their counts, while we have included all nouns.[7]

Situationality and Its Indicators

This term is used in a more general way than in Beaugrande and Dressler (1981); it covers all factors that make a text relevant to its communicative context.

Indicators of situationality shown in the second column of Table 7.4 revealed many interesting differences. Plenty of data in the relevant literature suggest that one of the most sensitive indicators of the dissolution of textual cohesion is the abundant use of irrecoverable proforms.[8] We consider this phenomenon under the heading of situationality because proforms are often formally identical with deictics such as *this* (which clearly belong to the core of situationality) and show functional parallels such as in pointing to the nonverbal context (deictics) versus the verbal context (proforms). Thus we distinguish anaphoric pronouns (which refer backward to previous verbal context), cataphoric pronouns (which refer forward), and "exophoric" pronouns (which refer neither backward to an existing antecedent nor forward to a verbal referent).

Such exophoric pronouns show up in rather different sorts of restricted communication. One of the clearest indicators of restricted code in the sense of the sociolinguistic theory of Bernstein (1971), for example, is the use of exophoric pronouns by lower class children at the beginning of schooling, as shown by Hawkins (1969) in England and by Pap and Pléh (1974) for Hungarian children. This is also characteristic of the discourse of schizophrenic patients (Rochester & Martin, 1979) and it is typical both of Broca's and Wernicke's aphasics.[9] In the example of the Broca's aphasic in Table 7.5, it is unclear whether the *Die* (the) (fem. def. article at the beginning of sentence 3) co-refers to *Katze* (cat) or *Mädchen* (girl) (which has neuter gender, but co-reference may be to natural sex, not to grammatical gender). See also *ihm* (him) and *sie* (her) in sentence 5. In both instances the therapist inquires about the identity of the co-referring pronouns and definite article.

Figure 7.4 shows the means of anaphoric and exophoric pronouns in the four groups of patients.[10] To our surprise, anaphoric pronouns were used more frequently than exophoric, but the difference was not significant ($F < 1$). Similarly, the smaller overall number of proforms produced by Broca's aphasics did not reach significance when the number of proforms was compared between the groups ($F < 1$).

There was, however, a strong correlation between aphasia type and the type of proform ($F_{3,12} = 5.06$, $p < 0.02$). As Figure 7.4 clearly shows, this correlation is caused by anomic patients using more anaphoric pronouns and global patients using more exophoric pronouns. When anaphoric pronouns are treated separately, the type of aphasia has a significant main effect ($F_{1,12} = 3.48$, $p < 0.05$), caused by the superiority of the anomic group.

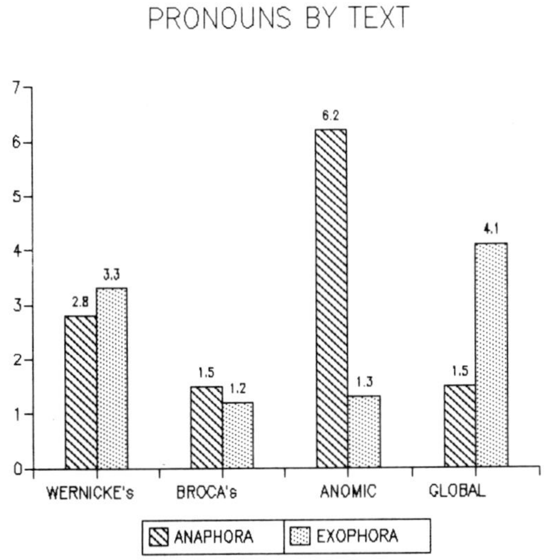

FIGURE 7.4 Differential use of pronouns according to aphasia type.

Pronouns

One group of exophoric pronouns consists of deictics and of incorrectly used anaphorics, which reveals a disturbance of co-reference. Moreover, posterior lesion aphasics often confuse the characters of a plot (dramatis personae, see Dressler, 1980a; Nespoulous, 1980, p. 21), which results in incorrect use of anaphorics. Thus, our results do not agree with Ulatowska and colleagues' observation (1981, p. 355, point 6): "All subject narratives contained all of the participants in the action." Of course, reduction of participants is one problem, partial confusion of participants another one.

For example, one of our Wernicke's patients started recall of the *Donkey* story during the first test session in the following way:

"Na, da ist ein Esel gekommen ... und ... ah so, da ist der Esel mit einen einer der geizigen Hals."

(Well, there has come a donkey ... and ... ah well, there is the donkey with a a [acc.] the [nom.] stingy [acc./dat./gen.] neck [*Geizhals* (miser) = literally "stingy neck"].)

Later the same patient produced:

"Dann sind sie in Wald gegangen und dann sind sie ... dann hat der Esel endlich gegessse ... und dann ... zum Schluß hat dann der geizige Hals so geschrien und der Esel und der Esel hat es doch gann gegessen."

(Then they have gone into wood and then are/have they ... then finally the donkey has eaten ... and then ... at the end then the stingy neck has cried so much and the donkey and the donkey then has eaten it nevertheless.)

In this story recall, no further participants (characters, dramatis personae) occurred.

The story recall of the same Wernicke's patient during the second test session 1 month later was as follows:

"Ja das ist von einem Esel von ... und und da ist der Esel hingekommen, hat gefressen und dann sind ist auch noch ein anderer Esel gekommen ... äh äh eine Eselin und weil der der Esel soviel geschrien hat, ist dann diese Eselin gekommen und haben sie beide gefrech-gefressen und sind dann in den Stall gekommen."

Yes, that is of a donkey of ... and and there ... the donkey has come, has eaten and then are/have is/has come still another donkey as well ... eh eh a she-ass and since the the donkey has cried so much, then this she-ass has come and they both have [phonological paraphasia] eaten and then have come into the stable.")

Compare the story recall of a Broca's aphasic:

"Ein Bauer hat einen Esel ... ein Bf-Bärenfell angezogen und er ging von einen Acker zum anderen und den Bauern das wegnehmen und dann kam ein Bauer und f-wagt dem Tier aus auflauern und sag- sog- in einen grau Mantel an und die S- Pistole oder nein Gewehr und und wie der Esel herunterk- kam s- sah m- mah- ... glaubte der Esel, das ist eine Eselin und der Bauer nahm den Esel mit."

(A peasant has a donkey ... put on a bf-bear's hide and he went from one field to the other and the peasant [acc.] that take [inf.] away and then came a peasant and f-dares to lay in wait out/for the beast and say - suck - in a grey coat on and the s-pistol or his gun given and and as the donkey came down, saw, mak-, believed the donkey [nom]. that is a she-ass and the peasant seized the donkey.")

The previous study (Dressler, 1980a) showed the following results (in 12 normal controls, 6 fluent aphasics, and 6 nonfluent aphasics recalling the same story once) with regard to confusion of participants:

	Fluent	Nonfluent	Normal
Confusion without repair	16	1	—
Confusion with correct repair	7	3	2
Confusion with incorrect repair	8	—	—

Anomics

The superiority of the anomic group was especially characteristic in story recall. While in picture stories there was no relationship between aphasia and anaphora use, in story recall the means for the 4 groups were 2.5, 1.1, 6.7, and 1.7 ($F_{3,12} = 4.37, p < 0.05$). Anomics had less word-finding problems in story recall, so that the establishment of correct reference facilitates the establishment of correct co-reference (identification of identical reference) and thus the correct use of anaphoric proforms. Wernicke's patients, however, have—due to disturbance of selection (cf. Jakobson, 1964; Kaczmarek, 1984a; Luria, 1976; Peuser, 1978a, pp. 141ff)—problems in establishing co-reference and in using anaphoric proforms.

Moreover, the word-finding problems of anomics involved particularly nouns, and pronouns to a much lesser extent; therefore, we must expect the substitution of recurrent co-referent nouns with anaphoric pronouns. Picture stories trigger an increased use of deictics, so that an increased use of exophoric pronouns is to be expected.

Male patients used significantly more deictics than female aphasics, which fits their preference for description strategies (see Dresler, Wodak, & Pléh, 1984, p. 52).

In story recall there was a significant interaction between recovery and anaphora use as well ($F_{3,12} = 4.18, p < 0.05$). The meaning of this effect was the following: In anomic patients, the use of anaphoric pronouns increased specifically in recovery from the first to the second test session (5.5. vs. 7.9), while in the other groups no such effect was observed.

Full Noun Phrases

The mean number of full noun phrases (NPs with a nominal head) was much higher than the number of proforms (9.6 vs. 6.5, $F_{1,12} = 13.46, p < 0.005$). The overwhelming use of pronominal co-reference was much less characteristic of our patients than we had expected. Koll-Stobbe (1985a, p. 34; 1985b, p. 75) classified the exaggerated use of full NPs by aphasics ("renominalization") as a sign of their reduced capacity to use pronouns (cf. Freedman-Stern et al. 1984, p. 193).

Exophoric Pronouns

In regard to anaphoric versus exophoric proforms, it is worth considering two aspects of the results concerning the indicators of situationality. First, at variance with Berko Gleason et al. (1980), we did not find a general propensity in aphasic patients to exophoric pronominal use. In the Berko Gleason et al. data, 80% of the pronouns used by aphasics had no clear antecedents, while in our sample this was true of only 38% of the pronouns. A possible reason for this might be that we used more liberal coding criteria in deciding about the "phoricity" of pronouns.

Another difference between our and the Berko Gleason et al. (1980) data was that whereas they found an increased use of deictic expressions (*here, that,* etc.) in Wernicke's, we found no differences due to aphasia type in our sample. The only clear difference emerging from the comparisons involving deictic expressions was a difference between types of deixis used. While patients in general had the values 3.6 tokens for place deixis by story and 1.9 for time deixis, they produced only 0.9 object deictic expressions ($F_{2,24} = 13.04, p < 0.0001$).

CONJUNCTIONS[11]

Use of Conjunctions

Only the intersentential connectives (those in the second columnn of Table 7.4) will be considered here, since the intrasentential conjunctions (of the type John *and* Mary) were very rare. Not too surprisingly, AND relations (the default connection), were the most frequent ones. Their mean number in stories was 4.5; the mean number for BUT being 1.9 and for THEN 1.0; CAUSAL conjunctions were by far the least frequent ($F_{3,36} = 15.73, p < 0.0001$). Berko Gleason et al. (1980), who considered only Wernicke's patients, also noted the overwhelming use of AND in their stories in comparison with normal subjects.

The only relevant difference related to aphasia types was found in the use of AND: An aphasia × text type interaction was observed of ($F_{9,36} = 2.33, p < 0.05$). The explanation for this interaction might be similar to our subsection on anomics: In anomic patients, in connection with their greater fluency in recall, the number of AND relations expressed increases in recalls compared with picture stories, from 4.2 to 7.2, whereas in the other groups the change is much less (e.g., Broca's, 4.1 to 5.2; global, 2.7 to 4.0). Interestingly, Wernicke's were the only patients who again had more conjunctions in picture stories (mean number 4.3) than in story recall (mean number 3.6), although this tendency was not yet statistically significant.

Conjunctions and Function Words

Generally, conjunctions are included in the class of grammatical or function words, and disturbance of this class is considered a typical symptom of Broca's aphasia (agrammatism/dysgrammatism; telegraphic style in more severe cases) (cf. Caplan, 1983a; Goodglass, 1976; Kean, 1979; Lesser, 1978, pp. 135ff; Peuser, 1978a, pp. 128ff). In our Broca's texts, however, as in the German part of the CLAS project (Stark & Dressler, in press), coordinating conjunctions (*and, but,* etc.) are much less disturbed than the other function words (articles, pronouns, auxiliary verbs).

Kaczmarek (1984a, p. 51, Tables 10 and 12, row 8) obtained the following Polish results (percentages of all words used): normal controls, 8.6%; Wernicke's, 8.6%; anomic, 8.7%; Broca's, 11%. Thus, Broca's aphasics used (relatively) many more conjunctions than did normal subjects. So much for "conjunctions being lost in telegraphic speech"!

The long-standing neglect of the special role of conjunctions (connectives) among function words stems from the neglect of text linguistics in aphasiology. Auxiliary verbs play a role in sentence grammar only, articles and pronouns primarily in sentence grammar and only secondarily in textual cohesion (particularly co-reference). Therefore telegraphic style cannot be a primary disturbance of the text level (viz., of cohesion), but a secondary consequence of a primary disturbance of the (sentence-grammatical) class of function words.

In contrast, the coordinating conjunctions have the primary textual function of connecting sentences (cohesion) and of signaling the kind of semantic coherence[12] that holds between connected sentences. Thus, agrammatism is primarily a disturbance of sentence grammar and not of the text level.

Reduction of Conjunctions

The main disturbance of conjunctions in aphasic text production consists of impairment of the overt differentiation of relationships between propositions, so that the precise type of semantic/pragmatic coherence becomes opaque. Even when patients become more fluent, they reduce the use of conjunctions to a few simple connectives (cf. Freedman-Stern et al., 1984, p. 196), particularly *"and,"* which expresses mere connection and thus is vague in respect to the exact kind of semantic relation expressed (cf. Dijk, 1977b; Halliday & Hasan, 1976, pp. 226ff; Lang, 1976; Schiffrin, 1986). The substitution of coordinating conjunctions with very few connectives (particularly the default connective) represents a reduction of types but not of tokens and results in underdifferentiation.

Koll-Stobbe's (1985a) qualitative analysis resulted in her claim that aphasics cannot use conjunctions systematically for text organization (e.g., as boundary signals between paragraphs or other textual chunks).

Sex Differences in the Use of Conjunctions

Female patients use many more conjunction tokens than do male aphasics (11.4 vs. 5.6 per text, $F_{1,14} = 5.39, p < 0.05$), and also more conjunction types (significant only for AND and CAUSAL), a fact interpreted by Dressler et al. (1984, p. 53) as due to sex-specific socialization (unimpaired in aphasia).

Use of Verb Tenses

The variable use of verb tenses (cf. Beaugrande & Dressler, 1981, pp. 69ff; Reinhart, 1984) might be a sensitive indicator of the formal organization of discourse. First, one could expect to find more verbal forms referring to past events in story recall than in picture stories if aphasics are sensitive to the temporal structure of events, since picture stories are based on immediate perceptual situations. On the other hand, the well-known grammatical difficulties of Broca's and global aphasics would predict an almost exclusive (or at least preferential) use of the formally simpler and semantically unmarked present tense.

In accordance with these expectations, the picture stories previously described contain only present tense forms, whereas there is a preponderance of perfect tense forms in the story recalls given in the section on general fluency.

Table 7.7 shows the use of the three most important tenses according to aphasia and text type. A four-way ANOVA based on these data (aphasia × therapy × text × tense) had clearly shown the overall superiority of the present tense (tense main effect $F_{2,24} = 20.75, p < 0.0001$), together with a strong text × tense interaction ($F_{6,72} = 19.37, p < 0.0001$). The meaning of this interaction can be clearly seen in the table: In story recall the use of perfect and imperfect tenses increased at the expense of the present tense. Thus, aphasic patients are sensitive to the requirements of discourse concerning tense organization.

This sensitivity, however, was much less evident in Broca's than in other aphasia patients. As the text × aphasia interactions in Table 7.7 show, the interaction that indicates these group differences was evident both for the decrease of present tense and the increase of past tenses in story recalls. Naturally also, the present tense may be used as narrative tense ("historical present"), but there is no reason why only Broca's aphasics should show a preference for the historical present. Moreover, normal subjects use the historical present for stylistic purposes at culminating points of a story or for rendering the account more vivid (cf. Quasthoff, 1979, p. 5). However, no such stylistic effects can be detected in texts produced by Broca's aphasics. Thus we stick to the traditional interpretation of aphasics substituting nonpresent tense forms with the unmarked and simpler present tense forms.

TABLE 7.7. Mean Number of Different Verb Tenses According to Text Types and Aphasia Types

Tense	Wernicke's	Broca's	Anomic	Global	$F(3,13)$	Text × aphasia		Text × tense
							$F(3,36)$	$F(9,36)$
Present tense								
Picture	17.4	7.7	10.8	8.2	1.57	n.s.	21.70	3.03
Recall	3.9	4.3	4.3	2.6		0.0001		0.01
Perfect tense								
Picture	1.2	0.4	0.7	0.2	1.75	n.s.	6.02	1.18
Recall	5.2	1.6	8.4	1.1		0.002		n.s.
Imperfect tense								
Picture	0.2	0.4	0.1	0.2	<1	n.s.	9.67	2.24
Recall	2.2	1.8	5.6	3.2		0.0001		0.05

In the colloquial speech of southern Germany, Austria, and Switzerland, the perfect tense replaces the imperfect (except the auxiliary *sein* [to be]). Therefore we expect aphasics to use the imperfect tense only in recalls of written standard texts that contain imperfect tense forms. This is true both for the patients of the CLAS project (Stark & Dressler, in press) and for our patients. Note that the text of our *Donkey* story consists of the imperfect tense (plus one instance of the pluperfect) and the *Rail* story consists of imperfect tense plus three pluperfect and one perfect tense form.

DISTURBANCES

The six categories of disturbances[13]—mostly related to hesitations and thus to problems in planning—were first compared in a four-way ANOVA treating disturbances themselves as a within-subject factor with six levels. As the means for different disturbances show in Table 7.8, the incidence of different disturbances had a wide range ($F_{5,60} = 18.80, p < 0.0001$).

Disturbances can be arranged into three groups on the basis of overall frequency: (a) pauses; (b) repetitions,[14] incomplete constructions, and wrong words; and (c) lexical and grammatical corrections (repair). It is very clear that corrections, which are rather frequent disturbance/hesitation phenomena in normal speech (cf. Levelt, 1983a, p. 288; 1983b), decrease in aphasia. This phenomenon can be compared with the category of successive approximation (see chapter on phonology).

As the lower line in Table 7.8 shows, Wernicke's aphasics (i.e., fluent aphasics without the word-finding problems of the anomics) produced the highest number of disturbances.

There was an interaction between the type of aphasia and the type of disturbance ($F_{15,60} = 1.97, p < 0.05$). Several factors can account for this. First, according to the ANOVAS performed for each disturbance category separately, the Wernicke's group had a higher mean only in the incidence of pauses ($F_{3,12} = 3.91, p < 0.05$) and of lexical corrections ($F = 3.37, p <$

TABLE 7.8. Various Disturbances

Disturbance	Mean number of disturbances				Overall mean	Disease F(3,12)
	Wernicke's	Broca's	Anomic	Global		
Pause	15.3	9.3	8.6	4.2	9.4	
Repetition	8.6	3.1	3.6	2.0	4.3	
Incomplete	5.8	3.5	2.2	4.6	4.0	
Wrong word	6.2	4.0	1.4	5.7	4.3	
Grammatical corrections	1.9	0.8	0.8	0.6	1.0	
Lexical corrections	2.6	1.1	1.6	0.6	1.5	
Sum	40.4	21.8	18.2	17.7	3.16	0.06

0.05). Incidentally, this effect was due to the hesitations of Wernicke's aphasics in picture stories; it disappeared in story recall, in which Wernicke's patients were less fluent.

The higher frequency of pauses in Wernicke's patients also remains if we take into consideration the differences due to fluency. When we weight pauses with the number of verb and noun tokens in the given text, we obtain a mean ratio of 0.74 in Wernicke's, 0.50 in Broca's, 0.31 in anomic, and 0.46 in global patients. This difference, however, fails significance ($F_{3'12}$ = 2.19, n.s.).

If we take a look at the columns, we find that in Wernicke's patients a high number of pauses and repetitions is characteristic, in Broca's patients the relatively high number of wrong words is characteristic, and in global patients there is a high incidence of wrong words and incomplete constructions.[15]

As to sex differences, men produced many more wrong words than women (Dressler et al., 1984, p. 55).

Story Recall

Table 7.9 summarizes the overall data on recall. It can be seen that, owing to their higher fluency evidenced in the formal analysis, the anomic group recalled more content units, (cf. the leftmost column of Tables 7.2, 7.3) of the story (cf. also Joanette et al., 1986). This difference was, however, significant only in the second round of tests, after therapy.

As to additions, there were no significant differences among the groups, although global aphasics produced less additions: Fluent aphasics produced more additions, but fewer than claims about redundant, super-

Table 7.9. Mean Number of Units Recalled and Additions Made in the *Donkey and Rails* Stories

	Aphasia type					
Story	Wernicke's	Broca's	Anomic	Global	$F(3,12)$	p
Recall						
Donkey 1	2.2	5.0	8.2	4.3	2.28	n.s.
Rails 1	3.0	4.5	7.7	4.0	1.21	n.s.
Donkey 2	2.8	4.0	11.0	2.6	3.09	0.07
Rails 2	3.2	4.5	11.5	3.3	4.39	0.05
Mean	2.4	4.5	9.6	3.6	4.12	0.05
Additions						
Donkey 1	1.4	1.0	1.7	1.7	1	n.s.
Rails 1	2.0	1.7	1.5	1.3	1	n.s.
Donkey 2	2.4	1.2	1.7	1.0	1	n.s.
Rails 2	0.8	3.2	1.7	1.7	1	n.s.
Mean	2.0	1.8	2.2	1.4	1	n.s.

fluous words or logorrhoe in Wernicke's aphasia and about circumlocutions of anomics[16] might suggest.

Table 7.10 indicates the number of patients who recalled a given "sentence" (19 sentences in *Donkey,* 18 in *Rails;* see Tables 7.2, 7.3) and the number of patients who produced additions at a given place. Although the small numbers do not allow a detailed statistical comparison, it can be seen that recall is selective. In both stories, patients tended to recall crucial events while ignoring less crucial ones. This is in keeping with the results reported by Engel (1977), Dressler (1980a), Ulatowska et al. (1981, p. 352), Mierzejewska and Grotecki (1982a) (for normal subjects cf. Pléh, 1986).

The order of the text chunks (orientation, complication, solutions coda), according to the methodology of Labov & Waletzky (1967; cf. Tables 7.2, 7.3), was well preserved in recall (for the frequency of omissions according to text chunk see Dressler, 1980a), as was the order of the "sentences," (cf. the segmentation in Table 7.3).[17] This preservation of sequential order seems to reflect retention of a cognitive rather than of a linguistic capacity (cf. Levelt, 1981, pp. 306, 313).

What can we learn from story recall for text comprehension[18] by aphasics? First, many aphasics understand texts better than isolated words or sentences (as often used in tests), because textual redundancy

TABLE 7.10. Frequency of Recall of the Separate Units of Each Text and Frequency of Additions Tied to the Given Unit

Donkey 1 and 2					*Rails* 1 and 2				
Sentence	No. of patients recalling		No. of patients making additions		Sentence	No. of patients recalling		No. of patients making additions	
1.	10	7	4	2	1.	3	1	2	0
2.	3	4	2	3	2.	6	6	4	3
3.	10	6	2	1	3.	4	6	2	1
4.	7	7	1	0	4.	1	2	0	0
5.	3	3	2	2	5.	3	2	1	1
6.	0	3	0	1	6.	2	4	0	1
7.	1	1	0	0	7.	1	1	1	0
8.	4	5	2	3	8.	1	6	1	2
9.	3	2	1	1	9.	2	1	0	0
10.	5	5	1	0	10.	3	2	1	0
11.	6	5	0	0	11.	2	3	1	2
12.	4	5	0	2	12.	4	3	1	1
13.	4	5	1	0	13.	4	5	3	1
14.	5	5	2	2	14.	7	5	1	1
15.	2	5	2	3	15.	4	3	0	2
16.	3	3	0	2	16.	7	5	2	1
17.	6	5	1	1	17.	5	6	2	0
18.	6	5	1	1	18.	4	5	0	0
19.	1	4	1	4					

compensates for wrong perception or processing of single words or sentences (cf. Brookshire & Nicholas, 1984, pp. 31ff; Kotten, 1982; Stachowiak, Huber, Poeck, & Kerschensteiner, 1977; for normal subjects cf. Linell, 1983, pp. 185ff). This explains why aphasics are able to assign adequate titles to stories read to them without a title (Engel, 1977).

Also the retention of the original order of textual chunks and sentences (cf. above) in recall indicates a fair amount of text comprehension, at least of the more informative sentences.[19]

As to the comprehension of anaphoric pronouns (cf. Dijk & Kintsch, 1983, pp. 160ff; McKoon & Ratcliff, 1980), there was no significant correlation between relative achievement in recall (degree of retention) and the contrast between anaphoric pronouns and anaphorically repeated full noun phrases. For example, sentence 3 of the *Donkey* story "bedeckte *er ihn* mit einem Bärenfell" (*he* covered *him* with a bear's hide) was well recalled although *er* (he) substitutes for *der Müller* (the miller) and *ihn* (him) for *den Esel* (the donkey) (accusative). Thus, anaphoric pronouns do not seem to be understood much worse than anaphoric full noun phrases.

Since the other properties of story recall discussed previously do not involve text comprehension, we may conclude that moderately disturbed aphasics have problems in text production rather than in text comprehension as far as our text types are concerned; but there are more severe comprehension deficits in Wernicke's aphasia.

However, F. J. Stachowiak (personal communication, 1985) informed one of us (W.U.D.) of different results of tests run in Aachen and Bonn: There, texts that either had less cohesion or were cognitively more difficult were understood much more poorly, even by Broca's aphasics.

Differences due to Language Therapy

Although the results discussed to this point have also included some effects of therapy, the *main effects* of language therapy (including spontaneous recovery between the first and the second round of tests) will be presented here more systematically.

As Table 7.11 shows, therapy had a significant effect on relatively few indicators. These mainly indicate an increase in grammatical control of text organization. There was a decrease in incomplete constructions and wrong words as well as in word-finding difficulties (and subjective reactions connected with them).

Simultaneously, direct speech increased slightly in the picture stories. In connection with the latter finding, it is worth noting that Berko Gleason et al. (1980, p. 378) interpreted use of direct speech as a negative sign, as avoidance of the grammatically more complex indirect speech (used slightly more by their Broca's patients). In our sample, however, the use of direct speech was not related to the type of aphasia, and its increased use

TABLE 7.11. Differences of Mean Tokens Between First (=1) and Second (=2) Test Runs

Indicator	Test 1	Test 2	*F*(1,12)	*p*
All texts				
Direct speech	0.4	0.8	8.35	0.01
Subjective reactions	4.0	2.1	5.92	0.05
Incomplete constructions	4.4	3.6	3.57	0.08
Picture stories				
Direct speech	0.8	1.4	7.78	0.02
Subjective reactions	4.0	2.0	10.99	0.01
Verb tokens	14.3	11.5	4.28	0.06
Verb types	9.1	8.0	3.94	0.07
Story recall				
Word-finding difficulty	3.7	2.7	3.49	0.10
Incomplete constructions	4.2	3.1	3.20	0.10
Wrong words	5.0	3.1	5.04	0.05

in picture stories with recovery can be interpreted as indicative of higher adaptation to the task and as formation of compensatory devices. This interpretation is supported by the fact that increase in direct speech is not compensated for by decrease in indirect speech. Therefore, an increase in direct speech cannot be interpreted as replacement of a more complex construction (viz. indirect speech) by a simpler equivalent (viz. direct speech).

Anomic aphasics improved the most of all patients from the first to the second test run, particularly in overall fluency and in coherence of story recalls produced. Does this mean that anomics react more positively to therapy in general? (Cf. Gloning, Trappl, Heiss, & Quatember, 1969; Leischner, 1976; Lesser, 1978, p. 102; Peuser, 1978a, pp. 376ff.)

Of course, it is not clear how much of such improvements is due to the specific linguistic therapy administered to our aphasics between the first and second rounds of tests and how much to spontaneous recovery.[20] However, the leveling of sex-specific differences between the first and second rounds of tests should be attributed to therapy (Dressler et al., 1984): Sex-specific differences in language production are due to different primary and secondary socialization at home and in school, respectively, and are reinforced after school (tertiary socialization). These differences remained in our aphasics before therapy. However, speech therapy for aphasics is not sex specific but represents a fourth socialization, which does not reinforce sex-specific language performance. On the contrary, it has a harmonizing effect.

Conclusions

To summarize, the following differentiations of disturbances were observed on the text level:

1. Disturbances of text production were nonspecific.
2. There were secondary consequences of impaired sentence grammar such as in the use of tense forms (particularly by Broca's aphasics), in telegraphic style where cohesion is reduced, in reduced sentence complexity.
3. The degree of fluency was not text specific but due to cognitive impairments or linguistic disturbances on other levels than primarily the text level.
4. Disturbances of anaphoric co-reference apparently were rather text specific, that is, due both to a deficit in cohesion and to impairment of coherence in co-reference, particularly in Wernicke's aphasia. The general disturbance of grammatical function words on the level of sentence grammar, however, was typical of Broca's aphasia.
5. Reduction and underdifferentiation of conjunctions impairs coherence at least in the eye of the observer. But it is not yet clear whether this is a primary disturbance of semantic/pragmatic coherence or of lexical/syntactic means of cohesion.

Notes

[1]This chapter is an outcome of research cooperation between the universities of Vienna and Budapest, supported by the Austrian Fonds zur Förderung der Wissenschaftlichen Forschung (project 3632) and by the Hungarian Ministry of Education (grant 24-2-084). We thank Judith Frater and Judit Osman Sági (Budapest), Jacqueline Ann and Heinz Karl Stark, and Elisabeth Lindner for compiling the data. A first report has been published in Dressler and Pléh (1984) (cf. Dressler, Wodak, & Pléh, 1984).

[2]Since Kaczmarek's (1984a) two-page English summary is rather devoid of content, and since Polish is not read by many aphasiologists, we will cite numbers from his tables in detail.

[3]Project 3632 of the Fonds zur Förderung der Wissenschaftlichen Forschung. In the meantime 80 aphasics have twice undergone a test battery (conceived by Karl Gloning, Wolfgang U. Dressler, and Jacqueline Ann Stark) consisting of 32 subtests, four of which were used for this study.

[4]Originally we wanted to have four groups of equal size (based on standard neurological and neuropsychological classifications). However, a careful neurolinguistic analysis revealed that one of the original four global aphasics had to be reclassified as a Wernicke's aphasic. Fortunately, the resulting unequal distribution (five vs. four vs. four vs. three) does not matter for the statistical methods used. For the classification of our four aphasia types see Huber (1981); Poeck, Kerschensteiner, Stachowiak, and Huber (1975); Poeck (1983); cf. Benson (1979); Kertesz (1979); Marshall (1982).

[5]Cf. Benson (1979); Fillmore (1979); Huber (1981); Leischner (1979); Lesser (1978); Peuser (1977, 1978a,b); Poeck et al. (1975).

[6]Cf. Beaugrande and Dressler (1981); Dressler (1983); Petőfi (1983). Following our report (Dressler & Pléh, 1984), Koll-Stobbe (1985b) tried to distinguish linguistic (competence) and performance fluency.
[7]But compare Kaczmarek's results (1984a, p. 52, Table 12, first and third row) with the following percentages of nouns and verbs used by the respective group:

	Wernicke's	Anomic	Broca's
Nouns	17.8%	19.6%	23.5%
Verbs	15.2%	18.0%	18.0%

[8]For proforms as indicators of co-reference see Beaugrande and Dressler (1981; pp. 60ff); Halliday and Hasan (1976, pp. 31ff); Levelt (1983a, pp. 284ff).
[9]Berko Gleason et al. (1980); Dressler (1980a); Koll-Stobbe (1985a, pp. 13, 24ff, 1985b, pp. 75ff); Nespoulous (1980); Nespoulous and Lecours (1980); Ulatowska et al. (1981, 1983).
[10]Kaczmarek (1984a, p. 52, Table 12 second row) found the following global distribution of pronouns (percentages of all words used), Wernicke's: 25:1; anomics: 23.4; Broca's: 17.1.
[11]Cf. Beaugrande and Dressler (1981, pp. 71ff); Dijk (1977a; 1977b pp. 43ff,); Halliday and Hasan (1976, pp. 226ff); Schiffrin (1986).
[12]Cf. Dijk (1977a, chapter 3 & 4); Lang (1976). For aphasia cf. Koll-Stobbe (1985a, pp. 39ff).
[13]Cf. Buckingham (1979, pp. 247ff), Quinting (1971); and outside aphasia Fillmore (1979), McNeill (1979, pp. 216ff), Quasthoff (1979, 4.1).
[14]For an analysis of verbal perseverations see Stark (1984).
[15]Kaczmarek's (1985a, p. 71, Table 14, rows 5, 7) numbers for incomplete and elliptic constructions (put together are: Wernicke's, 43.5; Broca's, 33; anomics, 31.
[16]Cf. Bhatnagar (1980, p. 16), Luria (1976, IIb), Peuser (1978a, p. 289).
[17]Similar results are found in Dressler (1980a), Engel (1977), Huber & Gleber (1982), Nespoulous (1980), Nespoulous & Lecours (1980), Ulatowska et al. (1981, 1983b).
[18]For text comprehension in general see Dijk and Kintsch (1983); Rickheit & Kock (1983).
[19]In text processing the hearer concentrates on information-loaded words (cf. Linell, 1983, pp. 185ff), sentences, and greater textual chunks (cf. Walker & Meyer, 1980); Dijk & Kintsch, 1983; Beaugrande & Dressler, 1981, chapter 7; Reinhart, 1984, on the foregrounded story line).
[20]In the next years we will be able to compare systematically the improvements observed in 40 aphasics given therapy with results from a parallel group of 40 aphasics not given therapy during the interval between the two rounds of tests. On text therapy in general see Andresen and Redder, 1985.

8
Aspects of Automatic versus Controlled Processing, Monitoring, Metalinguistic Tasks, and Related Phenomena in Aphasia[1]

JACQUELINE A. STARK

People can be aware of their language at many different levels, from the automatic, vitually unconscious monitoring of their own speech to the rapid switching of languages by professional translators to the detailed analytic work of linguists. (Clark, 1978, p. 17)

Introduction

In aphasia research, tests designed to probe the "many different levels" of language processing have become more refined in the past decades. Lexical decision making, monitoring, masking, and other on-line tasks are continually being improved. Even data from so-called "simple" or classical language tasks such as repetition, spontaneous speech, and naming are now being reinterpreted along numerous dimensions. In this context the question arises, how can one make sense of the various—sometimes surprisingly contradictory—results? Related to this question is the entire issue of what "level" or aspects of language processing are really being tapped in a particular task. This chapter grew out of my efforts to piece together data from several apparently conflicting basic areas of aphasia research. The main issues to be addressed are the following:[2]

1. How can the differentiation controlled versus automatic processing be applied to aphasic language performance?

In association with question 1, the following two questions will also be addressed, but in less detail:

2. What is meant by the term "monitoring"? What does impaired self-monitoring performance tell us about the aphasic's language-processing abilities?
3. What aspects or "levels" of processing are tapped in metalinguistic tasks such as grammaticality judgments and lexical decision tasks?

An attempt will be made to deal with these questions separately.

Controlled and Automatic Processing from a Developmental Perspective

The distinction controlled/automatic processing can best be understood starting from a developmental perspective and normal language performance (cf. Brown, 1976; Karmiloff-Smith, 1986; Pick, 1931). The reason for using the developmental framework as a starting-point for this discussion is that—by analogy with use of aphasic language data as an important source for delineating the components of language production in normal language processing—in development we may see various aspects of language processing that have become so intermingled in the adult speaker that isolating the more automatic from the more conscious or controlled components is even more difficult. I do not intend to make statements with respect to the regression hypothesis, but rather to refer to the normal and developmental literature whenever particular aspects are considered informative and applicable to aphasia.

The issue of the language abilities or linguistic skills involved in automatic versus controlled processing has been discussed in the child language development literature in terms of stages or levels of linguistic and/or cognitive development (e.g., memory), in particular the development of language awareness/controlled processing/conscious access, and in terms of the acquisition and/or automatization of a complex skill such as reading.

Stages/Levels of Linguistic and/or Cognitive Development

Exemplary of the work on stages or levels of linguistic development is Nelson and Nelson's (1978) cognitive pendulum theory. In this theory a distinction is made between child-level changes and system changes. The authors proposed five stages that apply to system development.[3] Of these five, the fourth and fifth stage are relevant to the present discussion (p. 228):

Stage 4. Integration and consolidation of the rule structure (stable, coordinated rules)

Stage 5. Flexible monitoring and conscious extension (adaptive, conscious rule use)

Stage 4 covers a period of overrigidity during which the system becomes integrated and autonomous and also resistant to interference. It is at this time that "the child's abilities to reflect on and directly refer to the system and to monitor its operation advance" (p. 227). The final step of system changes is one of flexible extension in which the child is adaptive and shows "conscious" rule use. Nelson and Nelson stressed that the final fifth stage of mature and flexible rule application may or may not be observed in all cases. Essential for the fifth stage—if it does emerge—is that "for the first time in system development, a clear awareness of and ability to monitor how rules can be changed to suit context or task or mode of thought, a dimension on which further development of the system is likely" (p. 228). By stages 4 and 5 the child's linguistic system is stable and demonstrates mastery of many rules, that is, more controlled processing.

Planning and monitoring of cognitive processes involve reflection on the systems and structures themselves, and this reflection is aided by steady developmental periods. In these periods, previously acquired rules and concepts are repeatedly applied. Nelson and Nelson noted a pendulum swing at about 7 to 12 years of age, including the following:

1. With reference to information storage and retrieval, attention becomes highly concentrated on central task information.
2. In terms of "a higher-order system of conscious monitoring and planning, the child, regardless of his or her stage level for the system, may tend toward a relatively narrow scope for rules" (p. 265).

From the foregoing, the developmental process can be viewed as an advancement toward stable rule use, flexibility, and progression in differentiation on all levels of language processing, that is, toward more conscious access, awareness, or monitoring of linguistic units, which in turn results in or is an expression of an increasing automatization in linguistic processing. Conscious access is not to be equated totally with controlled processing. There is, however, a close relationship between the two concepts.

Unconscious Metaprocesses and Conscious Access

Karmiloff-Smith (1986) explored the relation between unconscious metaprocesses and those processes available to conscious access and verbal statement[4] within the framework of a recurrent three-phase model of language development.[5] Implicitly defined representations are distinguished from progressive representational explicitation at several levels of processing, which results in the possibility of conscious access. Several aspects of Karmiloff-Smith's process-oriented model are applicable to analysis of aphasic language performance, and in particular to the issue of controlled versus automatic processing.

According to Karmiloff-Smith, metaprocesses—which lie between acquisition processes and conscious statable awareness—are an unconscious, fundamental aspect of the way in which a developing child spontaneously works on linguistic representations outside normal input/output relations. Conscious access is not implied, for example, in representational organization, rather it is linked to other metaprocesses that are unconscious in nature.

Karmiloff-Smith posited four levels of representation on which she based her model of representational change:

1. Implicit knowledge (I): Knowledge that is not defined representationally. The components of a procedure run through in their totality and cannot be accessed or operated on separately.
2. Primary explicitation (E-i): On the second level, implicit knowledge is redescribed in E-i form. "Representational redescription means that the knowledge components of a procedure can now be operated on internally, i.e. they are accessible to the operation of metaprocedural processes which make possible the explicit defining of relationships across representations within each code. (p. 102)"
3. Secondary explicitation (E-ii): Within the same code any particular knowledge was originally coded in at the E-i level, a second redescription takes place, resulting in representations available for conscious access, that is, in E-ii representations.
4. Tertiary explicitations (E-iii): On this level, "the organism makes use of representational redescription to translate E-ii representations from one code into another" (p. 103). The result is an abstract code. Only at this level (E-iii) can multiple representations of the same knowledge—existing in different codes—become explicitly linked by means of a common code (cf. Hunt & Lansman, 1986). Redescription and explicitation on the third (E-ii) and fourth (E-iii) levels occur only after each three-phase cycle is completed. Metalinguistic data demonstrate that explicitly defined relationships (cf. note 4) ultimately become available to conscious access.

Self-repairs—which occur prior to conscious access—are indices of representational change. All representations that pass from I to E-i form may be automatically scanned as part of the metaprocedural operation. Conscious awareness results from representational redescription from E-i to E-ii/E-iii form.

With regard to the metalinguistic and repair data, Karmiloff-Smith found similar developmental patterns: Children become progressively sensitive to or aware of the mapping between linguistic markers and extralinguistic contexts. Karmiloff-Smith considered metalinguistic awareness to be the end product of representational explicitation and not a prerequisite for it. The content of consciousness is the result of a complex process of representational redescription and explicitation. She viewed consciousness as the developmentally highest level of representational explicitation.

Metaprocesses in Aphasic Disorders

Pertaining to the status of metaprocesses in various types of aphasic disorders, it may be that the metaprocedural operations are differentially set in motion or are impaired and thus not set in motion, that is, are inhibited. Another possibility is that the metaprocedural operations proceed well, but the results of these operations cannot be passed on for further linguistic processing. Further, the operation of metaprocedures can only be assessed by means of specific well-defined tasks. One potential explanation for many types of aphasic errors is that they stem from an overtaxing of the processing system due to metaprocedural operations, that is, due to the redescription of the phase 1 representations (I representations) into E-i form.

One indication that metaprocedural operations are, however, at work for the aphasic is when the aphasic makes self-repairs. The issue of self-repairs will be discussed in short. An analysis of other trouble-indicating behavior such as pauses, editing terms, and the entire issue of timing in language planning and production would shed light on the interaction of such behavior with assumed ongoing metaprocedural operations.

Distinguishing between implicitly defined and explicitly defined representations has implications for analysis of aphasic language production, namely, that the degree of severity of language impairment or the specific type of aphasic deficit may be correlated to differential impairment of the four levels of representation. Severely impaired aphasics might be described as having reduced overall performance or having performance in specific domains reduced to representations in the form of implicit knowledge. Examples from global aphasics illustrate this point.

Concerning secondary explicitation, an aphasic's language performance may indicate that he or she can achieve level E-i but not level E-ii due to the severity of the language impairment or the specific type of deficit. The second redescription does not take place, and thus representations do not become available for conscious access. Milberg and Blumstein's results (1981; Blumstein, Milberg, & Schrier, 1982) on semantic processing in aphasia, in particular by the Wernicke's group, can be cited in this context. The Wernicke's aphasics demonstrated semantic priming effects, that is, unconscious automatic semantic processing in lexical decision tasks. Perhaps these subjects can achieve only E-i level representations and not tertiary explicitation (i.e., E-iii level representations), which would be necessary in performing more "abstract" semantic judgment tasks, which showed impairment in Wernicke's aphasics. A possible interpretation of this is that there is no linkage (or linkage is reduced) among multiple representations.

Since the E-ii and E-iii levels of redescription and explicitation occur only after each three-phase cycle is completed for a particular aspect of the linguistic system, one could posit that there is a potential natural break-off point following the E-i level of knowledge representation for aspects of the linguistic system, and that complex dissociations in aphasic processing might be adequately described in terms of these four levels of representation.

Karmiloff-Smith posited that a child can be at different phases for different aspects of language: Certain aspects of a particular form may be treated metaprocedurally at the lexemic level and simultaneously the same form is treated metaprocedurally at the cross-lexemic level. The possibility that an aphasic demonstrates use of different levels for the same linguistic form would also explain some diverging results (e.g., modality-specific impairments or differential impairment of the same form on different levels. The agrammatic's use of articles (definite and indefinite)—if they are produced at all—appears to be intact on the text or discourse level but is impaired on the syntactic or sentence level (cf. Stark & Dressler, 1988, and chapter 6).

Dissociations between modalities for the same knowledge could therefore be postulated to stem from an impairment of the E-iii level of representation: Knowledge existing in different codes cannot be explicitly linked, that is, redescribed by means of a common abstract code. The aphasic's dissociations are in fact more often multiple ones and thus very complex to delineate (cf. Shallice, 1987).

In Karmiloff-Smith's model, the output of phase 3 is postulated to be generated from explicitly linked memory entries represented in E-i form. In aphasia, perhaps the memory entries in E-i form are not accessible or are not explicitly linked (cf. Shallice, 1987). The nonaccessibility, differentially impaired accessibility, or irretrievability of particular linguistic units, for example, of closed class items in Broca's aphasics, has been postulated by several authors to account for the agrammatic's deficits. With reference to the word-finding difficulty in anomic and other aphasia types, it could be that explicit definition of internal representational links exists; however, the forms cannot be generated from E-i-form explicitly linked memory entries. It might also be that the anomic's impairment derives from impairment of a deeper level, because the forms cannot be explicitly linked.

Karmiloff-Smith claimed that all representations that pass from I to E-i form may be automatically scanned as part of metaprocedural operations. Is this to be taken as evidence why certain representations may or may not be automatically scanned? That is, depending on whether or not the representations pass from I to E-i form, they will or will not be automatically scanned. And if they are not automatically scanned, can they be scanned by means of controlled processing? These questions serve as a starting point for an interpretation of the processing deficits in agrammatism, for which I shall offer a possible account in terms of automatic and controlled processing.

Although Karmiloff-Smith's model pertains to the child's cognitive development, it offers interesting reference points for analysis of various aphasic phenomena, for example, for analysis of the aphasic's major language symptoms in terms of the four levels of knowledge representation. In response to question 3, given at the beginning of this chapter, it will be shown that it is essential to have an explicit definition/description of the task demands in order to determine dissociations, in particular in terms of levels of knowledge representation.

In aphasia, impairment of the ability to explicitly define relationships across redescribed existing representations or the redescription itself might be impaired in specific ways determined by the type of aphasia or with reference to a particular task (cf. question 3). It could also be the case that the ability to switch from one code to another is impaired or that the number of codes available to the aphasic is reduced. Each of these points could be the topic of lengthy discussions. I have mentioned only aspects of Karmiloff-Smith's model that I assume are illuminating to aphasia research, in particular to research on automatic and controlled processing.

Whereas Karmiloff-Smith spoke of the development of conscious access to represented knowledge as a continual constructive process in which greater explicitation occurs and in which consciousness is considered to be the highest level developmentally of representational explicitation (cf. also Clark, 1978),[6] other authors have distinguished the types of processing right from the start in terms of varying developmental patterns.

Deliberate Versus Automatic Processing

Naus and Halasz (1979) suggested that developmental patterns of deliberate processing and automatic processing are quite different, that is, that they are operationally independent.[7] They discussed the issue with reference to the structure of semantic memory within the levels of processing framework (Craik & Lockhart, 1972; Cermak & Craik, 1979). The essence of their distinction is that deliberate memory tasks are those that involve the use of mnemonic strategies, that is, a voluntary plan purposely adopted by the subject to improve memory performance. In contrast, involuntary memory tasks are those in which memory is the unplanned product of a person's continuous interaction with a meaningful environment. When a stimulus is highly compatible with a particular level of semantic analysis, it may be impossible to prevent processing from occurring at that level. That is, processing takes place automatically. The authors mentioned that although these two types of processing are viewed as independent components, performance in any given task necessarily requires an interaction of both types.

The different developmental patterns for the two types of processing are held to be useful in differentiating them. Deliberate processing begins as conscious planful mnemonic activity designed to accomplish a given task. The mnemonic strategies become maximally efficient through practice and repetition, requiring fewer analyses and a minimum of processing to accomplish the same task. With respect to metamemory and deliberate memory processes, Naus and Halasz pointed out that their development seems highly interdependent—though the relationship between them is extremely complicated. Developmental changes in deliberate memory processing affect metamemory by mediating changes in semantic memory.

The development of automatic processes progresses in connection with that of the structure and contents of semantic memory. Automatic processes are determined by the properties of the stimulus with reference to semantic memory structures. Therefore, due to changes in semantic memory, corresponding changes result in the available automatic processes. According to Naus and Halasz, any model of memory must view memory as an active constructive process that operates on the basis of the current knowledge and semantic organization of the individual. The features of memory processing according to Naus and Halasz's dichotomy are summarized in Table 8.1.

Naus and Halasz drew attention to the similar distinction made by Shiffrin and Schneider (1977; Schneider & Shiffrin, 1977) between automatic and controlled (strategic) processing, and by Posner and Snyder (1975) and LaBerge and Samuels (1974) between limited-capacity, strategically controlled processes and unlimited-capacity, automatic processes. Naus and Halasz stressed that "while these conceptualizations are complementary to the automatic/strategic distinction in the[ir] present paper, the developmental literature further suggests that automatic processing may operate throughout the memory system rather than simply in low-level perceptual tasks as demonstrated in the human performance literature" (p. 277). Their assertion that automatic processing may operate throughout the memory system rather than only in low-level perceptual tasks (such as consistent mapping category search and visual detection tasks) has important consequences for an understanding of aphasic language deficits in contrast to "surprising" intact performance in specific areas of language processing.

TABLE 8.1. Characteristics of Memory Processing[a]

Deliberate
Voluntary, planful
Generated by subject in response to specific task demands
May or may not be conscious
Requires attention
Developmental trends demonstrated by production deficiencies and related to metamemory
Automatic
Involuntary, unplanned
Elicited by environmental stimuli and the contents of semantic memory
Unconscious
Typically does not require attention
Few developmental trends

[a]According to Naus and Halasz, 1979, p. 263

Moreover, if Naus and Halasz's assumption can be upheld that the two types of memory processing derive from different developmental patterns, that is, develop qualitatively differently, accounting for specific dissociations in aphasic language processing or memory performance would be more feasible on the basis of this distinction. For example, a dissociation between automatic and controlled voluntary production of the same linguistic forms would be when an aphasic can automatically produce an utterance but cannot voluntarily produce the same utterance by means of controlled processing (cf. question 2). Further, the whole issue of how automatic and controlled/voluntary processing are to be viewed emerges: Are they separate entities of a dichotomy deriving from different processes (right from the start of development)? Or are they to be viewed as two ends of a continuum?

In addition to Naus and Halasz, representative of the first view is Marcel (1983a,b). Although he took a completely different approach from that of Naus and Halasz, Marcel examined the relation of automatic nonconscious processing to conscious representations and intentional processes. He claimed that the conscious representation of something is often qualitatively different from its nonconscious representation. The essence of his view is that phenomenal percepts depend not only on nonconscious sensory analysis (or activity in such mechanisms), but also on certain further operations that render the form of the phenomenal representation qualitatively different. The intentional aspect of phenomenal experience derives from these further operations (Marcel, 1983b, p. 243). Thus, according to Marcel, conscious representations and nonconscious representations differ qualitatively and have different effects.

Classical Information-Processing Studies

Representative of the continuum view would be the classical information-processing studies on controlled and automatic processing, including those by Schneider and Shiffrin (1977), Shiffrin and Schneider (1977), Posner and Snyder (1975), Neely (1977), LaBerge and Samuels (1974), and Shallice (1972). In these studies the degree or amount of practice in relation to the task demands is an important factor in the development of automatic processing. A listing of the properties—demonstrating the aspects of progression, that is, change from controlled to automatic processing—various authors have attributed to both types of processing is given in Table 8.2.

Factors in Automaticity Development

From the rich literature of information-processing studies, LaBerge and Samuels' (1974) study is summarized here because of these authors' treatment of the factors that may influence the development of automaticity:

TABLE 8.2. Characteristics of Automatic and Controlled Processing

Automatic Processing

Definition

Activation of a learned sequence of elements in long-term memory, initiated by appropriate inputs and proceeding automatically without subject control, without stress on the capacity limitations of the system, and without necessarily demand for attention (Schneider & Shiffrin, 1977)

General Properties

Posner & Snyder (1975): Automatic spreading-activation process that (a) is fast acting, (b) occurs without intention or conscious awareness, (c) does not affect retrieval of information stored in semantically unrelated logogens to which it has not spread
Schneider & Shiffrin (1977): Automatic processes (a) are not hindered by capacity limitations of STS and do not require attention; (b) may sometimes be initiated under subject control, but once initiated all run to completion automatically; (c) require considerable training to develop and are most difficult to modify, once learned; (d) have speed and automaticity that usually keep their constituent elements hidden from conscious perception; (e) do not directly cause new learning in LTS; and (f) performance levels gradually improve as automatic sequence is learned.

Controlled Processing

Definition

Temporary activation of a sequence of elements that can be set up, modified, and utilized quickly and easily in new situations but that requires attention, is capacity limited, (i.e., uses up short-term capacity [usually serial in nature]), and is controlled by the subject (Schneider & Shiffrin, 1977)

General Properties

Posner & Snyder (1975): Limited-capacity attentional mechanism that (a) is slow acting, (b) cannot operate without intention and conscious awareness, and (c) inhibits retrieval of information stored in semantically unrelated logogens upon which it is not focused.
Schneider & Shiffrin (1977): Control processes (a) are limited capacity processes requiring attention; (b) have limitations based on those of STS (such as limited-comparison rate and limited amount of information that can be retained without loss); (c) can be adopted quickly, without extensive training, and can be modified fairly easily; (d) can be used to control flow of information within and between levels, and between STS and LTS; and (e) can show rapid development of asymptotic performance.

LTS = long term store; STS = short term store.

"One of the prime issues in the study of a complex skill such as reading is to determine how the processing of component subskills becomes automatic" (p. 293). For LaBerge and Samuels, the criterion for deciding when a skill or subskill is automatic is that its processing can be completed while attention is directed elsewhere.[8] Among the factors assumed to be decisive in the rate of growth of automaticity are practice (repetitions), distribution of learning (massed versus distributed practice), and presentation of feedback. With respect to feedback, LaBerge and Samuels maintained that, since the important growth of automaticity takes place after the subject has achieved accuracy, overt feedback for correct or incorrect responses may be considered redundant. By this stage of learning the child knows when he or she is correct or not. (Cf. Karmiloff-Smith [1986] on the role of positive feedback in the development of knowledge representation in contrast to the assumption of negative feedback in Marshall and Morton's [1978] model [called EMMA].)

LaBerge and Samuels indicated that two criteria—automaticity and accuracy—are used to evaluate the degree of learning of the processing that occurs at various stages in reading. At the accuracy level of performance, attention is considered necessary for processing. Attention is also required for the reorganization into larger (i.e, higher-order) units in reading. In contrast, at the automatic level of performance, attention is not assumed necessary for processing.

With the previously discussed aspects (e.g., of Karmiloff-Smith's developmental model, Naus & Halasz's views, and the characteristics of automatic/controlled processing listed in Table 8.2) in mind, I would like to address the aphasia literature. Since the features of the two types of processing listed in Tables 8.1 and 8.2 have been arrived at on the basis of various experiments, I would like to adopt those properties of automatic and controlled processing. I would like to add one restriction to the general properties: Although automatic processing is considered to operate unconsciously, whereas controlled processing is considered to operate intentionally with conscious awareness, I assume that the overall speed of language processing—even subsequent to brain damage—indicates that the "awareness" aspect of controlled processing is a matter of degree. That is, in normal language processing such rapid interaction/integration of the two types of processing is required that the differentiation according to fast/slow acting and unconscious/conscious is relative. In this context, an overall slowing down of processing is also relative. In other words, the entire process of producing/perceiving language has become so automatized over time in development and due to constant use, that the automaticity of the separate processing types reduces the differences between them with reference to speed of processing and amount of awareness necessary to operate. Differences between the two types of processing are none the less real; however, they must be seen in the proper perspective.

It can be assumed that the adult aphasic premorbidly possessed a "complete" linguistic system in which explicitly defined relationships were available to conscious access, that is, levels I to E-iii can be assumed with regard to the language knowledge and skills of each patient before onset of illness. Under normal conditions, a great deal of the average healthy speaker's language processing is more or less automatic. In general, I assume that, aside from the necessity of controlled processing in the phase of formulating a thought/idea (ideation),[9] more controlled processing becomes necessary when the speaker/hearer runs into difficulties or when the speaker is dealing with complex topics or semantically processing at a "deeper level" of interpretation. For the aphasic, I suggest that automatic processing is either reduced, inhibited, or disinhibited in characteristic ways. The interaction/integration between automatic and controlled processing is thus qualitatively different in the various aphasia types, resulting in specific processing deficits. Thus, these deficits can in turn be interpreted with reference to the distinction between automatic/controlled processing. (I shall return to this point in short with respect to agrammatism/paragrammatism.)

That automatic processing is affected in brain-damaged patients has often been regarded as or linked to one of the general indicators or nonlocalizing symptoms of focal brain damage, which are so difficult to describe in an adequate manner—for example, general slowing in performance, longer reaction times, and so on. Although these nonspecific symptoms are so difficult to separate from the specific focal, localizing symptoms, application of the automatic/controlled distinction is informative in determining and understanding the specific processing deficits (cf. Stark, 1984).

The aforementioned studies from the literature on development and processing in healthy persons provide background for the aphasia studies and data. The aphasia literature on this subject is not as comprehensive as the studies on healthy people, although an increase in interest is observed. As will become evident, few of the studies on automatic versus controlled processing are experimental in nature. Rather, they consist of descriptions of aspects of the aphasic's performance with regard to automatic and/or controlled processing being intact, reduced, or impaired. Another topic in the aphasia literature is the relation between automatization and neuroanatomy.

The Automatic/Controlled Processing Distinction in Aphasia Research

Any aphasiological discussion would be incomplete without referring briefly to the classical aphasia literature, especially to the work of A. Pick. In his comprehensive treatment of diverse topics in aphasiology, Pick also dealt with the issue of automatic processing versus voluntary processing with respect to normal development and aphasia. From Pick's ideas, I mention only a few that are relevant to the present discussion.

Pick viewed "Einstellung" (attitude, determining tendency)—the term for certain manifest processes not demonstrable in consciousness—as a predominantly automatic and unconscious process that can hardly or only deficiently be substituted by a voluntary act, if at all (cf. Pick, 1931, p. 1449). Pick also drew attention to the detrimental effect of interfering with the automatic process of grammaticalization—the automatic processes often being better than the voluntary (cf. p. 1474). In a discussion of the economy hypothesis of agrammatism, Pick stressed that with the least expenditure of work, aphasics automatically adapt their best available linguistic means to express themselves as clearly as possible under the circumstances. A speaker calls special attention to those essential parts of the almost entirely present "unitary" thought for transfer to the executive apparatus. Other aspects put forward by Pick pertaining to automatic/controlled processing will be mentioned at the appropriate places in this text.

In an essay on consciousness and pathology of language, Brown (1976) interpreted jargon, semantic paraphasia, stereotypy, and echo responses—with reference to his model of cognitive organization—as forms of aphasic language characterized by "deficient insight." Several of Brown's remarks bear upon the distinction automatic/controlled processing (volitional speech). For example, Brown interpreted the differences and transition between stereotypic and volitional speech as follows: The stereotypy evolves from complete automaticity without awareness, through modification and then blocking, which is at first partial and incomplete. The stereotypy may alternate with some volitional speech at a later stage. The final stage reveals a transition: The stereotypy, which is signaled by the return of volitional speech, is completely inhibited.

The echo reaction is considered to be closely related to stereotypy. Echo reactions and semantic jargon are also discussed in term of four stages. With reference to echo reactions, the fourth stage is normal repetition, whereas with reference to semantic jargon, the fourth stage is anomia. From Brown's discussion of the aphasic language forms, it appears that lack of awareness can more or less be equated with automaticity. For Brown, volitional behavior always incorporates purposefulness (e.g., controlled accessing of a word by the anomic).

Whitaker's Brain Model of Automatization

Whitaker (1983) reflected on automatization in a discussion of a brain model of automatization, which he termed the "concentric-ring" model. He viewed the development of automatization in part as a process of "focalization," that is, of using less brain, and in part as a process of "localization," that is, of shifting functions to the perisylvian/perirolandic core (p. 199). Whitaker maintained that the cortex surrounding the Sylvian fissures is responsible for the automatized components of language. He divided the acquired behaviors into automatized and volitional behaviors, although he stressed that these two types are better described as ends of a continuum (p. 199):

← Automatized ———————————————— Volitional →
habitual ——— practiced ——— familiar ——— variable ——— novel

In his classification the automatized behaviors are characterized as structured or formulaic acts, which exhibit a well-defined path through the neural network; they are "executed with a minimum of attention, a high level of consistency and a low energy demand in a rapid and timely manner" (p. 199). In contrast, the volitional acts are described as acts that demand more focal attention.

Speech and language are necessarily composed of complex interactions of automatized and volitional acts, at several different levels. A working premise for Whitaker is that language processing "must incorporate packages or chunks of automatized skills or acts at each linguistic level: phonological, syntactic and semantic" (p. 199). He stressed that the process of automatization of components of speech and language does not render these components unavailable to attentional mechanisms (p. 203). In normal language use, however, one does not attend to or analyze these components for language use to proceed "smoothly, efficiently and in a reasonable time frame" (p. 203). LaBerge and Samuels (1974) also maintained that "during the execution of a complex skill, it is necessary to coordinate many component processes within a very short period of time. If each component process requires attention, performance of the complex skill will be impossible, because the capacity of attention will be exceeded" (p. 293).

In a discussion of a case of isolation of the language function (patient H.C.E.M.), Whitaker (1976, p. 51) delineated a neurolinguistic account of language in terms of three levels—speech, automatic, and volitional language—which is reproduced in Table 8.3. H.C.E.M.'s linguistic behavior was described as being intact with regard to levels (I) and (II); level (III), however, was severely impaired. That is, only the aspects of automatic language were correctly produced by the patient. The importance of

TABLE 8.3. Neurolinguistic Framework of Levels of Language Functions[a]

Level I	Accurate auditory perception Accurate verbal production	Speech
Level II	Intact phonological organization (phonemic patterns, stress, and intonation, etc.); overlearned aspects of grammatical organization which become automatic (late rules of syntactic agreement, function words, etc.); probably certain semantic features of lexical items in addition to phonological ones and certain overlearned phrases and verbal automatisms	Language (automatic, nonvolitional)
Level III	Cognition, intellectual functions, and creative aspects of language	Language (creative, volitional)

such a case as this is that a clear dissociation between automatic and volitional (controlled) processing is apparent.

Whitaker (1983) also discussed examples of aphasia and dementia that demonstrate dissociations between automatic and volitional language. Of the 10 case examples discussed, only 4 are cited here briefly to illustrate how this distinction has been used in the aphasia literature.

Case 1. Patient with apraxia of speech, who produced phonological-articulatory errors. Analysis of the errors reveals that the phonological pattern—which is assumed to be retrieved automatically—cannot be retrieved.

Case 2. Broca's aphasic with agrammatism. An impairment of automatized sentence-level routines is postulated for the deficit in language production. This patient demonstrated a "... higher level impairment in automatized language, [which affects] the level of surface syntactic markers such as the articles, forms of the verb 'to be,' some prepositions, auxilary verbs and the like" (p. 202).

Case 3. Foreign accent syndrome. Loss of the level of automatization of motor-articulatory patterns is involved. This results in the mispronunciation of segments and syllables; the patient thus sounded foreign.

Case 4. In the previously mentioned case (H.C.E.M.) discussed by Whitaker (1976, p. 51), the patient had an extensive lesion and showed global impairment of volitional speech and language, in the context of preserved automatized aspects of speech and language (cf. Table 8.3), echolalia, and verbal completion.

In commenting on Schwartz, Marin, and Saffran's (1979) study, in which the authors contrasted the performance on a particular task of a presenile demented patient with that of an agrammatic patient, Whitaker (1983) observed that: "The contrast between the performance of the agrammatic patient who knows what the task requires but does not have the automaticized elements available to perform it and the demented patient who does not really understand the task but does have the automaticized elements available with which to do it, is quite striking" (p. 208).

On the basis of Whitaker's four examples, the generalization that presents itself is that what is to be considered the main impairment of the patient—whether a sentence-level, phonological, or semantic processing deficit—is a reduction/loss in automatization for that particular area of language processing. In contrast, in the case of dementia, the description of language abilities is given in terms of those that are still intact, that is, that function automatically.

Whitaker also discussed the issue of automatization in relation to patients who received the Wada test before neurosurgery for epilepsy. The results were that the grammatical function words and the syntactic structure of the sentence, as well as the articulation patterns associated with the function words, were the first to return to normal functioning, whereas other units of language, for example, verbs, nouns, and adjectives, returned later (cf. Whitaker, 1983, p. 210). In this context, the similarity of units of language that return first after the sodium amytal clears versus the language units that return later, and the transparent levels (levels 1 to 3) versus the opaque semantic level (level 4) discussed by Perfetti (1979) is noteworthy (cf. discussion of my question 3). Whitaker's explanation for this pattern is that the cortical regions that support automatized functions, the perisylvian/perirolandic core, are cleared of amytal first, followed by the volitional ones. Thus, the automatic aspects of language processing return first.

Pertaining to brain structure, Whitaker posited (a) that the perisylvian/perirolandic core of the brain is the most heavily myelinated and the most differentiated and (b) that, whereas the maturation of the cortex proceeds outwards from the perisylvian/perirolandic core, the process of automatization works in reverse, that is, inward to this core.

Very few aphasiologists have dealt with the topic of automatization in such great detail. Whitaker's neuroanatomical ideas on automatization are speculative, although interesting with respect to the automatic/volitional aspects of language. With reference to agrammatic Broca's aphasia, the dissociations discussed in the literature are more complex and must therefore be analyzed in a more differentiated manner (e.g., agrammatic language production, asyntactic comprehension in the presence of intact grammaticality judgments) than just considering them to be a reduction in automatic sentence-level routines (cf. for example, Caramazza & Berndt, 1985; Coltheart, 1987). If it turns out that a description in terms of a reduction of automatic sentence-level routines applies, it will still be necessary, however, to show (a) what the interaction between the modalities/tasks is and (b) how/in what manner the sentence-level routines are reduced in their automatization. Except for the data on metalinguistic tasks, for example, those of Linebarger et al. (1983), of Milberg and Blumstein (1981), of Blumstein et al. (1982), and of Tyler (1985, 1987), to be discussed with reference to question 3, experimental findings that explicitly pertain to the automatic/controlled distinction in accounting for the deficits and intact processing are lacking in the aphasia literature.

Controlled and Automatic Processing in Agrammatism: A Single Case Study

Recent discussions of agrammatism indicate that the agrammatic deficits are more complex than just speaking of them—across the board—as a reduction in automatic sentence-level routines (cf. Coltheart, Sartori, & Job, 1987). From the various publications, I would like to illustrate the application of automatic/controlled distinction with reference to a case study of Broca's aphasia by Nespoulous and colleagues (1985). From the various case studies discussed in the aphasia literature, I single out their case study because the authors explicitly referred to the automatic/controlled distinction in accounting for their patient's deficits/dissociations among sentence production, sentence comprehension, and metalinguistic tasks. I shall refer to other studies and my own observations for further clarification (cf. Stark & Dressler, 1988).

Nespoulous et al. suggested that their patient's basic underlying deficit of sentence production was not a "central" one, because performance on sentence comprehension and metalinguistic tasks was not impaired. The deficit is further described as not being syntactic at the "level of knowledge." They claimed "that the deficit is absent from any task involving more 'local' processing, such as [written] sentence completion tasks, thus indicating that 'conscious,' 'restricted' and 'strategic' processing is still available to him, a type of (limited-capacity) processing which is obviously unusable in all sentence and discourse production tasks, the latter requiring the 'automatic activation' of unconscious processes (Posner & Snyder, 1975) which are thus assumed to be at fault in our patient" (p. 29). Their application of the controlled versus automatic processing distinction and the proposal that the deficit is not syntactic at the level of knowledge is interesting. However, the pattern of dissociations their patient demonstrates appears to be even more complex. In Karmiloff-Smith's (1986) model, for example, four various levels of knowledge representation are postulated. Which level of knowledge Nespoulous et al. are referring to is not explicitly stated.

Nespoulous and colleagues' agrammatic patient's good performance on metalinguistic tasks is limited to written language tasks including grammaticality judgments and categorization of triads, that is, these authors report only on written/visual grammaticality judgments. Therefore, it is not clear whether the rather good performance of agrammatic Broca's aphasics on auditory grammaticality judgment tasks found by Linebarger et al. (1983) was also demonstrated by their patient or whether good performance was restricted to the written grammaticality judgments.

Oral sentence completion (story completion test) was described by Nespoulous et al. as being impaired in the same manner as all other sentence production tasks. In contrast, written sentence completion did not show impairment. (The difference in complexity between the written and oral sentence completion tasks is noteworthy: requiring the patient to write in a missing word (e.g., Cloze test) in comparison to requiring oral completion of a sentence for which at most the subject noun phrase is supplied.) Thus, on the surface the dissociation their agrammatic patient shows is rather primarily a dissociation between orally produced and written language. I posit that the dissociation between conscious/controlled and automatic processing must therefore be elucidated with respect to the oral/written language functions in the following way:

In all language tasks—especially with reference to the aphasic—a complex combination and interaction of automatic and voluntary processing is necessary. On the surface, restricted conscious processing does not seem so available to the patient of Nespoulous et al. either. Otherwise one would expect an intact performance, for example, in the oral reading of sentences/discourse. In this task the patient theoretically can locally, consciously, and strategically process words, that is, can read one word at a time, especially since he or she is not under a time constraint. However, their patient's performance on oral reading of text and on reading sentences with several personal pronouns was described as massively disturbed. Although performance on single word reading was accurate, performance on a task of vertical reading was not, and was very interesting. When reading aloud separate words—which actually built up to form a sentence—the patient apparently realized he was reading a sentence by about the third or fourth word. At that point, errors began to be made that were similar to those made in oral sentence production.

Conscious, restricted, strategic processing is definitely usable in all sentence and discourse production tasks. Moreover, it would seem even more necessary when automatic processing is inhibited, reduced, or impaired. An indication that conscious, controlled processing was also affected is that the patient of Nespoulous et al. made errors even when focusing his attention on the form to be produced both in oral sentence production tasks (i.e., in so-called "on-line," time-constrained tasks) and in tasks without any time constraints. The dimension fluency also relates to the concept of automatization in that when fluency is greatly reduced, all language processing becomes more conscious.

In analogy with this point, LaBerge and Samuels (1974) pointed out with respect to reading that every time a word requires attention the reader is made aware of that aspect of the reading process. Moreover, the slower the rate of learning to read, the more the learning reader becomes aware of the component stages. An example is given of learning to read blends: "If a good deal of attention is required for him to be accurate in sounding letter patterns, then 'blending' will be more difficult to perform owing to the total number of things he must attend to and hold in short-term memory" (p. 319). The role of repetition is also considered in this context: "To perceive an entirely new word or other combination of strokes requires considerable time, close attention and is likely to be imperfectly done . . . In either case, repetition progressively frees the mind from attention to details, makes facile the total act, shortens the time, and reduces the extent to which consciousness must concern itself with the process" (Huey, 1908, p. 104, cited by LaBerge & Samuels, 1974).

To return to Nespoulous and colleagues' agrammatic aphasic, sentence repetition was also impaired—he could neither automatically repeat the target sentence nor consciously attend to the stimulus and correctly repeat it. Therefore, I claim that the combination of intact and impaired language processing displayed by this patient requires another interpretation. That is, although I agree that the agrammatic's deficits can be described with reference to the automatic/controlled distinction, I interpret the role of these two types of processing differently.

Even when attention is focused on producing particular forms one by one, this patient did not correctly produce an utterance. I would like to interpret this in another way: Since the patient is concentrating on particular aspects of processing, that is, is processing in a very controlled manner, the automatic processing the patient might otherwise be able to make use of or demonstrate is inhibited. The overall slowing down of processing due to concentrated use of controlled processing is also reflected by reduced fluency or rate of production. In other words, I assume that either the automatic processing, involved in producing an utterance is inhibited right from the start and, unconsciously, controlled processing immediately takes over, or controlled processing immediately takes control and the automatic processing—whether otherwise reduced, inhibited, or whatever—does not have a chance to automatically contribute to the conscious production of an utterance. There is a chain reaction effect. However, it is difficult to determine what is the cause and what is the effect in ongoing language production. The result is clear: Interaction/integration between the two forms of processing does not function/develop adequately.

The Production Activation Model and Agrammatism/Paragrammatism

A summary of the characteristics of automatic and controlled processing postulated on the basis of detection, category search, categorization tasks, and so on has been provided in Table 8.2. However, I would like to analyze the agrammatic's performance in greater detail with reference to a model, namely, the production activation model put forward by Hunt and Lansman (1986), which was developed to handle problem solving, that is, to handle complex tasks more comparable to natural language processing than the tasks on which, for example, Shiffrin and Schneider (1977, etc.) based their hypotheses. Two ideas are basic to the Hunt–Lansman model:

1. A semantic network to activate the elements of long term memory
2. A production system to manipulate information in working memory

According to this model, a production is a pattern–action pair. A stimulus initiates two different concurrent forms of information processing, namely:

Controlled. This form depends on the execution of a sequence of productions. It involves the interaction between a set of productions stored in long-term memory and a blackboard area that contains information about the current situation.

Automatic. This form involves the spread of activation from one production, that is, from one node in a semantic network, to its associates within long-term memory. Although indirect dependencies exist, the spread of activation is independent of the presence of information in working memory.

In controlled processing, at each step in the sequence part of a production pattern is recognized as being part of the present stimulus complex. The stimulus complex includes information in working memory. The following actions can be taken: An action that will change the configuration of working memory, an action that will initiate an overt response, or an action that will do both. This process then continues: The new configuration of working memory serves as a trigger for further pattern recognitions and actions. The blackboard is described as consisting of external sensory channels and working memory. The pattern segment of each production is continuously compared with information in the blackboard area. The production is executed only if a match is found.

Computations within a cycle, that is, finite steps of time, are functionally in parallel. Within a cycle, at most one semantic, auditory production may be selected for execution. It is assumed that the larger the patterns the production can use, the fewer the productions required to process a single message. Patterns are stated in terms of features on a single channel. Controlled responding, which is based on decisions made about the current stimulus complex, is determined by the working memory system.

Underlying automatic, highly overlearned mental activity is the semantic network. It is possible that information is passed from production to production by spreading of activation, without pattern recognition being involved. All productions simultaneously convey information about their levels of activation. A decay mechanism is postulated to avoid the unlimited spreading of activation. In addition, to prevent constant repetition of a production, the activation level is assumed to be reduced once its action is taken.

The distinctions presented in Table 8.2 between controlled, conscious, and automatic and often unconscious processing approximate Hunt and Lansman's distinction between arousal of a production by recognition of its pattern part and arousal of a production by semantic activation, respectively. Hunt and Lansman stressed that although complex reasoning is based on both controlled and automatic processing, verbal protocols reveal only the products of conscious reasoning. Such protocols, therefore, do not provide direct information about automatic processing. Reaction time and accuracy are considered to be sensitive to the effects of semantic activation.

Having presented the bare essentials of Hunt and Lansman's production activation model, I would like to continue my account of the processing difficulties manifest in agrammatic aphasics in general and, in particular, the deficits that the patient of Nespoulous et al. demonstrated.

I suggest that the agrammatic's language performance can be summarized as follows: The main impairment of the patient of Nespoulous et al. (and my patients tested to date) is on the morphosyntactic level(s) of processing. In particular, performance on all tasks requiring oral responses above the word level appears to be impaired, in contrast to performance on language tasks that tap written language and remain within this modality. In other words, the ability to perform more complex tasks requiring intensive interaction and constant switching between automatic and controlled processing in oral production and in intermodal production shows impairment.

Since all of the sentence/discourse oral production tasks depend on this complex interaction and constant switching between the two types of processing, which result in the execution of a sequence of productions, the agrammatic will show impaired performance on these tasks. The agrammatic has difficulty executing the sequence of productions due to decreased efficiency in the interactions between/among the set of productions in long-term memory and the blackboard area. The continuous comparisons between long-term memory and the information in the blackboard area, in particular syntactic information (i.e., the working memory system) lead to overtaxing of the agrammatic Broca's processing abilities. Stark and Dressler (1988) have also demonstrated that the probability that an agrammatic makes an error is correlated with the length of the utterance: The longer the utterance, the greater the possibility that it will be incorrect. Automatic processing appears to be intact in the Nespoulous patient if it is allowed to function (i.e., is not inhibited). Due to the overtaxing caused by controlled responding, the process of pattern recognition is always evoked. In turn, the automatic passing of information from production to production by spreading of activation, without the process of pattern recognition, is undermined. Arousal of a production by semantic activation thus becomes virtually impossible in sentence/discourse production tasks, due to the aforementioned overtaxing caused by controlled processing of morphosyntactic information. Further, it is assumed that due to reduced efficiency in morphosyntactic processing in oral production, the patterns that production can use are also smaller in size. This results in more (rather than fewer!) productions required to process/produce a single message, which further overtaxes the processing system. The vicious circle is thus complete: The pattern segment continuously compared in the blackboard area is smaller and more comparisons are necessary.

For the patient of Nespoulous et al., performance of all tasks based only on written language (no constant switching of oral to graphic responses and vice versa) is more or less intact. Interaction between the productions appears to function well and the size of the patterns for production in these tasks can be assumed to be large. I assume, therefore, that automatic processing can be considered to function adequately in these tasks, because controlled processing does not constantly interrupt or inhibit it. The agrammatic's good performance on these written language tasks is thus due not to an impairment of automatic processing, but rather to the possibility of automatically processing the stimuli in such tasks.

The interaction of automatic and controlled processing is apparent in the aforementioned vertical reading task: Automatic processing, that is, the spreading of activation from one production, (=word) to another, worked well to the point when controlled processing became necessary. The patient could not suppress processing from one form (=word) to another, and when he realized that the words he was reading were parts of a sentence, controlled processing took over and automatic processing was inhibited. On the other hand, the aphasic's good word-level reading and naming performance can be considered the result of the semantic activation of words in long-term memory. Since only one short production is required, an overtaxing of the system does not occur.[10] The decay mechanism or reduction in activation level after an action is made, that is, an object is named, does not affect performance on such a task.

Auditory sentence comprehension was also intact in the Nespoulous patient. I interpret the dissociations between auditory comprehension and oral production of sentences reported in the literature and also in this patient (cf. also Miceli, Mazzucchi, Menn, & Goodglass, 1983) as follows: Depending on whether the aphasic can automatically process the sentences or the interaction between controlled and automatic processing is not overtaxed, the aphasic will be able to auditorily or graphically process the sentences correctly as required by such a task. (It is important to stress that a sentence–picture matching or an object manipulation comprehension task does not require a lengthy oral response.) The size of the productions correctly processed will depend on the type and structure of the sentence to be produced and on the degree of the severity of the language impairment. Stark and Wytek's results discussed in this volume (chapter 6) do not confirm this dissociation between oral agrammatic production and auditory comprehension. The agrammatic Broca's aphasics demonstrated syntactic deficits on auditory sentence comprehension. That is, their language processing broke down due to overtaxing of the processing system: Controlled processing of morphosyntactic information (e.g., expressed by articles) would ordinarily have been done by automatic processing. However, this automatic processing was inhibited/impaired. Or, due to a constant switching between automatic and controlled processing in (re)constructing the relations of the units of the spoken sentence to one another—which becomes necessary in reversible active/passive/topicalized sentences—processing broke down. The language units ordinarily processed by automatic processing are exactly the ones necessary to understand the sentence correctly, for example, to choose the correct drawing in a sentence–picture matching task. If the automatic processing is inhibited in this task, the working memory system determines controlled responding. The decisions to be made about the current stimulus complex ((morpho) syntactic structure) are thus carried out by a system not specialized for the automatic processing of highly overlearned language units, that is, of the function words.

The preceding remarks refer to the appearance or occurrence of processing difficulties—when the processing system becomes overtaxed, processing breaks down—and to the interaction between automatic and controlled processing. I have not discussed the form or type of the deficits, that is, whether forms are omitted or substituted. Both of these types of deficits are found in agrammatic utterances. I would like to put forward a tentative interpretation of these different types of performance or error: When automatic processing, for example, of the articles, is inhibited, a form (article, pronoun, auxiliary verb) will be omitted. There are, of course, several reasons for this inhibition. For example, two forms are simultaneously activated and they inhibit each other (cf. Hunt & Lansman, 1986). Automatic processing would normally result in the correct and quick selection and production of the form(s). If controlled processing takes over or dominates from the start (not allowing a complex interaction of automatic and controlled processing), a correct form can still be produced if the overall processing is momentarily not overtaxed and the controlled processing is successful at producing a form usually automatically produced; or an incorrect form is produced due to a momentary overtaxing of overall processing, or because controlled processing simply cannot accomplish the production of such a function word. Several reasons for this possibility can also be posited.

Controlled and Automatic Processing in Recovery from Aphasia

The above remarks concerning whether a form will be substituted or omitted also apply to the agrammatic's recovery process over time. Initially, the agrammatic's telegram style reveals numerous omissions of the closed-class, function-word vocabulary, and the verb is produced in the infinitive form. This could be due to the initial (near) total inhibition of automatic processing, which particularly affects the closed-class items. Table 8.3 shows that exactly those aspects of grammatical organization—the rules of syntactic agreement, function words, and so on—are affected in agrammatic aphasics.

If automatic processing is inhibited, there is a vacancy (=omission), controlled processing successfully takes over (=correct production), or controlled processing takes over but is not successful (=substitution). I assume that the production of these overlearned aspects of grammatical structure is primarily achieved by automatic processing. That is, over time in normal language development, these aspects are relegated to automatic processing because of their role in sentence processing. Initially, in development conscious/controlled processing was necessary to produce these forms (cf. note 8). Over time the forms became more and more automatic, which made room for more "complex" aspects to be consciously processed. This would explain why controlled processing cannot adequately accomplish aspects normally automatically processed and substitutions are produced. If this were not the case, one would expect correct forms to be produced when focal attention is directed at them. However, this does not occur in the agrammatic's spontaneous production or in specific tasks requiring oral production.

In light of the above remarks concerning recovery, I view the "development" of agrammatism differently from Heeschen (1985). Heeschen claimed that the Broca's aphasic is not agrammatic right from the start, that is, immediately post onset, but rather must learn to become agrammatic by trial and error. In this context, Pick (1931, p. 1472) asserted that there are two types of motor agrammatism. The first type is present immediately post onset. The second type develops over time as the aphasic becomes adjusted to the language impairment. Pick, however, considered the decrease in "diaschisis" to play a role in the development of the second type.

In my opinion, there are neither two types of agrammatism, due to the aforementioned reasons, nor does the Broca's aphasic all of a sudden become agrammatic in recovery. In recovery, the agrammatic does show changes and also at times great fluctuations in language performance. However, both of these aspects can be accounted for in terms of the automatic/controlled processing distinction. The impact of diaschisis—albeit that this concept is far from understood—on language processing can also be understood as an inhibition of automatic processing. Depending on the ititial degree of severity of the language impairment, the agrammatic's language processing will demonstrate either total inhibition of automatic processing (=omissions, correct telegram style; cf. Isserlin, 1936), in the context of an overtaxed controlled processing system, both minimal automatic processing and increased controlled processing. Controlled processing in this case is excessive in attempting to make up for the minimal automatic processing; its being excessive hinders automatic processing to a greater extent. The aforementioned problem of cause and effect can once again be cited. The result will be a mixture of correct and incorrect production of function words, and so on.

With reference to Heeschen's theory of agrammatism, the terms "compensatory strategies," "avoidance," and "adaptation" do not seem to imply the organism's automatic, unconscious immediate response to the situation without awareness at a higher level—which I consider to the point. The efficiency of the aphasic's linguistic/cognitive processing system necessarily depends on many simultaneously active factors (cf. also the general discussion of Stark and Wytek in chapter 6). The agrammatic's variation in the type of structures used and the form of utterances attempted documents a striving for a more adequate production (cf. Stark & Dressler, 1988), and not a conscious avoidance of particular forms or an adaptation to a constrained, reduced form. The more complex the syntactic constructions the aphasic attempts to produce, the more often the results will be faulty. In this context, I regard spontaneous speech, sentence and text production as the most natural language tasks requiring an integration of automatic and controlled processing, and at the same time the most demanding for the agrammatic: for example, the expression of one's (at times very personal) thoughts on a particular topic. Analysis of changes in language processing, for example, spontaneous speech, over time in recovery is important for an understanding of the interaction/integration of automatic and controlled processing.

With reference to Whitaker's (1983) remarks on the return of language functions following the administration of sodium amytal in the Wada test, the fact that the lesion producing agrammatism is in the region of Broca's area (anterior, prerolandic), it could be hypothesized that a lesion in this area results in an inhibition/impairment of automatic language processing of morphosyntactic information (cf. Benson, 1979).[12]

The automatic language functions listed in Table 8.3 encompass exactly those aspects that are impaired in agrammatics. By describing the agrammatic's language-processing deficits as I have done above—albeit in general terms—with respect to the automatic/controlled distinction, I think that Goodglass and Menn's (1985) criticism that no single-factor explanation of agrammatism can be correct can be reconsidered (cf. also Coltheart, 1987, and the contributions on agrammatism in that volume). Moreover, their assertion pertaining to the term "syntax," in particular that it seems questionable that this term can translate into a single process, could thus be reinterpreted according to the automatic/controlled distinction. I do not claim that impairment of a single rule or process results in agrammatism, rather that the distinction between automatic and controlled processing can provide a basis for analyzing the aphasic's language behavior in a more coherent manner.

Agrammatism Versus Paragrammatism

Goodglass and Menn (1985) and Heeschen (1985) drew attention to the similarities between agrammatism and paragrammatism. Goodglass and Menn claimed that instead of assuming that the usual approach—treatment of the similarities as surface responses to different underlying causes (cf. also Isserlin, 1936)—is correct, the following approach might be more fruitful: "Perhaps the grammatical similarities of anterior and posterior aphasias are underlying and the differences are due to particular processing problems (for example, sentence initiation difficulties) that are not grammatical, and to compensatory strategies arising in response to these problems" (Goodglass & Menn, 1985, p. 21).

The language aspects regarded as automatic in Table 8.3 are posited to be automatic for all speakers, including agrammatic and paragrammatic aphasics alike. In these aphasics, one does not expect a de novo organization of automatic/voluntary language functions according to new principles or concepts. Of course, the other possibility, that de novo the automatic functions exchange places with the voluntary ones, cannot be totally ruled out. The question is, why should this or would this occur in the context of a processing system reduced in efficiency due to brain damage? (Cf. chapter 6, Stark and Wytek's hierarchy of complexity/difficulty of the various sentence types tested. The hierarchy of difficulty holds for all aphasics; the particular processing deficits characteristic of the various aphasia types, however, result in different error patterns.)

I am assuming that the same language functions that were automatic premorbidly remain automatic. Those language functions that were controlled/voluntary remain controlled/voluntary, regardless of aphasia type. I suggest that the difference one can expect in language processing, in particular the differences between the Broca's and Wernicke's aphasics, will thus necessarily be in terms of how they differentially process language automatically versus voluntarily/controlled, that is, how their automatic/controlled processing operates. Thus, I assume that although similar hierarchies have been posited for agrammatics and paragrammatics with reference to specific language categories/functions, underlying qualitative differences in how these language aspects are processed exist:

Agrammatic. Inhibition of automatic processing in specific language tasks, especially in those requiring integration of controlled and automatic processing

Paragrammatic. Disinhibition of automatic processes and simultaneous impairment of controlled processing

Thus, I assume that in paragrammatism the interaction between automatic and controlled processing is differentially affected, that is, is qualitatively different from the interaction between these two in agrammatism. The fluent paragrammatic's automatic processing is disinhibited, the spread of activation at times being even excessive, perhaps due to the action of interfering stimuli, whereas voluntary, controlled processing—the interaction between a set of productions stored in long-term memory and the blackboard (working memory and external sensory channels)—is impaired. In Wernicke's aphasia, impaired controlled processing results in (or is an expression of) a combination of auditory/graphic comprehension deficits, lexical retrieval, and phonological processing deficits.

In terms of the aforementioned production activation model (Hunt &

Lansman, 1986), the first step in controlled processing is an evaluation of the match between the stimulus and each of the patterns in long-term memory. A "simple" pattern recognition can already be a problem for the Wernicke's aphasic. The level of activation is posited to be used in determining which production is to be executed when a stimulus complex contains several patterns. However, in Wernicke's aphasia the regulation of activation levels can be considered to be impaired: The incorrect or less adequate unit of memory assumes control of action because its level of activation exceeds that of other, more adequate units. The level of activation among several patterns thus interferes with the appropriate pattern in the environment. The selection of the pattern within a single modality (or code) is based on comparisons with one another to determine which one is selected.

According to the Hunt and Lansman model, two selection conditions require (a) that the pattern's activation is above a preset threshold that is characteristic of the pattern, and further (b) that the activation level of the selected production must exceed the activation level of any other pattern. Thus, I assume that, if the activation levels are not (exactly) controllable, the pattern with the highest activation level will not necessarily be the "selected," adequate pattern but rather the most powerful one whose activation level is greater.

A strong restriction of the production activation model is that patterns are stated in terms of the features in a single channel, and it is therefore not possible to define a pattern in terms of a multimodal stimulus complex. In order for the systems to react to multichannel stimulus complexes, the components of these complexes must be recoded to internal stimuli in the semantic code. Only then is a response to such multichannel stimulus complexes possible (cf. Karmiloff-Smith's [1986] E-iii level of tertiary explicitation). Thus, in Wernicke's aphasia, this recoding either is impossible or is impaired, depending on the degree of severity of the lexical semantic processing difficulties. The working memory system is posited to determine controlled responding, based on decisions made about the current stimuli complex. It becomes clear that the Wernicke's patients' decisions about the current stimuli complex will necessarily be deficient either before the stimuli complex reaches working memory or due to a reduced working memory, which in turn may be the result of overtaxing of the processing system (cf. question 2 on monitoring at the beginning of this chapter).

The disinhibition of automatic processing in long-term memory—which as previously mentioned does not directly depend on the presence of information in working memory or does not involve pattern recognition—necessarily has a detrimental effect on controlled processing. This is exactly the situation that presents itself when the spread of activation from one production to another gets the upper hand due to disinhibition. The decay mechanism can also be considered to be impaired because the activation levels are not reduced after a computation cycle. A great number of phonological/lexical/semantic perseverations produced by Wernicke's aphasics can also be cited in this context. Thus, deficits both in the semantic network underlying automatic activity and in the production system, that is, in the manipulation of information in working memory, are qualitatively different from those in agrammatic Broca's aphasia. An overtaxing of the processing system is demonstrated in both aphasia types; however, the cause(s) of the overtaxing is (are) different.

Fluency in Controlled/Automatic Processing

In the very logorrheic Wernicke's aphasic fluency is intact or even increased. The influence of fluency on grammatical form in terms of a facilitatory effect when fluency is high is not only a positive one (cf. Goodglass & Menn, 1985, p. 25; cf. note 10). With reference to fluency, I suggest that although the preserved rate of production, rhythm, and intonation of speech aids in producing longer runs of speech, the sum of these features also has a detrimental effect on the paragrammatic: The disinhibited production of automatic language functions cannot be controlled or consciously monitored (i.e., repaired) by the severely impaired aphasic. As previously mentioned, since the production of automatic functions of language (function words, e.g., articles, determiners, pronouns, and verb inflections, etc.) cannot be successfully taken over by controlled processing—these functions being automatic ones—the paragrammatic produces forms fluently. However, they are often incorrect forms, due to disinhibition of automatic and impairment of controlled processing. Depending on the predominant type of the deficits the Wernicke's aphasic has (phonological and/or semantic), controlled processing is totally occupied with the production/retrieval of the correct forms. Achieving awareness of the errors—prearticulatory or postarticulatory—is thus even more difficult because of the normal or even increased rate of production in the context of the specific processing difficulties. In the case of jargon aphasia, controlled processing totally overtaxes the system. If it were not for the (sometimes correct) automatic production of the function words, the researcher would not be able to recognize/reconstruct certain language units in this type of aphasia.

Therefore, it holds not only that fluency—redefined by Goodglass and Menn (1985) as the ability to initiate and maintain a continuous stream of speech (p. 26)—interacts with agrammatism but that it also interacts with paragrammatism. The negative influence of fluency becomes less, in correlation with the paragrammatic's slowing down in the rate of production, the more controlled the processing. The opposite holds for the agrammatic Broca's aphasic, an increase in fluency being associated with a reduction in inhibition of automatic processing, that is, an increase in automatic processing is assumed to result in more correct language production. (This will be the case if controlled processing can be maintained at a certain level, allowing automatic processing to contribute to language processing.) It is my opinion that further research on why certain language aspects are automatically processed, that is, are automatic language functions, and also defining a hierarchy of these automatic language functions and how the linguistic forms become more explicitly represented (e.g., in terms of Karmiloff-Smith's [1986] four levels of knowledge representation, etc.), will resolve several problems in relation to the "cognitive operations of the various devices that signal syntactic relationships" (cf. Goodglass & Menn, 1985, p. 21; Coltheart, 1987, pp. 22–23). Moreover, an important issue is to determine the cross-linguistic differences of these automatic functions. Analysis of data from the Cross Linguistic Aphasia Study (Menn, Obler, & Miceli, 1988) could provide a starting point for such an analysis in the 14 languages investigated in that study.

These remarks are speculative and incomplete. It is hoped that future treatment will delve into this highly complex subject to disentangle aspects of automatic processing from those of controlled processing. The most important question is how these two types of processing can be empirically tested. The automatic/controlled processing distinction has been suggested to account for various contrasting results. An important issue for future research is how the production/perception dissociations can be reconciled in an encompassing systematic account of the aphasic's language processing in terms of the two types of processing.

Monitoring

The automatic/unconscious–controlled/conscious processing distinction also relates to the second question, namely, self-monitoring. Although this term has already been adverted to in the discussion of stages of language development, it has not been explicitly defined. Laver (1973) defined monitoring as follows: "I have used the term 'monitoring' to refer to the neural function of detecting and correcting errors in the neurolinguistic program . . . I am not thinking of the use of sensory feedback to control speech-movements directly." (p. 137). "That is, monitoring is the reception and processing of sensory reports on myodynamic execution for the purpose of detecting and correcting errors" (p. 138). Monitoring in the sense of monitoring for target items (e.g., as in on-line gaiting tasks) is briefly discussed under on-line monitoring (cf. Tyler, 1985, 1987).

Laver's definition of self-monitoring is better understood within his framework of the four main functions involved in the generation of any speech utterance. These are (a) ideation, (b) neurolinguistic program planning, (c) myodynamic execution, and (d) monitoring. With regard to these four functions, Laver pointed out that the "activities of scrutiny and revision are not the monopoly of the monitoring function, but an integral characteristic of all the brain's processes for constructing and controlling speech programs" (1973, p. 134). Constructing the neurolinguistic program in turn involves the organization of a program for the selection of lexical items in accordance with the semantics of the idea, the grammatical arrangements, and the phonological aspects.

Since the planner and monitor have so many aspects in common, Laver suggested that the two functions can be considered different manifestations of a common major function termed the "central control function." This central control function is "able to make decisions at the highest level, with access to the idea, to all types of long- and short-term memory storage concerned with speech production and to all levels of the process of generating a particular utterance" (1973, p. 141). The purpose of the monitor is thus to edit the initial program by correcting overt errors, while the purpose of the planner is to detect errors and correct them before the myodynamic execution of the program. (Cp. the attention of Laver to Hockett's distinction between overt and covert editing.) Laver (1980) asserted that not correcting an error is not to be equated with not detecting the error (cf. also Levelt, 1983b). Another point stressed by Laver is that conscious awareness is not considered a necessary part of the monitoring process (cf. Clark, 1978).

With reference to how the speaker detects an error, Levelt (1983b) discussed two theories:

1. Production-based theory of monitoring. The speaker is considered to have direct access to particular components of the production process (albeit by means of comprehension!). Levelt classified Laver's (1980) theory of monitoring as production based.
2. Comprehension based, that is, the perceptual theory of monitoring. In this theory the speaker is assumed not to have access to the components of production, but rather to the final result of the process. Levelt preferred this theory with reference to his own data.

Levelt postulated that three phases are involved in making a self-repair: (a) the monitoring of one's own speech and the interruption of the flow of speech when trouble is detected, (b) a phase characterized by hesitation, pausing, and the use of so-called "editing" terms, such as "uh," and (c) a last phase consisting of making the repair. He stressed that the structural relation between the original utterance and the repair determines the linguistic well-formedness of the repair, not the speaker's respecting the integrity of constituents. That is, the speaker must have access to structural properties of the original utterance. Levelt differentiated repairs from covert repairs.

An interesting finding of Levelt's study is that trouble detection improves toward the end of constituents. This could be explained by the fact that the processing system is coming to the end of a production and, for example, (controlled) processing is less taxed than it was in initiating the production. Levelt pointed out that speakers have little access to their speech production process. For this reason, he considered self-monitoring to be based on parsing one's inner or overt speech.

Various definitions of the term "monitoring" refer to it as being a more or less automatic process. However, there is a gradation according to the linguistic aspects or the level of language being monitored. Clark (1978) presented a hierarchy of different types of awareness with reference to the child's development of monitoring functions. Of the various monitoring functions Clark discussed, I mention only three of them (listed in order from simpler, i.e., earlier, to more complex, i.e., later developed): The monitoring of one's own ongoing utterances with reference to form and function—which is considered a prerequisite for spontaneous repairs; checking the result of one's utterance; and reflecting on the product of an utterance, that is, reflecting on language structure independent of its actual use, for example, in grammaticality judgments or judgments of semantic anomaly, and so on.

Monitoring by Aphasics

According to Clark (1978), the idea behind development of such a hierarchy is that the study of what children are aware of provides a way of finding out what their conception of language is. In analogy with this, an understanding of the types of linguistic awareness or monitoring functions in aphasia would provide information on the aphasic's intact processing abilities and impairments. The main assumption I would like to put forward is that the types of monitoring carried out by or not possible for an aphasic are a direct reflection of the "primary" impairment, as judged by differential monitoring. This means that if an aphasic systematically monitors (detects and/or corrects errors in) ongoing language production in terms of specific aspects of language processing, whereas he or she does not monitor other specific aspects, the presence/absence of detecting/correcting errors provides information about the aphasic's processing abilities. An understanding of the aphasic's monitoring abilities will in turn bring us closer to isolating components of automatic versus controlled processing.

In Stark (1984), a case study of transcortical sensory aphasia (M.H.) was interpreted. M.H.'s monitoring performance was shown to mirror the extent and type of her processing abilities and difficulties. M. H. auditorily monitored her own speech output with reference to the phonological aspects: She detected and corrected all phonological paraphasias and uncertainties immediately. However, she did not detect her semantically anomalous productions, that is, semantic paraphasias and semantic jargon. Her deficient monitoring was exactly for those linguistic domains that showed impairment in production and comprehension tasks. At that time, her monitoring performance was considered to support the idea of a central impairment in retrieving lexical items from the lexicon and in the overall processing of semantic information. Although her syntactic processing was intact, she produced semantically inadequate and anomalous utterances and she did not detect or correct any semantic errors, even semantic jargon. With reference to her language performance, one can posit that she automatically unconsciously detected and overtly corrected errors pertaining to level I (and often language aspects of level II, which can be described with reference to syntax and without reference to meaning) (cf. Table 8.3). However, she was not aware of semantic errors, which can be correlated to level III. She neither automatically corrected the semantic errors nor showed any overt evidence of conscious awareness of her errors, for example, making repairs or other trouble-indicating behavior. Self-monitoring performance could thus be viewed as an indicator of type of aphasic processing deficits as well as of the degree of their severity.

I claim that in aphasia the following combinations of self-monitoring performance are possible:

1. In a severe, central, specific language impairment, self-monitoring will be impaired exactly with regard to those aspects of language processing that in turn will reveal a similar type of performance (i.e., impairment) in various other language tasks (e.g., jargon aphasia). In the very severe case there will therefore be no evidence of automatic (unconscious) detecting of these errors or inadequacies (i.e., no repairs).
2. In recovery and in moderate or mild language impairment, self-monitoring and other language performance will fluctuate with reference to those aspects of language processing that are impaired. Depending on the complexity of the task and on the momentary condition of the processing system, trouble-indicating behavior (e.g., filled or unfilled pauses) will reveal that an error was detected and attempts at correcting the error will be present. The aphasic will automatically and overtly correct an error, unconsciously at times and at other times consciously, by means of controlled processing, for example, successive approximations.
3. On the basis of language data from a case of 'initial global aphasia recovering into a Broca's aphasia,' a third type of performance can be posited. In this aphasic (K.L.), a (near) total dissociation between automatic and controlled processing was observed: Controlled processing was not possible in any language task. On the other hand, automatic processing functioned well—when it could be called into action by means of certain tasks. For example, on-line monitoring of other speaker's language production was possible.

K. L., a 45-year-old, female, commercial high school graduate, suffered a left cerebrovascular accident. Angiography showed an occlusion of the left internal carotid artery. Computed tomography scan at 10 days post onset showed a large hypodense zone in the left frontocentral, anterior temporal, insula, and basal ganglia areas. Two slices from the CT scan are shown in Figure 8.1. Extensive language testing began 3 weeks post onset. The Aachen Aphasia Test (AAT) was administered several times. Results from three tests—at 5 to 6 weeks, at 10 weeks, and at 4 months post onset—are given in Figure 8.2.

Spontaneous, self-initiated speech was totally absent at the time of the first testing. At 4 weeks post onset, K. L. produced two recurring utterances; later several others were added to her repertoire. The results of the first AAT indicated a global aphasia—all language modalities were severely impaired. At 10 weeks post onset the type of aphasia was not definitely classifiable: most accurately K.L. could be considered a global aphasic in recovery. At 4 months post onset—although her aphasia had

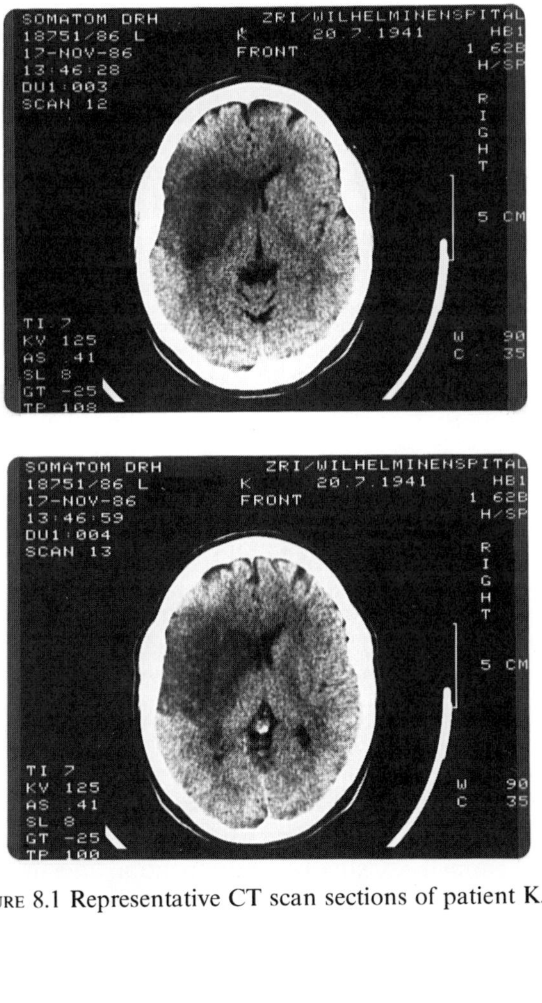

FIGURE 8.1 Representative CT scan sections of patient K. L.

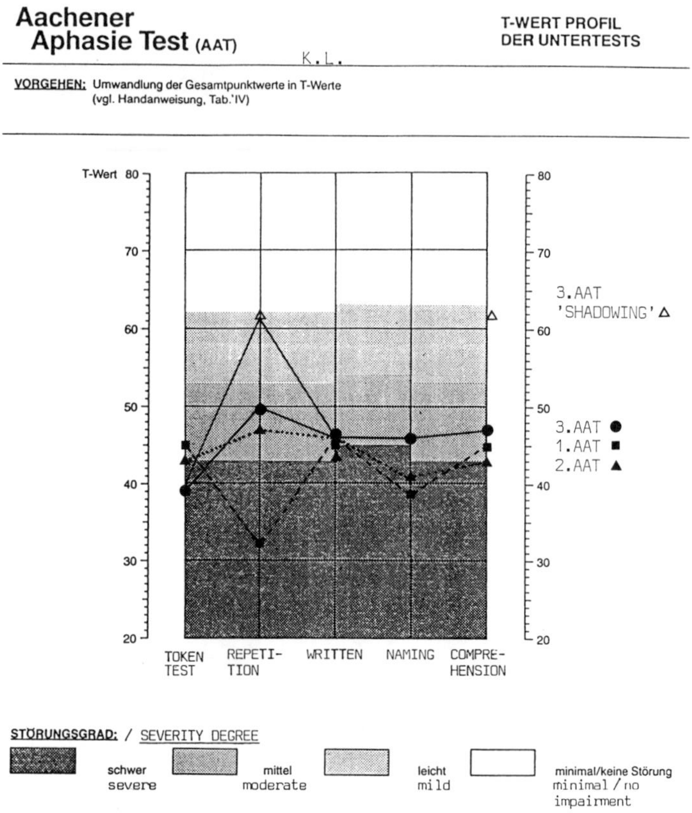

FIGURE 8.2 Aachen aphasia test profiles of patient K. L.

been classified as Broca's moderately impaired on the basis of the third AAT—her language performance was not that of a typical agrammatic Broca's aphasic. Her linguistic performance appeared comparable to that seen in transcortical motor aphasia; however, she was too impaired (moderately) in all modalities (included in the AAT), including repetition. Her repetition performance, however, showed less impairment. Her spontaneous speech slowly improved; the recurring utterances were produced less often. From the onset of her aphasia she did not demonstrate any articulatory difficulties with what she actually produced.

K. L. displayed very interesting language performance, which I would like to describe in terms of her monitoring functions: K. L. showed a near total dissociation between automatic and controlled processing. In the context of severely reduced spontaneous speech, she displayed moderate impairment of repetition, excellent shadowing abilities, and extensive completion phenomena. Using normal repetition and shadowing a comparison of the AAT repetition results (from the third test) revealed the difference between the two types of linguistic behavior. Utterances begun by another speaker were very often completed, quite irrespective of the content. At times K. L. spontaneously completed almost every utterance. The linguistic structure of the completed utterances varied greatly. The utterances were not formulaic in form.

I would like to attribute K. L.'s completion phenomena and shadowing to intact automatic processing. More controlled language processing was initially absent and later highly constrained: Confrontation naming, picture descriptions, sentence production tasks, and so on were not possible on request or spontaneously, but were possible when another speaker started the utterance. In recovery, the dissociation between automatic and controlled processing remained striking. In this context, due to the extent of the lesion, the neurologists were surprised about her language performance and improvement.

Quite early in the recovery process, K. L. was thus able to monitor another speaker's speech well. In order to monitor, she must have had access to some structural properties of the ongoing utterance, which enabled her to continue and to complete the utterance, often quicker than the other speaker. Since her self-initiated language performance was severely impaired, I would like to claim that her controlled processing was initially totally inhibited or impaired, and the language she produced was by means of automatic processing. Syntactic and semantic information must have been available to her, as judged by the syntactically correct and semantically adequate completions. Otherwise, she could not have shadowed and completed utterances with such accuracy or so quickly. (Shadowing latencies are presently being analyzed.)

Monitoring in Agrammatism

With regard to the previous discussion of agrammatic processing deficits, if the agrammatic is severely impaired, his or her attention will be so intensively directed at, for example, oral production (i.e., the person will be processing in such a controlled manner) that monitoring of morphosyntactic information will not be possible. The ability to self-monitor articulation may also be impaired; however, self-monitoring with respect to semantic information is assumed to be intact and will proceed automatically, if the processing system is not entirely overtaxed due to the morphosyntactic processing demands: The interaction/integration of the various linguistic levels becomes critical (cf. chapter 6).

In the process of recovery from aphasia, or with reference to moderate/mild agrammatic impairment, when automatic and controlled processing "interact" to a certain degree, the agrammatic will be able to detect morphologial and syntactic errors and will also sometimes correct or repair them. That is, the partially recovered, i.e. improved agrammatic will automatically produce repairs, or on the basis of successive controlled attempts at processing morphosyntactic information will arrive at a correct form, or may give up attempting after a few unsuccessful trials. It is thus assumed that if automatic processing is not completely inhibited (i.e., is functioning), repairs of syntactic and morphological information will be attempted or produced.

Monitoring Studies on Aphasia

The above remarks pertain to when self-monitoring should operate and why self-monitoring will break down. Monitoring in the sense of reflecting on language structure independent of its actual use will be discussed with reference to the third question stated at the beginning of this chapter. I would like to briefly consider aspects pertaining to monitoring behavior in aphasia discussed in the literature.

Marshall and Morton (1978) stated that their awareness operator "EMMA" (=even more mysterious apparatus) either operates or does not. Further, they asserted that there are no degrees of awareness, although the type and extent of information about normal language processing to which EMMA has access does vary. Their definition of awareness is thus an EMMA that is functioning: "Awareness arises from the operation of error-detecting mechanisms which have access to subparts of the output of primary production and comprehension systems" (p. 237). Their awareness operator is thus ubiquitous. I agree with the idea that anywhere in the language production process the aphasic will or will not detect/correct an error. However, the momentary processing demands will play an essential role in determining success.

In a study of the aphasic's self-monitorng functions in sentence (naming) performance, Schlenck, Huber, and Willmes (1987) differentiated two types of monitoring function: (a) repairs, that is, self-correction or modification of parts of the preceding utterance, and (b) prepairs, that is, forms of searching behavior that are not preceded by an error and that aim at the following utterance. Both repairs and prepairs are further classified as trouble-indicating behavior, in contrast to language systematic errors. With respect to all aphasic groups (Broca's, Wernicke's, and anomic), prepairs were made much more frequently than repairs. This finding is viewed by the authors as evidence that postarticulatory monitoring is impaired, whereas prearticulatory monitoring is intact in these aphasics. Prepairs were more common in aphasics with relatively good comprehension, aphasics with poor production, and also in aphasics with both good comprehension and poor production.

The Wernicke's aphasics' relative frequency of prepairs was not significantly different from that of Broca's and anomics. Schlenck et al. (1987) claimed that the Wernicke's comprehension deficit did not prevent patients from making prepairs, as would be expected if prepairs were covert repairs. In my opinion, a tentative explanation of why there are more prepairs is that the prepairs may be more automatically detected and also responded to automatically. In contrast, repairs are assumed to require more controlled processing: (conscious) substitution of the incorrect/inadequate linguistic form (lexical, syntactic). Postarticulatory monitoring would be more taxed because the aphasic may already be working on or "preparing" the next production (cf. Hunt & Lansman, 1986). The production of oral language—depending on the task—demands a certain amount of controlled processing. Therefore, if an error is not detected and responded to prearticulatorily, chances of its being detected and repaired decrease.

The overall status of prepairs is, however, more difficult to interpret in ongoing language production. With reference to the Schlenck study, one difficulty in analyzing the same overall patterns in Broca's and Wernicke's aphasics is that the authors left out phonemic paraphasias from the analysis. They considered phonemic paraphasias to be tied to the word at which they occurred and not to ongoing language production. This is not necessarily the case. Another difficulty with their analysis is that they attempted to correlate the monitoring performance with auditory comprehension performance on the Aachen Aphasia Test. However, the AAT is not sensitive enough to detect specific syntactic processing deficits, especially in Broca's aphasics. Therefore, a comparison of these two performances is not very useful.

With respect to whether a monitor is production and/or comprehension based, I assume that it is rather a question of the *type of errors/deficits that the aphasic displays,* whether or not these errors will be detected. Moreover, it will depend on the momentary state of the processing system, whether the errors will be (successfully) repaired. As previously mentioned, I view the monitoring function to be both production and comprehension based. Where/when an error is detected in language processing will thus depend on an interaction of both production and comprehension in the overall processing context. I suggest further, that the momentary type of processing (automatic/controlled) correlates with the detection/correction of an error. Analysis of repair/prepair data is planned in relation to automatic and controlled processing by aphasics.

Metalinguistic Tasks

In the previous discussions, the dissociations between automatic and controlled processing were discussed with reference to the aphasic's performance on specific tasks and the assumed underlying deficits of, for example, Nespoulous and colleagues' agrammatic patient and patients M. H. and K. L. In response to the third question raised in the introduction, namely, what aspects are being tapped in metalinguistic tasks (i.e., tasks that require the aphasic to reflect on particular aspects of language use), I will limit my remarks to data discussed in the aphasia literature on grammaticality judgments, lexical decision tasks, and on-line monitoring tasks.

When the results from the various tasks fit together to provide a unitary description of the deficit(s), a unitary description is less problematic to formulate. However, such a description is particularly difficult when results from one task contrast with valid results from other tasks described in the literature. In this context, the aphasic's performance on metalinguistic tasks can be described as displaying a very interesting pattern. At times, generalizations from specific results to other processing issues are highly speculative or ambiguous. With reference to the previous discussions, I would like to address particular results reported on grammaticality judgments, lexical decisions, and on-line monitoring for target words with my main interests being the ability actually tapped by the task and with reference to the automatic/controlled processing distinction.

Grammaticality Judgment Tasks

Linebarger, Schwartz, and Saffran's (1983) results on an auditory grammaticality judgment task, in which agrammatics' sensitivity to grammatical structure was investigated, provide an excellent example of "surprising" results. (It must, however, be stressed that Isserlin [1936] and Salomon [1914] already called attention to this phenomenon in agrammatism!)

In the Linebarger et al. study, agrammatics were notably sensitive to structural information, that is, their syntactic knowledge was significantly spared. These results were considered surprising, because the agrammatic's deficit had been described—until that time—as a syntactic processing deficit. The syntactic deficit hypothesis was based on data from sentence production tasks, auditory comprehension, and so on that showed that syntactic processing was impaired in the various tasks employed. That is, the syntactic theory of agrammatism posits that agrammatics show impairment on those tasks requiring processing of syntactic information (function words, word order, etc.). The agrammatics' good performance on a grammaticality judgment task, therefore, was taken by Linebarger et al. as evidence that the Broca's aphasics were able to perform complex syntactic analyses of sentences. The syntactic abilities that Linebarger et al. assumed their test tapped include the following: awareness of subcategorization requirements, sensitivity to the function word vocabulary, and the ability to handle discontinuous syntactic dependencies.

The authors discussed various counterarguments regarding their results, in particular in attempting to explain their aphasics' poor performance on tag questions and reflexive sentences. Linebarger et al. attributed the poor performance on these two sentence types to "shallow decoding of the lexical content of the subject noun phrase, given the hypothesized tradeoff between syntactic and semantic processing" (p. 389). A trade-off between syntactic and semantic processing posits that aphasics can achieve their best performance in only one domain. The authors concluded their discussion by stating that in arriving at a grammaticality judgment, due to a limited immediate memory span, the agrammatic cannot backtrack to recover relevant information when processing has been too "shallow" in building up descriptions of the input.

I would like to propose a different interpretation of the agrammatics' good performance on grammaticality judgments: It can best be accounted for by assuming that this task taps automatic processing. Therefore, the agrammatics' good performance on this task can be regarded as evidence for intact automatic processing. The demand of the auditory grammaticality judgment task is that the aphasic accepts a sentence as grammatical ("yes") or as not grammatical ("no"). If one recalls the discussion of Nespoulous and colleagues' agrammatic with reference to metalinguistic tasks, I posited that if the task does not require oral production (above the word level) or constant switching between automatic and controlled processing, that is, between oral and graphic modalities, language performance would be more or less intact. That is, if automatic processing were not inhibited and the aphasic could respond by automatic processing, the language performance would show less impairment. I assume that in the grammaticality judgment task the agrammatic is able to syntactically process the stimuli by means of automatic processing.

With reference to the poorer performance on tag questions and reflexive sentences, it could be that automatic processing is interrupted because controlled processing is called into action from the need for further syntactic processing to determine whether person, number, and gender agree. Because these two sentence types require retracing of elements, an interruption of automatic processing could result. In contrast, the other sentence constructions are usually processed automatically, unless this processing is interrupted. An interruption in automatic processing—due to general fluctuation in performance—could also be posited as the reason for the agrammatic aphasic's occasional incorrect judgments on other sentences types.

Linebarger et al. discussed the notion of "shallow processing" in accounting for their results. In this context, Perfetti's (1979) dichotomy of levels of language seems comparable. His breakdown according to transparent/opaque has interesting consequences for the analysis of processing levels and task demands in grammaticality judgments. In his analysis, the levels are partially ordered according to transparency, from most transparent (prelinguistic, level 1; phonological, level 2; and syntactic, level 3) to normally opaque (propositional, level 4) to sometimes opaque and often transparent (referential, level 5; thematic, level 6; and functional, level 7).

Perfetti provided a distinction between transparent and opaque processing levels and between controlled/selective and automatic processing in order to elaborate on levels of language in language awareness (i.e., consciousness of linguistic forms as forms).

Attention is assumed to be focused ordinarily on meaning (level 4). Meaning is, however, opaque, whereas form is transparent. Thus, the levels of language involving semantic relations (i.e., meaning) are the focus of attention, and superficial levels such as phonology (level 2) and syntax (level 3) are transparent. The levels of language are considered to be available to conscious perception. The allocation of attention is considered to be controlled processing, which in turn is considered to be responsive to language structures in natural language understanding. The transparent forms of language are thus held to be relatively automatically processed, whereas the semantic processes (levels 4 through 7) are the focus of attentional selection. Perfetti's transparent levels can be considered roughly comparable to Whitaker's (1976) automatic, nonvolitional language functions (cf. Table 8.3). Thus, with reference to grammaticality judgments, this task can be considered to tap automatic processing of transparent levels. More important, the agrammatics' good performance on such a task can be taken as substantial evidence that the agrammatic can automatically process transparent levels of language.

In a recent publication, Schwartz, Linebarger, Saffran and Pate (1987) discussed results from a semantic anomaly judgment test administered to various aphasia types including agrammatic Broca's. Their aim was to investigate whether agrammatics' comprehension difficulties derive from faulty mapping from syntactic functions to thematic roles. As in the Linebarger et al. (1983) study, the agrammatics showed sensitivity to syntactic structure. Their deficit was posited to lie "in the utilization of syntactic information for the assignment of thematic roles, particularly where the syntactic relationship between the verb and its noun arguments is not transparently evident in surface structure" (p. 85). Without going into the details of this study, I cite it as another study that sheds light on the automatic/controlled processing distinction. Schwartz et al. suggested that "the vulnerability to nontransparent mappings may be a more pervasive problem in exploiting the output of a 'shallow' parse for semantic interpretation" (p. 107). If this is the case, they considered their results to provide strong support "for the psychological reality of parsing, as distinct from semantic interpretation" (p. 107).

I would like to postulate that perhaps their notion of parsing, (i.e., processes of recovering grammatical functions) is comparable to automatic processing, and their notion of semantic interpretation (i.e., processes of assigning thematic roles) is roughly equitable with controlled processing. Pertaining to "nontransparency," Schwartz et al. posited that the loss of transparency creates specific difficulties for the Broca's and conduction aphasics' sentence interpretation. In my terms, the loss of transparency possibly results from a switch from automatic to controlled processing (or from constant switching) that creates an overtaxing of the overall process of language processing. The complexity of the linguistic stimuli is also a decisive factor in overall processing. According to Schwartz et al., the non-transparent mappings may be a problem of exploiting the output of a shallow parse for semantic interpretation. With reference to their results, Perfetti's (1979) distinction between transparent (syntactic) and opaque (semantic) once again finds application.

Lexical Decision Tasks

Proceeding to a different metalinguistic task, Milberg and Blumstein (1981) and Blumstein, Milberg, and Schrier (1982) administered a visual and an auditory lexical decision task, respectively, to Broca's, Wernicke's, conduction, and global aphasics. The demands of this task require the aphasic to determine whether the stimulus is a word or is not. The stimuli were preceded by semantically related, unrelated, or nonword primes. The aphasics were also given a further metalinguistic task, namely, a semantic judgment task that consisted of word pairs from the lexical decision task.

For the present discussion, the important issue to be considered is what is actually being tapped by such metalinguistic lexical decision tasks. In brief, to anticipate an answer to this question, the results from the lexical decision task appear to tap automatic processing in aphasics of various types.

The results of the lexical decision task in both modalities revealed that the Wernicke's, Broca's, conduction, and global aphasics showed significantly shorter latencies in making real-world identifications when the stimuli were preceded by semantically related words (also superordinate and coordinate associates), than when preceded by semantically unrelated words. That is, the aphasics—even those with severe comprehension deficits—were sensitive to semantic facilitation effects in a lexical decision task. In contrast, the Wernicke's and global aphasics performed (very) poorly on the semantic judgment task in which they were required to state whether or not the two words of each pair were related or similar to each other.

At first glance, the results from the lexical decision task appear surprising—in particular those from the Wernicke's aphasics in contrast to results from other tasks, such as semantic judgments. However, in accounting for their results, Blumstein et al. (1982) pointed out an important aspect: Since semantic facilitation—as evidenced in the lexical decision task—is possible, "semantic information appears to be available to the aphasic patient as long as no overt semantic manipulation or judgment is required' (p. 313). Furthermore, "when patients are required in a metalinguistic task to have access to and directly manipulate semantic information, then deficits become apparent" (p. 313). This is exactly what happened to some of the more severely impaired aphasics in the semantic judgment task: Their processing broke down.

With reference to automatic and controlled processing, the authors pointed out that their results show that: "With regard to lexical processing in aphasia, it may well be that the automatic activation of semantic features is spared while the conscious access to this information in the retrieval of a specific lexical entry is impaired. Such access may require a spared ability to make use of or categorize the semantic features that are consciously or automatically activated even when a linguistic stimulus is presented" (p. 314). In the context of problems inherent in the use of both metalinguistic and repair data, Karmiloff-Smith (1986) drew attention to the distinction between direct (e.g., is "x" a word?) and indirect (e.g., notion of sentence) metalinguistic questioning. She stressed that the problems may have less to do with the possession of knowledge of a particular linguistic concept and more with the way in which such knowledge is represented and accessed. The results of Blumstein et al. demonstrate this distinction.

The importance of Milberg and Blumstein's (1981) and Blumstein et al.'s (1982) investigations is that they further demonstrate the relevance of the automatic/controlled distinction to aphasia research. These experimental results show that there can be a dissociation between automatic and controlled processing: Aphasics with very severe language impairments retain stored semantic information that may be inaccessible to conscious semantic decision making during metalinguistic tasks. However, Milberg and Blumstein stressed that the Wernicke's aphasics' longer latency of response is an indication that they have some impairment in the automatic activation of the semantic system (cf. the discussion of paragrammatism).

A word of caution is also given by Milberg and Blumstein with reference to the use of metalinguistic tasks, namely, that metalinguistic tasks provide a more limited picture of the lexical-semantic abilities of Wernicke's aphasics than what may be justified. This point demonstrates the importance of considering the aphasic's performance on many various tasks to arrive at a comprehensive understanding of the processing abilities.

On-line Monitoring Tasks

Tyler (1985,1987) discussed aspects of real-time processing of spoken language comprehension in aphasia within the framework of the model proposed by Marslen-Wilson and Tyler (1981). From the many issues and experiments discussed, I mention briefly only those that are pertinent to the present discussion. Tyler (1987) reported on results from on-line data, for example, monitoring for target words in normal and semantically anomalous prose and in scrambled strings. A deficit in real-time processing is considered to be reflected by the monitoring performance. In a case study of an agrammatic Broca's aphasic (D. E.), Tyler suggested that D. E.'s responses showed that he was able to use some syntactic information to construct a syntactic representation. D. E. showed a facilitation in normal prose, which was considered to be due to structural information. Tyler viewed such overall facilitation as evidence for a general measure of an aphasic's ability to use structural information.

With respect to the effects of word position in semantically anomalous prose, D. E.'s use of syntactic information to construct a syntactic representation was, however, viewed as deviant: D. E. was not able to use some aspects of syntactic information that are necessary for constructing a structural representation of an entire utterance (i.e., "global syntactic representations").

Results from five other agrammatics indicated that they were able to construct a syntactic representation that spans an utterance. The nonagrammatic and Broca's aphasics who produced only one to two word utterances could not "take advantage of larger scale syntactic structure" (Tyler, 1987, p. 158); however, they were able to construct "local syntactic" groupings.

I would like to interpret these monitoring tasks as tapping primarily automatic language processing, and further, that the agrammatics' results on these tasks support the claim that automatic processing is intact in agrammatism—if it is allowed to operate. The same applies to D. E.'s performance. In the nonagrammatics and aphasics who produced one to two word utterances, automatic processing would appear to be (totally) inhibited or severely reduced to automatic processing of shorter sequences of speech, that is, smaller syntactic groupings. In these aphasics, automatic processing broke down and controlled processing began. A disruption in processing hindered automatic processing from continuing. In my opinion, Tyler's claim that such overall facilitation is evidence for a general measure of an aphasic's ability to use structural information can rather be cited as evidence for a measure of automatic processing that runs "through to completion or until [it] fails[s] in some way" (Tyler, 1987, p. 145). Tyler's results are interesting with respect to the distinction between automatic and controlled processing. Further elaboration of these issues is planned.

Summary

In this chapter I have tried to bring together various issues that I believe are essential in aphasia research. Future research on automatic and controlled processing will bring us closer to an understanding of the aphasic's processing abilities and allow us to reinterpret "contrasting" results. I would like to stress that I do not view automatic processing as simpler, more superficial, or less "creative" than controlled processing. Rather, the two types are different, and they complement each other in normal language processing. Aphasic deficits demonstrate how essential the smooth integration between both types of processing is for efficient language production and comprehension. Further, the importance of being aware of what is being tested by a task and how the results can be interpreted adequately cannot be overemphasized. What can be learned about both types of processing and their interaction will enable the researcher/therapist to develop more adequate test material and to provide a better therapy program based on this distinction.

Notes

[1]Special thanks to Ruth Kramer Ostrin for her constructive comments. This chapter was written after chapter 6 of this volume. Various issues discussed in that chapter are being reevaluated in terms of the automatic/controlled processing distinction.

[2]Moreover, it must be emphasized that concentration on specific aspects of language processing for the purpose of discussing those aspects results in insufficient attention being given to other equally important issues. Simplification/reduction of the entire process to the selected aspects is by no means intended. The complexity and interaction of various components/levels of processing is assumed at all times.

[3]Applicable to both types of change is that the cognitive pendulum shifts back and forth in two ways (rapid versus limited and stable versus unstable growth). The pendulum also shifts within systems and between systems, whereby the across-system changes modulate the intrasystem changes.

[4]In contrast, the term "explicit" refers to accessible, verbally encoded knowledge. For Karmiloff-Smith the notion "meta" is not restricted to conscious accessibility.

[5]The three-phase cycles are defined by Karmiloff-Smith as recurrent cycles of processes which take place over and over again as the various aspects of the linguistic system develop. They can be summarized as follows: At phase 1 the surface output for a single linguistic form is mainly driven by external stimuli: a one-to-one mapping between the specific linguistic form and the particular context for which it is used in the adult model's output. Phase 1 representations are in the form of compiled procedures, whereby the contents of these procedures cannot be addressed. Generalization across tasks does not take place during this phase, because it would require operating on primary explicitation (E-i) representations (see text for explanation), not only on implicit (I) representations. In phase 2, a metaprocess is invoked to evaluate the internal state of any part of the organism. The child concentrates on gaining control over the organization of internal representations stored independently during phase 1. By phase 3 there is a stability and consolidation concerning the explicit definition of internal representational links. For further elaboration of Karmiloff-Smith's model, such as systemic grouping, refer to the publication.

[6]Development of the child's awareness of various language aspects is also discussed by contributors to the volume on child's conception of language (cf. Sinclair, Jarvella, & Levelt, 1978).

[7]Hagen (1979) disagreed that Naus and Halasz (1979) have demonstrated that different developmental patterns exist.

[8]Shallice (1972) commented on this aspect in the context of his model of the dual aspects of consciousness, in particular with reference to an action system: It requires only selector input at the beginning of its operation and can operate with little or no selector input. "Moreover, it explains why one is not conscious of processes connected with lower levels of skills, as these would always be directly controlled by never-dominant effector units. It also helps to explain why skills, initially performed under conscious control, can be performed later without conscious control. If one accepts the idea that learning a skill involves the formation of a neural system of increasing redundancy, then initially the corresponding action system would require maximum activation, with practice it would function satisfactorily with less" (p. 391).

[9]Ideas have so-called "Bewusstheitscharakter" (conscious component). However, prior to formulation of an idea unconscious processes have operated, which then suddenly lead to the idea/thought. This applies to the situation in which an idea is understood as a verbal "solution" to a problem.

[10]An agrammatic patient of mine reported that when she spoke about something "without thinking about it," that is, when she just blurted it out without trying to arrive at a grammatical structure before uttering the words, her utterances or phrases were more often correct. That is, when she allowed herself to produce more "automatically" the results were more correct than when her processing system operated in a very controlled manner. (Cf. Stark & Dressler, 1988, for an analysis of Mrs. Braun's agrammatic deficits.)

[11]The agrammatic's difference in performance in naming nouns versus verbs could possibly derive from the differential role of these parts of speech, for example, in sentence production and comprehension, and thus to the type of processing: Nouns can be considered to be more automatically processed by the Broca's aphasic than verbs. Because of the function of the verb in language processing, verbs are assumed to involve a greater interaction between controlled and automatic processing or to involve more controlled processing (cf. Miceli, Silveri, Villa, & Caramazza, 1984). Other evidence pertaining to possible differences in processing is offered by Tyler (1987, p. 153): "When listeners encounter a verb, part of the lexical representation which they access includes the syntactic and semantic restrictions on the arguments which the verb can take." See also Stark and Dressler, 1988.

[12]In this context, the relation of Broca's aphasia to transcortical motor or dynamic aphasia—which results from prefrontal damage or damage to the supplementary motor cortex—can be described as follows: In this type of aphasia the initiation of language production is more impaired than in Broca's aphasia. Automatic processing thus seems to be reduced or inhibited with reference to initiation of speech, in contrast to initiation and continuation of language production in Broca's aphasia. However, when a "language initiating" threshold is overcome, the transcortical motor aphasic correctly produces the necessary forms automatically. The problem is in starting to produce language in the first place.

References

Ahutina, T. V. (1975). Nejrolingvističeskij analiz dinamičeskoj afazii. Moscow: Izdatel'stvo Moskovskogo Universiteta.

Alajouanine, T., Ombredane, A., & Durand, M. (1939). *Le syndrome de la désintegration phonétique dans l'aphasie.* Paris: Masson.

Albert, M. L., Goodglass, H., Helm, N. A., Rubens, A. B., & Alexander, M. P. (1981). *Clincial Aspects of Dysphasia.* Vienna: Springer-Verlag.

Andresen, H., & Redder, A. (1985). Aphasie: Kommunikation von Aphatikern in Therapiesituationen. *Osnabrücker Beiträge zur Sprachtheorie (OBST), 32.*

Barkai, M. (1980). Aphasic evidence for lexical and phonological representations. *Afroasiatic Linguistics, 7,* 163–187.

Baudouin de Courtenay, J. (1972, 1886). On pathology and embryology of language. In E. Stankiewicz (Ed.), *A Baudouin de Courtenay Anthology* (pp. 727–724). Bloomington, Ind.: Indiana University Press.

Beaugrande, R. - A. de, & Dressler, W. U. (1981). *Einführung in die Textlinguistik.* Tübingen: Niemeyer. *Introduction to Text Linguistics.* London: Longman.

Benson, D. F. (1979). *Aphasia, alexia and agraphia.* New York: Churchill Livingstone.

Berg, T. (1985). *Die Abbildung des Sprachproduktionsprozesses an einem Aktivationsflußmodell: Untersuchungen an deutschen und englischen Versprechern.* Unpublished doctoral dissertation, Technical University, Braunschweig.

Berko Gleason, J., Goodglass, H., Obler, L., Green, E., Hyde, M. R., & Weintraub, S. (1980). Narrative strategies of aphasic and normal speaking subjects. *Journal of Speech and Hearing Disorders, 23,* 370–382.

Berndt, R., & Caramazza, A. (1980). A redefinition of the syndrome of Broca's aphasia. *Applied Psycholinguistics, 1,* 225–278.

Berndt, R. S., Caramazza, A., & Zurif, E. (1983). Language functions: Syntax and semantics. In S. J. Segalowitz (Ed.), *Language functions and brain organization* (pp. 5–28). New York: Academic Press.

Bernstein, B. (1971). *Class, codes and control.* London: Routledge.

Bhatnagar, S. C. (1980). *A neurolinguistic analysis of paragrammatism.* Edmonton, Saskatchewan: Linguistic Research Inc.

Bisazza, J. A., & Sasanuma, S. (1984). Compound formation by Japanese aphasics. *Annual Bulletin RILP, 18,* 179–195.

Blumstein, S. (1973). *A phonological investigation of aphasic speech.* The Hague: Mouton.

Blumstein, S. (1978). Segment structure and the syllable in aphasia. In A. Bell & J.

B. Hooper (Eds.), *Syllables and segments* (pp. 189–200). Amsterdam: North Holland.

Blumstein, S. (1981). Phonological aspects of aphasia. In M. Taylor-Sarno (Ed.), *Acquired Aphasia* (pp. 129–159). New York: Academic Press.

Blumstein, S., Cooper, W. E., Goodglass, H., Statlender, S., & Gottlieb, J. (1980). Production deficits in aphasia: A voice-onset time analysis. *Brain and Language, 9,* 153–170.

Blumstein, S. E., Cooper, W. E., Zurif, E. B., & Caramazza, A. (1977). The perception and production of voice-onset time in aphasia. *Neuropsychologia, 15,* (pp. 371–383). England: Pergamon Press.

Blumstein, S. E., Katz, B., Goodglass, H., Shrier, R., & Dworetsky, B. (1985). The effects of slowed speech on auditory comprehension in aphasia. *Brain and Language, 24,* 246–265.

Blumstein, S. E., Milberg, W., & Schrier, R. (1982). Semantic processing in aphasia: Evidence from an auditory lexical decision task. *Brain and Language, 17,* 301–315.

Blumstein, S. & Shinn, P. (1984). The spectral characteristics of stop consonants provide important clues to the nature of place of articulation production in Broca's aphasia: A reply to W. Ziegler, *Brain and Language, 23,* 171–174.

Borrell, A., & Nespoulous, J. -L. (1977). A psycholinguistic analysis of several substitution phenomena in paraphasic speech. *International Journal of Psycholinguistics, 4,* 13–30.

Bowerman, M., & Eling, P. (1983). Annual Report Nr. 4. Max Planck Institute for Psycholinguistics, Nijmegen, Holland.

Brookshire, R. H. (1978). Auditory comprehension in aphasia. In D. F. Johns (Ed.), *Clinical management of neurogenic communication disorders* (pp. 103–128). Boston: Little, Brown.

Brookshire, R. H., & Nicholas, L. E. (1984). Comprehension of directly and indirectly stated main ideas and details in discourse by brain-damaged and non-brain-damaged listeners. *Brain and Language, 21,* 21–36.

Brown, J. W. (1976). Consciousness and pathology of language. In R. W. Rieber (Ed.), *The neuropsychology of language: Essays in honor of Eric Lenneberg* (pp. 67–93). New York: Plenum Press.

Buckingham, H. W. (1979). Linguistic aspects of lexical retrieval disturbances in the posterior fluent aphasias. In H. Whitaker & H. Whitaker (Eds.), *Studies in neurolinguistics: Vol. 4* (pp. 269–291). New York: Academic Press.

Buckingham, H. (1980). On correlating aphasic errors with slips-of-the-tongue. *Applied Psycholinguistics, 1,* Applied Psycholinguistics, 1, 199–220.

Buckingham, H. (1982). Critical issues in the linguistic study of aphasic speech. *Brain and Language, 8,* 313–337.

Buckingham, H. (1983). Apraxia of language versus apraxia of speech. In R. Magill (Ed.), *Memory and control of action* (pp. 275–292). Amsterdam: North Holland.

Buckingham, H., & Kertesz, A. (1974). A linguistic view of fluent aphasia. *Brain and Language, 1,* 43–62.

Buhr, R. D. (1976). Naming deficits in anomia and aphasia. Unpublished doctoral Dissertation, Brown University, Providence, Rhode Island.

Burns, M., & Canter, G. (1977). Phonemic behavior of aphasic patients with posterior cerebral lesions. *Brain and Language, 4,* 492–507.

Cairns, H. S. & Cairns, C. E. (1976). *Psycholinguistics: A cognitive view of language.* New York: Holt, Rinehart & Winston.

Canter, G., Trost, J., & Burns, M. (1985). Contrasting speech patterns in apraxia of speech and phonemic paraphasia. *Brain and Language, 23,* 204–222.

Caplan, D. (1983b). Notes and discussion. A note on the "word-order problem" in agrammatism. *Brain and Language, 20,* 155–165.

Caplan, D., Baker, C., & Dehaut, F. (1985). Syntactic determinants of sentence comprehension in aphasia. *Cognition, 21,* 117–175.

Caplan, D., & Futter, C. (1986). Assignment of thematic roles to nouns in sentence comprehension by an agrammatic patient. *Brain and Language, 27,* 117–134.

Caramazza, A. (1982). A comment on Heeschen's "Strategies of decoding actor-object relations by aphasic patients." *Cortex, 18,* 159–160.

Caramazza, A. (1986). On drawing inferences about the structure of normal cognitive systems from the analysis of patterns of impaired performance: The case for single-patient studies. *Brain and Cognition, 5,* 41–66.

Caramazza, A. (1987). Some aspects of language processing revealed through the analysis of acquired aphasia: The lexical system. *Reports of the cognitive neuropsychology laboratory* (John Hopkins University), *24.*

Caramazza, A. & Berndt, R. S. (1978). Semantic and syntactic processes in aphasia. *Psychological Bulletin, 85,* 898–918.

Caramazza, A., & Berndt, R. S. (1985). A multi-component deficit view of agrammatic Broca's aphasia. In M. L. Kean (Ed.), *Agrammatism* (pp. 27–63). Orlando, Fla.: Academic Press.

Caramazza, A., & Zurif, E. B. (1976). Dissociation of algorithmic and heuristic processes in language comprehension: Evidence from aphasia. *Brain and Language, 3,* 572–582.

Cermak, L. S., & Craik, F. I. M. (Eds.) (1979). *Levels of processing in human memory.* Hillsdale, N.J.: Lawrence Erlbaum.

Cerwenka, Maria (1975). *Phonetisches Bilder- und Wörterbuch.* Vienna: Jugend und Volk Verlag.

Clark, E. V. (1978). Awareness of language: Some evidence from what children say and do. In A. Sinclair, R. J. Jarvella, & W. J. M. Levelt (Eds.), *The child's conception of language* (pp. 17–44). New York: Springer-Verlag.

Clark, E., & Hecht, B. (1982). Learning to coin agent and instrument nouns. *Cognition, 12,* 1–24.

Clark, H. H. & Clark, E. V. (1977). *Psychology and language: An introduction to psycholinguistics.* New York: Harcourt, Brace & Jovanovich.

Cohen, R., Kelter, S., & Schäfer, B. (1977). Zum Einfluß des Sprachverständnisses auf die Leistungen im Token Test. *Zeitschrift für klinische Psychologie, 6,* 1–14.

Cohen, R., Kelter, S., & Woll, G. (1980). Analytical competence and language impairment in aphasia. *Brain and Language, 10,* 331–347.

Coltheart, M. (1987). Functional architecture of the language-processing system. In M. Coltheart, G. Sartori, & R. Job (Eds.). *The cognitive psychology of language* (pp. 1–25). Hillsdale, N.J.: Lawrence Erlbaum.

Coltheart, M., Sartori, G., & Job, R. (Eds.) (1987). *The cognitive psychology of language.* Hillsdale, N.J.: Lawrence Erlbaum.

Comrie, B. (1981). *Language universals and linguistic typology. Syntax and morphology.* Oxford: Basil Blackwell.

Coseriu, E. (1967). Sistema, norma y habla. In E. Coseriu (Ed.), *Teoria del lenguaje y lingüística general* (pp. 11–113). Madrid: Gredos.

Craik, F. I. M. & Lockhart, R. S. (1972). Levels of processing: A framework for memory research. *Journal of Verbal Learning and Verbal Behavior, 11,* 671–684.

Crystal, D. (1980). *Introduction to speech pathology.* London: Arnold.

Crystal, D. (1984). *Linguistic encounters with language handicap.* Oxford: Blackwell.

Cutler, A. (1981). Degrees of transparency in word formation. *Canadian Journal of Linguistics, 26,* 73–77.

Cutler, A. (1983), Lexical complexity and sentence processing. In G. Flores d'Arcais & R. Jarvella (Eds.), *The processing of language understanding* (pp. 43–79). Chichester: Wiley.

Cvetkova, L. S. (1966). Narušenije analiza literaturnogo teksta u bolnih s poraženiem lobnih dolej mozga. In A. R. Luria (Ed.), *Lobnie doli i regulacija psihičeskih processov.* Moscow: Izdatel'stvo Moskovskogo Universiteta.

Deal, J. L., & Darley, F. L. (1972). The influence of linguistic and situational variables on phonemic accuracy in apraxia of speech. *Journal of Speech and Hearing Research, 15,* 639–653.

De Bleser, R. (1987). The communicative impact of nonfluent aphasia on the dialogue behavior of linguistically unimpaired partners. In F. Lowenthal & F. Vandamme (Eds.), *Pragmatics and education* (pp. 273–285). New York: Plenum Press.

De Bleser, R., & Bayer, J. (1986). German word formation and aphasia. *Linguistic Review, 5,* 1–40.

De Renzi, E. & Vignolo, L. A. (1962). The token test: A sensitive test to detect receptive disturbances in aphasics. *Brain, 85,* 665–678.

Deutsch, W. A. (1985). Halbautomatische Verfahren zur Formantfrequenzmessung. *Wiener linguistische Gazette, 35–36,* 95–103.

Dijk, T. A. van (1977a). Connectives in text grammar. In T. A. van Dijk & J. Petöfi (Eds.), *Grammars and descriptions* (pp. 11–63). Berlin: de Gruyter.

Dijk, T. A. van (1977b). *Text and context. Explorations in the semantics and pragmatics of discourse.* London: Longman.

Dijk, T. A. van, & Kintsch, W. (1983). *Strategies of discourse comprehension.* New York: Academic Press.

Dik, S. C. (1980). *Studies in functional grammar.* New York: Academic Press.

Dittmar, N. (1973). Soziolinguistik. Frankfurt: Athenäum.

Dixon, J., & Brown, E. (1979). The BMPD-Statistical Software-P Series. Berkeley: University of California Press.

Dogil, G. (1981). Elementary accent systems. In W. Dressler (Ed.), *Phonologica 1980* (pp. 89–99). Innsbruck: Innsbrucker Beiträge zur Sprachwissenschaft.

Dogil, G. (1985). Theory of markedness in nonlinear phonology. *Wiener linguistische Gazette, 24,* 3–21.

Donegan, P., & Stampe, D. (1979). The study of natural phonology. In D. Dinnsen (Ed.), *Current approaches to phonological theory* (pp. 126–173). Bloomington: Indiana University Press.

Dressler, W. (1972). On the phonology of language death. *Proceedings of the 8th Regional Meeting, Chicago Linguistic Society,* 448–457.

Dressler, W. (1973). Die Anordnung phonologicher Prozesse bei Aphatikern. *Wiener linguistische Gazette, 4,* 9–20.

Dressler, W. (1974). Aphasie und Theorie der Phonologie. *Incontri Linguistici, 1,* 9–20.

Dressler, W. (1975). Methodisches zu Allegroregeln. In W. Dressler & F. Mareš (Eds.), *Phonologica* (1972) (pp. 219–234). Innsbruck: Institut für Sprachwissenschaft.

Dressler, W. (1977a). *Grundfragen der Morphonologie.* Vienna: Austrian Academy of Sciences.

Dressler, W. (1977b) Morphonological disturbances in aphasia. *Wiener linguistische Gazette, 14,* 3–11.

Dressler, W. (1978). Phonologische Störungen bei der Aphasie. In H. Mierzejewska (Ed.), *Badania lingwistyczne nad afazią* (pp. 11–21). Warsaw: Ossolineum.

Dressler, W. (1979a). Experimentally induced phonological paraphasias. *Brain and Language, 8,* 19–24.

Dressler, W. (1979b). On a polycentristic theory of word formation. *PICL, 12,* 426–429.

Dressler, W. U. (1980a). Disturbi linguistici del riassunto nell'afasia. *Acta Phoniatrica Latina II, 1,* 19–22.

Dressler, W. (1980b). Qualitative Merkmale phonologischer Paraphasien als Diagnosehilfe. In K. Gloning & W. Dressler (Eds.), *Paraphasie* (pp. 53–62) Munich: Fink.

Dressler, W. (1982). A classification of phonological paraphasias. *Wiener linguistische Gazette, 29,* 3–16.

Dressler, W. U. (1983). Textlinguistik unter Berücksichtigung der Patholinguistik. In W. Kühlwein (Ed.), *Texte in Sprachwissenschaft, Sprachunterricht, Sprachtherapie* (pp. 15–23), Tübingen: Narr.

Dressler, W. U. (1984a). Philologie und Aphasiologie. Ein Beitrag zu Theorie und Methodik der Patholinguistik. *Anzeiger der Österreichischen Akademie der Wissenschaften, 120,* 268–285.

Dressler, W. (1984b). Explaining natural phonology. *Yearbook of Phonology, 1,* 29–50.

Dressler, W. (1985). *Morphonology*. Ann Arbor, Mich.: Karoma Press.

Dressler, W., & Hufgard, J. (1980). *Études phonologiques sur le breton sud-bigouden.* Vienna: Akademie der Wissenschaften.

Dressler, W., Magno Caldognetto, E., & Tonelli, L. (1986). Phonologische Fehlleistungen und Paraphasien im Italienischen und Deutschen. *Grazer linguistische Studien, 16,* 43–57.

Dressler, W., Mayerthaler, W., Panagl, O., & Wurzel, W. (1987). *Leitmotifs in Natural Morphology.* Amsterdam: John Benjamins.

Dressler, W., Moosmüller, S., & Stark, H. (1985). Sociophonology and aphasia. In W. Dressler & L. Tonelli (Eds.), *Natural Phonology from Eisenstadt* (pp. 45–52). Padua, Italy: Clesp.

Dressler, W., & Pléh, C. (1984). *Zur narrativen Textkompetenz bei Aphatikern.* In W. Dressler & R. Wodak, (Eds.), *Normale und abweichende Texte* (pp. 1–45). Hamburg: Buske.

Dressler, W., & Stark, J. (1976). Störungen der Textkompetenz bei Aphasie. In W. Meid & K. Heller (Eds.), *Textlinguistik und Semantik* (pp. 265–268). Innsbruck: Institut für Sprachwissenschaft.

Dressler, W., & Stark, H. (1981). Phonologische Verstärkungsprozesse in Paraphasien. Paper presented at the Jahrestagung der Deutschen Arbeitsgemeinschaft für Aphasieforschung und Aphasietherapie. November, 1981, West Berlin.

Dressler, W., & L. Tonelli (Eds.), (1985). *Natural Phonology from Eisenstadt.* Padua, Italy: Clesp.

Dressler, W., Tonelli, L., & Magno Caldognetto, E. (1987). Analisi contrastiva dei lapsus e delle parafasie fonologiche rispetto alla sillaba. In W. Dressler & C. Grassi (Eds.), *Parallela III. (pp. 54–60).* Tübingen: Narr.

Dressler, W., & Wodak, R. (1982). Sociophonological methods in the study of sociolinguistic variation in Viennese German. *Language in Society, 11,* 339–370.

Dressler, W. U., & Wodak, R. (Eds.) (1984). *Normale und abweichende Texte.* Hamburg: Buske.

Dressler, W., & Wodak, R. (1986). Disturbed texts. In J. Petöfi (Ed.), *Text connectedness from psychological point of view* (pp. 141–149). Hamburg: Buske.

Dressler, W., Wodak, R., & Pléh, C. (1984). Geschlechtspezifisches Sprachverhalten von Aphatikern auf der Textebene. In W. Dressler & R. Wodak (Eds.), *Normale und abweichende Texte* (pp. 47–63). Hamburg: Buske.

Dronkers, N. (1982). Formulaicity in aphasic language. Paper presented at the Formulaicity in Language conference, University of Maryland, College Park, Maryland. July, 1982.

Edwards, M. (1984). *Disorders of articulation.* New York: Springer-Verlag.

Eisenberg, P. (1986). *Grundriss der deutschen Grammatik.* Stuttgart, West Germany: J. B. Metzlersche Verlagsbuchhandlung.

Eling, P. (1986). Recognition of derivations in Broca's aphasics. *Brain & Language, 28,* 346–356.

Ellis, A. W. (1980). Errors in short-term memory: The effects of phoneme similarity and syllable position. *Journal of Verbal Learning and Verbal Behavior, 19,* 624–634.

Engel, D. (1977). *Textexperimente mit Aphatikern.* Tübingen: Narr.

Fillmore, C. J. (1979). On fluency. In C. J. Fillmore, D. Kempler, & W. S. Wong (Eds.), *Individual differences in language ability and language behavior* (pp. 85–101). New York: Academic Press.

Fillmore, C. J., Kempler, D., & Wong, W. S. (Eds.) (1979). *Individual differences in language ability and language behavior.* New York: Academic Press.

Fradis, A., & Calavrezo, C. (1976). Phoneme elisions and additions in aphasia. *Revue Roumaine de linguistique, 21,* 653–664.

Frazier, L. (1982). Shared components of production and perception. In D. Caplan, M. Arbib, & J. C. Marshall (Eds.), *Neural models of language processes* (pp. 225–236). New York: Academic Press.

Freedman-Stern, R., Ulatowska, H., Baker, T., & DeLacoste, C. (1984). Disruption of written language in aphasia: A case study. *Brain and Language, 22,* 181–205.

Freud, S. (1891). *Zur Auffassung der Aphasien: Eine kritische Studie.* Vienna: Deuticke.

Freyd, P., & Baron, J. (1982). Individual differences in acquisition of derivational morphology. *Journal of Verbal Learning, 21,* 282–295.

Friederici, A. (1985). Levels of processing and vocabulary types: Evidence from on-line comprehension in normals and agrammatics. *Cognition, 19,* 133–165.

Friederici, A. (1982). Syntactic and semantic processes in aphasic deficits: The availability of prepositions. *Brain and Language, 15,* 249–258.

Fromkin, V. (Ed.) (1973). *Speech errors as linguistic evidence.* The Hague: Mouton.

Gandour, J., & Dardarananda, R. (1984). Voice onset time in aphasia: Thai. II Production. *Brain and Language, 23,* 177–205.

Garnham, A., Shillock, R., Brown, G., Mill, A., & Cutler, A. (1982). Slips of the tongue in the London-Lund corpus of spontaneous conversation. *Linguistics, 19,* 805–817.

Garnsey, S. M., & Dell, G. S. (1984). Some neurolinguistic implications of prearticulatory editing in production. *Brain and Language, 23,* 64–73.

Garrett, M. F. (1982). Remarks on the relation between language production and language comprehension systems. In D. Caplan, M. Arbib, & J. C. Marshall (Eds.), *Neural models of language processes* (pp. 209–236). New York: Academic Press.

Givon, T. (1984). *Syntax. A functional-typological introduction: Vol. 1.* Amsterdam: John Benjamins.

Glass, A. V., Gazzaniga, M. S., & Premack, D. (1973). Artificial language training in global aphasics. *Neuropsychologia, 11,* 95–103.

Gloning, K., Trappl, R., Heiss, W. D., & Quatember, R. (1969). Eine experimentell-statistische Untersuchung zur Prognose der Aphasie. *Nervenarzt, 40,* 491–494.

Glozman, Ž. M. (1974). K voprosu o narušenii morfologičeskoj struktury reči pri afazii. *Voprosy Psihologii, 5,* 81–87.

Goodglass, H. (1976). Agrammatism. In H. Whitaker & H. Whitaker (Eds.), *Studies in Neurolinguistics: Vol. 1* (pp. 237–260). New York: Academic Press.

Goodglass, H. (1983). Word retrieval for production. In M. Studdert-Kennedy (Ed.), *Psychobiology of language* (pp. 129–138). Cambridge, Mass.: MIT Press.

Goodglass, H., Blumstein, S., Gleason, J. B., Hyde, M. R., Green, E., & Statlender, S. (1979). The effect of syntactic encoding on sentence comprehension in aphasia. *Brain and Language, 7,* 201–209.

Goodglass, H., Gleason, J. B., & Hyde, M. R. (1970). Some dimensions of auditory language comprehension in aphasia. *Journal of Speech and Hearing Research, 13,* 595–606.

Goodglass, H., & Kaplan, E. (1972, 1983). *The assessment of aphasia and related disorders.* Philadelphia: Lea and Febiger.

Goodglass, H. & Menn, L. (1985). Is agrammatism a unitary phenomenon? In M. L. Kean (Ed.), *Agrammatism,* (pp. 1–26). Orlando, Florida: Academic Press.

Gutstein, S. P. (1982). Language functions as indicators of fluency. Paper presented at summer meeting of the Linguistic Society of Amcrica, University of Maryland, College Park, Md., August 1982.

Guyard, H., Sabouraud, O., & Gagnepain, J. (1981). A procedure to differentiate phonological disturbances in Broca's aphasia and Wernicke's aphasia. *Brain and Language, 13,* 19–30.

Hagen, J. W. (1979). Development and models of memory: Comments on the papers by Brown and Naus and Halasz. In L. S. Cermak & F. I. M. Craik (Eds.), *Levels of processing in human memory* (pp. 289–297). Hillsdale, New Jersey: Lawrence Erlbaum.

Halliday, M. A. K., & Hasan, R. (1976). *Cohesion in English.* London: Longman.

Hamburg-Wechsler-Intelligenztest für Kinder (1966). Edited by C. Bondy, the Psychology Institute of the University of Hamburg. Bern: Verlag Hans Huber. (Original copyright: The Psychological Corporation, New York)

Harmes, S., Daniloff, R:G., Hoffman, P.R., Lewis, J., Kramer, M. B., & Absher, R. (1984). Temporal and articulatory control of fricative articulation by speakers with Broca's aphasia. *Journal of Phonetics, 12,* 367–385.

Hartung, W. (1977). Zum Inhalt des Normbegriffs in der Linguistik. In W. Hartung (Ed.), *Normen in der sprachlichen Kommunikation* (pp. 9–69). Berlin: Akademie Verlag.

Hawkins, J. A. (1983). *Word order universals.* New York: Academic Press.

Hawkins, P. (1969). Social class, the nominal group and reference. *Language and Speech, 12,* 125–135.

Hayes, B. (1984). The phonology of rhythm. *Linguistic Inquiry, 15,* 33–74.

Head, H. (1926). *Aphasia and kindred disorders of speech.* Cambridge: Cambridge University Press.

Heeschen, C. (1980). Strategies of decoding actor-object-relations by aphasic patients. *Cortex, 16,* 5–19.

Heeschen, C. (1985). Agrammatism versus paragrammatism: A fictitious opposition. In M. L. Kean (Ed.), *Agrammatism* (pp. 207–248). Orlando: Academic Press.

Heilman, K.M. & Scholes, R. J. (1976). The nature of comprehension errors in Broca's, conduction and Wernicke's aphasia. *Cortex, 12,* 258–265.

Herdan, G. (1966). *The advanced theory of language as choice and chance.* New York: Springer-Verlag.

Hilgard, E., Atkinson, R., & Atkinson, R. (1971). *Introduction to psychology.* New York: Harcourt Brace.

Hogg, R., & McCulley, C. B. (1987). *Metrical phonology: A coursebook.* New York: Cambridge University Press.

Hooper, J. B. (1980). Child morphology and morphophonemic change. In J. Fisiak (Ed.), *Historical Morphology* (pp. 157–188). The Hague: Mouton.

Houston, S. (1969). A sociolinguistic consideration of black English of children in northern Florida. *Language, 45,* 599–607.

Huber, W. (1981). Aphasien. *Studium Linguistik, 11,* 1–21.

Huber, W., & Gleber, J. (1982). Linguistic and nonlinguistic processing of narratives in aphasia. *Brain and Language, 16,* 1–18.

Huber, W., Poeck, K., Weniger, D., & Willmes, K. (1983). *Aachener-Aphasie-Test (AAT).* Göttingen: Hogrefe.

Hunt, E., & Lansman, M. (1986). Unified model of attention and problem solving. *Psychological Review, 93,* 446–461.

Isserlin, M. (1936) Aphasie. In O. Bumke & O. Foerster (Eds.), *Handbuch der Neurologie: Vol. 6* (pp. 626–806). Berlin: Springer-Verlag.

Jackson, K. (1967). *A historical phonology of Breton.* Dublin: Dublin Institute for Advanced Studies.

Jakobson, R. (1939). Le développement phonologique du language enfantin et les cohérences correspondantes dans les langues du monde. Résumés of the 5th International Congress of Linguists, Brussels.

Jakobson, R. (1941). *Kindersprache, Aphasie und allgemeine Lautgesetze.* Uppsala, Sweden: Almquist.

Jakobson, R. (1964). Toward a linguistic typology of aphasic impairments. In A. V. S. de Reuck & M. O'Connor (Eds.), *Disorders of language* (pp. 21–42). London: Churchill.

Jakobson, R. (1968). *Child language, aphasia and phonological universals.* The Hague: Mouton.

Jakobson, R. (1971). *Studies on child language and aphasia.* The Hague: Mouton.

Jarvella, R., & Meijers, G. (1983). Recognizing morphemes in spoken words. In G. Flores d'Arcais & R. Jarvella (Eds.), *The process of language understanding* (pp. 81–112). Chichester: Wiley.

Joanette, Y., Goulet, P., Ska, B., & Nespoulous, J. -L. (1986). Informative content of narrative discourse in right-brain-damaged right handers. *Brain and Language, 29,* 81–105.

Joanette, Y., Keller, E., & Lecours, A. R. (1980). Sequences of phonemic approximations in aphasia. *Brain and Language, 11,* 30–44.

Johnson, D. E. (1977). On relational constraints on grammars. In P. Cole & J. M. Sadock (Eds.), *Syntax and semantics: Vol. 8, Grammatical relations* (pp. 151–178). New York: Academic Press.

Johnston, R., Goldberg, L., & Mathers, P. (1984). Coarticulation: Theory to therapy. In R. G. Daniloff (Ed.), *Articulation assessment and treatment issues* (pp. 31–49). San Diego: College Hill Press.

Jones, E. V. (1984). Word order processing in aphasia: Effect of verb semantics. In F. C. Rose (Ed.), *Advances in neurology: Vol. 42, Progress in aphasiology* (pp. 159–181). New York: Raven Press.

Kaczmarek, B. (1984a). Mózgowe mechanizmy formowania wypowiedzi stownych. Lublin, Poland: Uniwersitet Marii-Curie Skzodowskiej.

Kaczmarek, B. (1984b). Neurolinguistic analysis of verbal utterances in patients with focal lesions of frontal lobes. *Brain and Language, 21,* 52–58.

Karmiloff-Smith, A. (1986). From meta-processes to conscious access: Evidence from chldren's metalinguistic and repair data. *Cognition, 23,* 95–147.

Kean, M. -L. (1977). The linguistic interpretation of aphasic syndromes. *Cognition, 5,* 9–46.

Kean, M. -L. (1979). Agrammatism: A phonological deficit? *Cognition, 7,* 69–83.

Kean, M. -L. (Ed.) (1985). *Agrammatism.* Orlando: Academic Press.

Keenan, E. L., & Comrie, B. (1977). Noun phrase accessibility and universal grammar. *Linguistic Inquiry, 8,* 1, 63–99.

Keller, E. (1978). Parameters for vowel substitution and Broca's aphasia. *Brain and Language, 5,* 265–286.

Keller, E. (1981). Competence and performance in aphasia within a performance model of language. *Cortex, 17,* 349–356.

Keller, E. (1984). Simplification and gesture reduction in phonological disorders of apraxia and aphasia. In J. C. Rosenbek, M. R. McNeil, & A. E. Aronson (Eds.), *Apraxia of speech* (pp. 221–256). San Diego: College Hill Press.

Kent, R. D. (1983). The segmental organization of speech. In P. F. MacNeilage (Ed.), *The production of speech* (pp. 57–89). New York: Springer-Verlag.

Kent, R. D. & Minifie, F. D. (1977). Coarticulation in recent speech production models. *Journal of Phonetics, 5,* 115–133.

Kent, R. D., & Rosenbek, J. C. (1982). Prosodic disturbance and neurologic lesion. *Brain and Language, 15,* 259–291.

Kertesz, A. (1979). *Aphasia and associated disorders: Taxonomy, localization and recovery.* New York: Grune and Stratton.

Kertesz, A. (1985). Aphasia. In J. A. M. Frederiks (Ed.), *Handbook of clinical neurology, Vol. 1 (45)* (pp. 287–331). Amsterdam: Elsevier Science Publishers.

Kilani-Schoch, M. (1982). *Processus phonologiques, processus morphologiques et lapsus dans un corpus aphasique.* Bern, Switzerland: Lang.

Kilani-Schoch, M. (1983). Troncation ou insertion dans les liaisons françaises: quelques données aphasiques comme indices externes. *Folia linguistica, 17,* 445-461.

Kleist, K. (1934). *Gehirnpathologie.* Leipzig: Barth.

Kohn, S. (1984). The nature of the phonological disorder in conduction aphasia. *Brain and Language, 23,* 97-115.

Kohn, S., Schönle, P., & Hawkins, W. (1984). Identification of pictured homonyms: Latent phonological knowledge in Broca's aphasia. *Brain and Language, 22,* 160-166.

Kolk, H. H. J., & Friederici, A. D. (1985). Strategy and impairment in sentence understanding by Broca's and Wernicke's aphasics. *Cortex, 21,* 47-67.

Koll-Stobbe, A. (1984). Narrative communication type vs. narrative text type: Evidence from dysphasia. *LACUS, 10,* 483-492.

Koll-Stobbe, A. (1985a). *Textleistung im Komplex Bild - Sprache: Semantische Prozesse und linguistische Repräsentation am Beispiel der klinischen Empirie.* Tübingen, West Germany: Niemeyer.

Koll-Stobbe, A. (1985b). Aphatischer Sprachgebrauch. Ein Überblick aus der Perspektive der Textwissenschaft. *Osnabrücker Beiträge zur Sprachtheorie, 32,* 73-84.

Koll-Stobbe, A. (1986). Sprachliche Variation: Das Fluent versus Nonfluent Kontinuum aphasischer Rede aus der Sicht der Prozesslinguistik. In R. Mellies et al. (Eds.), *Erschwerte Kommunikation und ihre Analyse* (pp. 109-126). Hamburg: Buske.

Kotten, A. (1982). Textverständnis bei Aphasie. In W. Kühlwein (Ed.), *Texte in Sprachwissenschaft, Sprachunterricht, Sprachtherapie* (pp. 137-138). Tübingen, Germany: Narr.

Kotten, A. (1984). Phonematische und phonetische Probleme in Srachproduktion und Rezeption für die Aphasietherapie. In V. M. Roth (Ed.), *Sprachtherapie* (pp. 83-99). Tübingen, Germany: Narr.

LaBerge, D. & Samuels, S. J. (1974). Toward a theory of automatic information processing in reading. *Cognitive Psychology, 6,* 293-323.

Labov, W., & Waletzky, J. (1967). Narrative analysis: Oral versions of personal experience. In J. Helm (Ed.), *Essays on the verbal and visual arts* (pp. 12-44). Seattle: University of Washington.

Lang, E. (1976). *Semantik der koordinativen Verknüpfung.* Berlin: Akademie Verlag.

Lapointe, S. (1983). Some issues in the linguistic description of agrammatism. *Cognition, 14,* 1-39.

Lass, R. (1985). *Phonology: An introduction into basic concepts.* London: Cambridge University Press.

Laver, J. (1973). The detection and correction of slips of the tongue. In V. Fromkin (Ed.), Speech Errors as Linguistic Evidence (pp. 132-143). The Hague: Mouton.

Laver, J. (1977). Neurolinguistic aspects of speech production. In C. Gutknecht (Ed.), *Grundbegriffe und Hauptströmungen der Linguistik* (pp. 142-155). Hamburg: Hoffmann and Campe.

Laver, J. (1980). Monitoring systems in the neurolinguistic control of speech production. In V. A. Fromkin (Ed.), *Errors in linguistic performance* (pp. 287-306). New York: Academic Press.

Lavorel, P. M. (1986). Types and tokens in pathological discourse. In J. Petöfi (Ed.),

Text connectedness from psychological point of view (pp. 122–140). Hamburg: Buske.
Lebrun, Y. (1970). On the so-called phonemic patterning of language dissolution in aphasia. *PICL, 10,* 703–707.
Lebrun, Y. (1983). Issues in neurolinguistics. *Language Sciences, 2,* 241–248.
Lebrun, Y., Lenaerts, L., Goiris, K., & Demol, O. (1969). Aphasia and the concept of the phoneme. *Logopedie en Foniatrie, 41,* 127–135.
Lecours, A. R., & Caplan, D. (1975). Review of Blumstein 1973. *Brain and Language, 2,* 237–254.
Lecours, A. R., & Lhermitte, F. (1969). Phonemic paraphasias. *Cortex, 5,* 193–228.
Lehiste, I. (1965). *Some acoustic characteristics of dysarthric speech.* Basel: Karger.
Leischner, A. (1976). Aptitude of aphasics for language treatment. In Y. Lebrun & R. Hoops (Eds.), *Recovery in aphasics* (pp. 112–120). Amsterdam: Swets & Zeitlinger.
Leischner, A. (1979). *Aphasien und Entwicklungsstörungen. Klinik und Behandlung.* Stuttgart: Thieme.
Lempert, W. (1970). Der Zugang zu beruflichen Rollen-schichtspezifische Qualifikationen. besonders sprachliche Fähigkeiten. In Claessens, D. (Ed.) *Rolle und Macht, Grundfragen der Soziologie: Vol. 6* (pp. 108–119). Munich: Juventa.
Leodolter, R. (1975). *Das Sprachverhalten von Angeklagten vor Gericht.* Kronberg/Taunus (BRD): Scriptor.
Lesser, R. (1974). Verbal comprehension in aphasia: An English version of three Italian tests. *Cortex, 10,* 247–263.
Lesser, R. (1976). Verbal and non-verbal memory components in the token test. *Neuropsychologia, 14,* 79–85.
Lesser, R. (1978). *Linguistic investigations of aphasia.* London: Arnold.
Lesser, R. (1984). Sentence comprehension and production in aphasia: An application of lexical grammar. In F. C. Rose (Ed.), *Advances in neurology: Vol. 42* (pp. 193–201). New York: Raven Press.
Levelt, W. J. M. (1981). The speaker's linearization problem. *Philological Transactions of the Royal Society London, 295,* 305–315.
Levelt, W. J. M. (1983a). The speaker's organization of discourse. *PICL, 13,* 278–290.
Levelt, W. J. M. (1983b). Monitoring and self-repair in speech. *Cognition, 14,* 41–104.
Lindblom, B. (1983). Economy of speech gestures. In P. F. MacNeilage (Ed.), *The production of speech* (pp. 57–89). New York: Springer-Verlag.
Lindner, E. (1985). Untersuchungen zu Silbentheorien bei Aphasie. MA thesis, University of Vienna.
Linebarger, M. C., Schwartz, M. F., & Saffran, E. M. (1983). Sensitivity to grammatical structure in so-called agrammatic aphasics. *Cognition, 13,* 361–392.
Linell, P. (1983). How misperception arises. In F. C.-L. Elert (Ed.), *From sounds to words. Umea Studies in the Humanities, 60,* 179–191.
Luria, A. R. (1973). Two basic kinds of aphasic disorders. *Linguistics, 115,* 57–66.
Luria, A. R. (1974). *Neijropsihologija pamjati. Vol. 1.* Moscow: Pedagogika.
Luria, A. R. (1976). *Basic problems of neurolinguistics.* The Hague: Mouton.
Luria, A. R. (1982). *Sprache und Bewusstsein.* Cologne: Pahl-Rugenstein.

MacKay, D. (1974). Aspects of the syntax of behavior: Structure and speech rate. *Quarterly Journal of Experimental Psychology, 26,* 642–657.

MacKay, D. (1978). Derivational rules and the lexicon. *Journal of Verbal Learning and Verbal Behavior, 77,* 61–71.

MacNeilage, P. (1982). Speech production mechanisms in aphasia. In S. Grillner (Ed.), *Speech motor control.* New York: Pergamon Press.

MacWhinney, B. (1978). *The Acquisition of Morphophonology.* Chicago: Chicago University Press.

Magno Caldognetto, E., & Tonelli, L. (1985). Syllabic constraints on phonological speech errors in Italian. In W. Dressler & L. Tonelli (Eds.), *Papers in Natural Phonology from Eisenstadt* (pp. 73–88). Padua, Italy: Clesp.

Magno Caldognetto, E., Tonelli, L., & Luciani, N. (1987). Problemi di classificazione e distribuzione nell' analisi di parafasie e lapsus fonologici. *Acta Phoniatrica Latina, 9,* 51–59.

Marcel, A. J. (1983a). Conscious and unconscious perception: Experiments on visual masking and word recognition. *Cognitive Psychology, 15,* 197–237.

Marcel, A. J. (1983b). Conscious and unconscious perception: An approach to the relations between phenomenal experience and perceptual processes. *Cognitive Psychology, 15,* 238–300.

Marshall, J. C. (1982). What is a symptom-complex? In M. A. Arbib, D. Caplan, & J. C. Marshall (Eds.), *Neural models of language processes* (pp. 389–410). New York: Academic Press.

Marshall, J., & Morton, J. (1978). On the mechanics of EMMA. In A. Sinclair, R. J. Jarvella, & W. J. M. Levelt (Eds.), *The child's conception of language* (pp. 225–239). New York: Springer-Verlag.

Marshall, R. C. (1981). Heightening auditory comprehension for aphasic patients. In R. Chapey (Ed.), *Language intervention strategies in adult aphasia* (pp. 297–304). Baltimore: Williams & Wilkins.

Marslen-Wilson, W., & Tyler, L. K. (1980). The temporal structure of spoken language understanding. *Cognition, 8,* 1–71.

Marslen-Wilson, W., & Tyler, L. K. (1981). Central processes in speech understanding. *Philosophical Transactions of the Royal Society of London B, 295,* 317–332.

Martin, A. D., Wasserman, N. H., Gilden, L., Gerstman, L., & West, J. A. (1975). A process model of repetition in aphasia: An investigation of phonological and morphological interactions in aphasic error performance. *Brain and Language, 2,* 434–450.

McKoon, G., & Ratcliff, R. (1980). The comprehension processes and memory structures involved in anaphoric reference. *Journal of Verbal Learning and Verbal Behavior, 19,* 668–682.

McNeill, D. (1979). *The conceptual basis of language.* Hillsdale, N. J.: Erlbaum.

Menn, L., Obler, L. K., & Miceli, G. (1988). *Agrammatic aphasia: A cross-language narrative sourcebook.* Amsterdam: John Benjamins Publishing Company.

Meringer, R. (1908). *Aus dem Leben der Sprache: Versprechen, Kindersprache und Nachahmungstrieb.* Berlin: Behr.

Meringer, R., & Mayer, K. (1895). *Versprechen und Verlesen: Eine psychologische-linguistische Studie.* Stuttgart: Goeschen.

Miceli, G., & Caramazza, A. (1987). Dissociation of inflectional and derivational morphology. *Reports of the Cognitive Neuropsychology Laboratory* (Johns Hopkins University), *23.*

Miceli, G., Mazzucchi, A., Menn, L., & Goodglass, H. (1983). Contrasting cases of Italian agrammatic aphasia without comprehension disorder. *Brain and Language, 19,* 65–97.

Miceli, G., Silveri, C., Villa, G., & Caramazza, A. (1984). On the basis for the agrammatic's difficulty in producing main verbs. *Cortex, 20,* 207–220.

Mierzejewska, H. (1977). *Afatyczna dezintegracja fonetycznej postaci wyrazów.* Wroclaw, Poland: Ossolineum.

Mierzejewska, H., & Grotecki, W. S. (1982a). Zum informatorischen Wert aphatischer Texte. In H. Mierzejewska (Ed.), *Badania porównawcze afazji* (pp. 71–88). Wroclaw, Poland: Ossolineum.

Mierzejewska, H., & Grotecki, W. S. (1982b). Fonotaktyczne badania porownawcze tekstów afatycznych. In H. Mierzejewska (Ed.), *Badania porównawcze afazi* (pp. 59–69). Wroclaw, Poland: Ossolineum.

Mihailescu, L., Fradis, A., & Voinescu, I. (1968). Biphonematic groups in aphasics. *Revue Roumaine de Neurologie, 5,* 101–109.

Milberg, W., & Blumstein, S. E. (1981). Lexical decision and aphasia: Evidence for semantic processing. *Brain and Language, 14,* 371–385.

Minkowski, M. (1927). Klinischer Beitrag zur Aphasie bei Polyglotten, speziell im Hinblick auf das Schweizerdeutsche. *Schweizer Archiv für Neurologie und Psychiatrie, 21,* 43–72.

Mössner, A., & Pilch, H. (1971). Phonematisch-syntaktische Aphasie. *Folia Linguistica, 22,* 231–239.

Mugdan, J. (1977). *Flexionsmorphologie und Psycholinguistik.* Tübingen, West Germany: Narr.

Naumann, E., Kelter, S., & Cohen, R. (1980). Zum Einfluss amnestischer, semantischer und konzeptueller Faktoren auf die Leistungen aphasischer Patienten im Token Test. *Archiv für Psychiatrie und Nervenkrankheiten, 228,* 317–328.

Naus, M. J., & Halasz, F. G. (1979). Developmental perspectives on cognitive psychology and semantic memory structure. In L. S. Cermak & F. I. M. Craik (Eds.) *Levels of processing in human memory* (pp. 259–288). Hillsdale, N.J.: Lawrence Erlbaum.

Neely, J. H. (1977). Semantic priming and retrieval from lexical memory: Roles of inhibitionless spreading activation and limited-capacity attention. *Journal of Experimental Psychology: General, 106,* 226–254.

Nelson, K. E., & Nelson, K. (1978). Cognitive pendulums and their linguistic realization. In K. E. Nelson (Ed.), *Children's language: Vol. 1* (pp. 223–285). New York: Gardner Press.

Nespoulous, J.-L. (1980b). Linguistique et aphasie: intérèt d'une approche dynamique du discours aphasique. *Revue Neurologique, 138,* 637–650.

Nespoulous, J.-L., & Borrell, A. (1979). A propos des perturbations phonétiques et/ou phonémiques dans le discours aphasique. *La linguistique, 15,* 135–146.

Nespoulous, J.-L., Dordain, M., Perron, C., Bub, D., Caplan, D., Mehler, J., & Lecours, A. R. (1985). Agrammatism in sentence production without comprehension deficits: Reduced availability of syntactic structures and/or of grammatical morphemes? A case study. *Les Tapuscrits du Laboratoire Theophile–Alajouanine, Laboratory Working Papers, 1,* April 1985.

Nespoulous, J.-L., & Lecours, A. R. (1980a). Du trait au discours: les différents niveaux de structuration du langage et leur atteinte chez les aphasiques. *Grammatica, 7,* 1–36.

Nespoulous, J.-L., Joanette, Y., Béland, R., Caplan, D., & Lecours, A. R. (1984). Phonologic disturbances in aphasia: Is there a "markedness effect" in aphasic phonemic errors? In F. C. Rose (Ed.), *Advances in Neurology, Vol. 42* (pp. 203-214).

Nespoulous, J.-L., Lecours, A. R., & Joanette, Y. (1983). La dichotomie phonétique—phonémique a-t-elle une valeur nosologique? In P. Messerli, P. M. Lavorel, & J.-L. Nespoulous (Eds.), *Neuropsychologie de l'expression orale* (pp. 71-91). Paris: Editions du CNRS.

Niemi, J. (1983). Units of communication and aphasia: New languages, new perspectives. In F. Karlsson (Ed.), *Papers from the 7th Scandinavian Conference of Linguistics 10* (pp. 522-531).

Nuyts, J. (1982). Een psycholinguistische benadering van de fonologische aspekten van afasie. *Antwerp Papers in Linguistics, 26.*

Obler, L. K. (1980). Narrative style in the elderly. In L. K. Obler & M. C. Albert (Eds.), *Language of the elderly* (pp. 75-90). Lexington, Mass.: Heath.

Pap, M., & Pléh, C. (1974). Social class differences in the speech of six-year-old Hungarian children. *Sociology, 8,* 267-275.

Paradis, M. (1978). The stratification of bilingualism. In M. Paradis (Ed.), *Aspects of bilingualism* (pp. 165-175). Columbia, South Carolina. Hornbeam Press.

Paradis, M. (Ed.), (1983). *Readings on aphasia in bilinguals and polyglots.* Montreal: Didier.

Parisi, D. & Pizzamiglio, L. (1970). Syntactic comprehension in aphasia. *Cortex, 6,* 204-215.

Perfetti, C. A. (1979). Levels of language and levels of processing. In L. S. Cermak & F. I. M. Craik (Eds.), *Levels of processing in human memory* (pp. 159-181). Hillsdale, N.J.: Lawrence Erlbaum.

Petöfi, J. S. (1983). Aufbau und Prozess, Struktur und Prozedur. In J. Petöfi (Ed.), *Texte und Sachverhalte. Papiere zur Textlinguistik 42* (pp. 310-321). Hamburg: Buske.

Peuser, G. (1977). *Sprache und Gehirn: Eine Bibliographie zur Neurolinguistik.* Munich: Fink.

Peuser, G. (1978a). *Aphasie: Eine Einführung in die Patholinguistik.* Munich: Fink.

Peuser, G. (Ed.) (1978b). *Brennpunkte der Patholinguistik.* Munich: Fink.

Peuser, G., & Fittschen, M. (1977). On the universality of language dissolution: The case of a Turkish aphasic. *Brain and Language, 4,* 196-207.

Pick, A. (Thiele, R.) (1931). Aphasie. In A. Bethe (Ed.), *Handbuch der normalen und pathologischen Physiologie, 15,* (pp. 1416-1524). Berlin: Springer-Verlag.

Pilch, H., & Hemmer, R. (1970). Phonematische Aphasie. *Phonetica, 22, 231-239.*

Pléh, C. (1986). On formal- and content-based models of story memory. In L. Halasz (Ed.), *Studies on the psycholinguistics of literature.* New York: de Gruyter.

Poeck, K. (1983). What do we mean by "aphasic syndromes"? A neurologist's view. *Brain and Language, 20,* 79-89.

Poeck, K., Kerschensteiner, M., Stachowiak, F.-J., & Huber, W. (175). Die Aphasien. *Aktuelle Neurologie, 2,* 159-169.

Posner, M. I. & Snyder, R. R. (1975). Attention and cognitive control. In R. Solso (Ed.), *Information processing and cognition:* The Loyola symposium (pp. 55-85). Hillsdale, New Jersey: Lawrence Erlbaum.

Pullum, G. K. (1977). Word order universals and grammatical relations. In P. Cole & J. M. Sadock (Eds.), *Syntax and semantics: Vol. 8, Grammatical relations* (pp. 249–277). New York: Academic Press.

Quasthoff, U. (1978). The uses of stereotype in every day argument. *Journal of Pragmatics, 2,* 1–48.

Quasthoff, U. M. (1979). Linguistische Studien zu Erzählungen in Gesprächen. Habilitationsschrift, University of West Berlin.

Quasthoff, U. (1983). Formelhafte Wendungen im Deutschen: Zu ihrer Funktion in dialogischer Kommunikation. *Germanistische Linguistik, 5–6, 81,* 5–24.

Quinting, G. (1971). *Hesitation phenomena in adult aphasic and normal speech.* The Hague: Mouton.

Reinhart, T. (1984). Principles of gestalt perception in the temporal organization of narrative texts. *Linguistics, 22,* 779–809.

Reischies, F. M. (1984). Nicht-verbale Determination aphasischer Syndrome. Paper read at the 11th Annual Meeting of the Arbeitsgemeinschaft für Aphasieforschung und Aphasietherapie, Berlin-Steglitz, November.

Rekart, D. M. & Buckingham, H. W. (1979). La importancia de la dialectología en el estudio de la afasia: Un caso Cubano. Paper presented at the 4th Annual Symposium of Spanish Caribbean Dialectology, San Juan, Puerto Rico, Apr. 19–21.

Rickheit, G., & Kock, H. (1983). Interference processes in text comprehension. In G. Rickheit & M. Bock (Eds.), *Psycholinguistic studies in language processing* (pp. 182–206). Berlin: de Gruyter.

Ringen, J. (1975). Linguistic facts. In D. Cohen & J. Wirth (Eds.), *Testing linguistic hypotheses* (pp. 1–42). Washington, D.C.: Hemisphere.

Rochester, S., & Martin, J. R. (1979). *Crazy talk: A study of the discourse of schizophrenic speakers.* New York: Plenum Press.

Rosenbek, J., McNeil, M., & Aronson, A. (Eds.) (1984). *Apraxia of speech.* San Diego: College-Hill Press.

Sadowska, M. (1976). Afatyczna dezintegracja afrykat. *Polonica, 2,* 169–184.

Saffran, E. M., Schwartz, M. F., & Marin, O. S. M. (1980). Evidence from aphasia: Isolating the components of a production model. In B. Butterworth (Ed.), *Language production: Vol. 1* (pp. 221–241). New York: Academic Press.

Salomon, E. (1914). Motorische Aphasie mit Agrammatismus und sensorisch-agrammatischen Störungen. *Monatsschrift für Psychiatrie und Neurologie, 35,* 181–275.

Schaner-Wolles, C. (1981). Quelques aspects du langage des enfants mongoliens. In J. Rondal (Ed.), *Psycholinguistique et handicap mental* (pp. 150–166). Brussels: Mardaga.

Schaner-Wolles, C., & Dressler, W. (1985). On the acquisition of agent instrument nouns and comparatives by normal children and children with Down's syndrome: A contribution to natural morphology. *Acta linguistica Hungarica, 35,* 137–149.

Scherer, H. S. (1984). *Sprechen im situativen Kontext.* Tübingen, West Germany: Stauffenberg.

Schiffrin, D. (1986). Functions of *and* in discourse. *Journal of Pragmatics, 10,* 41–66.

Schlenck, K. J., Huber, W., & Willmes, K. (1987). "Prepairs" and repairs: Different monitoring functions in aphasic language production. *Brain and Language, 30,* 226–244.

Schneider, W. & Shiffrin, R. M. (1977). Controlled and automatic human information processing: I. Detection, search, and attention. *Psychological Review, 84,* 1–66.

Schnitzer, M. (1972). *Generative phonology—Evidence from aphasia.* University Park, Pa.: Pennsylvania State University Press.

Schnitzer, M., & Martin, J. E. (1974). Sequential constraint impairment in aphasia: A case study. *Brain and Language, 1,* 283–292.

Scholes, R. J. (1978). Syntactic and lexical components of sentence comprehension. In A. Caramazza & E. B. Zurif (Eds.), *Language acquisition and language breakdown* (pp. 163–193). Baltimore: Johns Hopkins University Press.

Schwartz, M. F., Linebarger, M. C., Saffran, E. M., & Pate, D. S. (1987). Syntactic transparency and sentence interpretation in aphasia. *Language and Cognitive Sciences, 2,* 85–113.

Schwartz, M. F., Marin, O. S. & Saffran, E. M. (1979). Dissociations of language in dementia: A case study. *Brain and Language, 7,* 277–306.

Schwartz, M. F., Saffran, E. M. & Marin, O. S. (1980). The word order problem in agrammatism, I: Comprehension. *Brain and Language, 10,* 249–262.

Selkirk, E. D. (1984). *Phonology and syntax: The relation between sound and structure.* Cambridge, Mass.: MIT Press.

Shallice, T. (1972). Dual functions of consciousness. *Psychological Review, 79,* 383–393.

Shallice, T. (1987). Impairments of semantic processing: Multiple dissociations. In M. Coltheart, G. Sartori, & R. Job (Eds.), *The cognitive psychology of language* (pp. 111–127). Hillsdale, N.J.: Lawrence Erlbaum.

Shankweiler, D., & Harris, K. S. (1966). An experimental approach to the problem of articulation in aphasia. *Cortex, 2,* 277–292.

Shattuck-Hufnagel, S. (1979). Speech errors as evidence for a serial-ordering mechanism in sentence production. In W. E. Cooper & E. C. T. Walker (Eds.), *Sentence processing: Psycholinguistic studies presented to Merrill Garrett* (pp. 295–342). Hillsdale, N.J.: Lawrence Erlbaum.

Shewan, C. M. (1980). Phonological processing in Broca's aphasics. *Brain and Language, 10,* 71–88.

Shewan, C. M. & Canter, C. J. (1971). Effects of vocabulary, syntax, and sentence length on auditory comprehension in aphasic patients. *Cortex, 7,* 209–226.

Shiffrin, R. M. & Schneider, W. (1977). Controlled and automatic human information processing: II. Perceptual learning, automatic attending, and a central theory. *Psychological Review, 84,* 127–190.

Shinn, P. & Blumstein, S. (1983). Phonetic disintegration in aphasia: Acoustic analysis of spectral characteristics for place of articulation. *Brain and Language, 20,* 90–114.

Sinclair, A., Jarvella, R. J. & Levelt, W. J. M. (1978) (Eds.), *The child's conception of language.* Berlin: Springer-Verlag.

Smith, P., & Sterling, C. (1982). Factors affecting the perceived morphemic structure of written words. *Journal of Verbal Learning and Verbal Behavior, 21,* 704–721.

Söderpalm, E. (1979). *Speech errors in normal and pathological speech.* Malmö, Sweden: Gleerup.

Söderpalm-Talo, E. (1980). Slips of the tongue in normal and pathological speech. In V. Fromkin (Ed.), *Errors in linguistic performance* (pp. 81–86). New York: Academic Press.

Stachowiak, F. -J. (1978). Some universal aspects of naming as a language activity. In H. Seiler (Ed.), *Language universals* (pp. 207–228). Tübingen, West Germany: Narr.

Stachowiak, F. -J. (1979). *Zur semantischen Struktur des subjektiven Lexikons.* Munich: Fink.

Stachowiak, F. -J., Huber, W., Poeck, K., & Kerschensteiner, M. (1977). Text comprehension in aphasia. *Brain and Language, 4,* 177–195.

Stampe, D. (1969). The acquisition of phonetic representation. *Papers from the 5th Regional Meeting,* Chicago: Chicago Linguistic Society, pp. 443–454.

Stampe, D. (1979). *A dissertation on natural phonology.* New York: Garland.

Stark, H. K., Bruck, J., & Stark, J. A. (in press). Verbal and nonverbal aspects of text production in aphasia. Paper presented at the First European Conference on Aphasiology, Vienna, October 4–6, 1987.

Stark, J. (1974). Aphasiological evidence for the abstract analysis of the German velar nasal [ŋ]. *Wiener linguistische Gazette, 7,* 21–37.

Stark, J. (1984). *Verbale Perseveration bei Aphasie: Ein neurolinguistischer Ansatz.* Unpublished doctoral dissertation, University of Vienna.

Stark, J. A., & Dressler, W. U. (1988). Agrammatism in German-speaking aphasics. In L. Menn, L. K. Obler, & G. Miceli (Eds.) *Agrammatic aphasia—A cross-language narrative sourcebook.* Amsterdam: John Benjamins Publishing.

Stemberger, J. (1983). *Speech errors and theoretical phonology: A review.* Bloomington, Ind.: Indiana University Linguistic Club.

Stemberger, J. (1984). Structural errors in normal and agrammatic speech. *Cognitive Neuropsychology, 1,* 281–313.

Stockwell, R. P. (1977). *Foundations of syntactic theory.* Englewood Cliffs, New Jersey: Prentice Hall, Inc.

Strachalska, B. (1978). Zaburzenia formacji slowotwórcych języka polskiego w afazji akustyczno-mnestycznej i ruchowej. In H. Mierzejewska (Ed.), *Badania lingwistyczne nad afazją* (pp. 203–210). Warsaw: Ossolineum.

Swinney, D. A. (1981). Lexical processing during sentence comprehension: Effects of higher order constraints and implications for representation. In T. Myers, J. Laver, & J. Anderson (Eds.), *The cognitive representation of speech* (pp. 201–209). Amsterdam: North Holland Publishing Company.

Tissot, R., Mounin, G., & Lhermitte, F. (1973). *L'agrammatisme.* Brussels: Dessart.

Traill, A. (1970). Transformational grammar and the case of an Ndebele speaking aphasic. *Journal of the South African Logopedic Society, 17,* 48–66.

Treiman, R. (1983). The structure of spoken syllables: Evidence from novel word games. *Cognition, 15,* 49–74.

Trost, J., & Canter, G. J. (1974). Apraxia of speech in patients with Broca's aphasia. *Brain and Language, 1,* 63–80.

Tyler, L. K. (1985). Real-time comprehension processes in agrammatism: A case study. *Brain and Language, 26,* 259–275.

Tyler, L. K. (1987). Spoken language comprehension in aphasia: A real-time processing perspective. In M. Coltheart, G. Sartori, & R. Job (Eds.), *The cognitive psychology of language* (pp. 145–162). Hillsdale, N.J.: Lawrence Erlbaum.

Ulatowska, H. K., & Baker, W. D. (1977). On the notion of markedness in linguistic systems: Application to aphasia. *Linguistica Silesiana, 2,* 91–103.

Ulatowska, H. K., Freedman-Stern, R., Weiss-Doyel, A., Macaluso-Haynes, S., & North, A. J. (1983b). Production of narrative discourse in aphasia. *Brain and Language, 19,* 317–334.

Ulatowska, H. K., North, A. J., & Macaluso-Haynes, S. (1981). Production of narrative and procedural discourse in aphasia. *Brain and Language, 13,* 345–371.

Ulatowska, H. K., Weiss Doyel, A. W., Freedman-Stern, R., & Macaluso-Haynes, S. (1983). Production of procedural discourse in aphasia. *Brain and Language, 18,* 315–341.

Van der Hulst, H., & Smith, N. (Eds.). (1985). *Advances in nonlinear phonology.* Dordrecht, Holland: Foris.

Voinescu, I., Vish, E., Sirian, S., & Maretsis, M. (1977). Aphasia in a polyglot. *Brain and Language, 4,* 165–176.

Walker, C. H., & Meyer, B. J. F. (1980). Integrating different types of information in text. *Journal of Verbal Learning and Verbal Behavior, 19,* 263–275.

Watamori, T., & Sasanuma, S. (1976). The recovery process of a bilingual aphasic. *Journal of Communication Disorders, 9,* 157–166.

Weigl, E. (1979). Neurolinguistische Untersuchungen zum semantischen Gedächtnis (Benennen und Benennungsstörungen). In M. Bierwisch (Ed.), *Psychologische Effekte sprachlicher Strukturkomponenten* (pp. 269–331). Berlin: Akademie Verlag.

Weigl, E., & Bierwisch, M. (1970). Neuropsychology and linguistics: Topics of common research. *Foundations of Language, 6,* 1–18.

Weinrich, H. (1976). *Sprache in Texten.* Stuttgart: Klett.

Weniger, D., & Beck, G. (1985). Unterschiedliche Ausprägung der aphasischen Symptome in Mundart und Hochsprache. In C. L. Naumann (Ed.), *Dialekt und Sprachstörungen* (pp. 1–22). Hildesheim, West Germany: Olms.

Wepman, J. M. (1972). Aphasia therapy: A new look. *Journal of Speech and Hearing Disorders, 37,* 203–214.

Whitaker, H. A. (1970). Linguistic competence: Evidence from aphasia. *Glossa, 4,* 46–54.

Whitaker, H. A. (1971a). *On the representation of language in the human brain.* Edmonton, Saskatchewan: Edmonton Linguistic Research, Inc.

Whitaker, H. A. (1971b). Neurolinguistics. In W. O. Dingwall (Ed.), *Survey of linguistic science* (pp. 137–244). College Park, Md.: University of Maryland.

Whitaker, H. A. (1972). Unsolicited nominalizations. *Linguistics, 78,* 62–71.

Whitaker, H. A. (1976). A case of isolation of the language function. In H. A. Whitaker & H. A. Whitaker (Eds.), *Studies in neurolinguistics: Vol. 2* (pp. 1–58). New York: Academic Press.

Whitaker, H. A. (1983). Towards a brain model of automatization: A short essay. In R. A. Magill (Ed.), *Memory and control of action* (pp. 199–214). Amsterdam: North Holland.

Whitaker, H. A., & Selnes, O. A. (1978). Token test measures of language comprehension in normal children and aphasic patients. In A. Caramazza & E. B. Zurif (Eds.), *Language acquisition and language breakdown* (pp. 195–210). Baltimore: Johns Hopkins University Press.

Williams, S., & Seaver, E. (1986). A comparison of speech sound durations in three syndromes of aphasia. *Brain and Language, 29,* 171–182.

Wodak, R. (1985). *Language behavior in groups.* Berkeley/Los Angeles: University of California Press.

Wurzel, W., & Boettcher, R. (1979). Konsonantenkluster, phonologische Komplexität und aphasische Störungen. In M. Bierwisch (Ed.), *Psychologische Effekte sprachlicher Strukturkomponenten* (pp. 401–445). Berlin, DDR (or East Berlin): Akademie Verlag.

Ziegler, W., & Cramon, D. v. (1985). Anticipatory coarticulation in a patient with apraxia of speech. *Brain and Language, 26,* 117–130.

Ziegler, W., & Cramon, D. v. (1986). Timing deficits in apraxia of speech. *European Archives of Psychiatry and Neurological Sciences, 236,* 44–49.

Zurif, E. B. (1980). Language mechanisms: A neuropsychological perspective. *American Scientist, 68,* 305–311.

Zurif, E. B., & Caramazza, A. (1976). Psycholinguistic structures in aphasia: Studies in syntax and semantics. In H. A. Whitaker & H. A. Whitaker (Eds.), *Studies in neurolinguistics: Vol. 1* (pp. 261–292). New York: Academic Press.

Index